THE MIRACLE FINDERS

THE MIRACLE FINDERS

The Stories Behind the Most Important Breakthroughs of Modern Medicine

DONALD ROBINSON

David McKay Company, Inc.

New York

Library of Congress Cataloging in Publication Data

Robinson, Donald B   1913-
  The miracle finders.

  Bibliography: p.
  Includes index.
  1. Medicine—History. 2. Medical innovations—
History. 3. Medical research personnel—Biography.
I. Title.
R149.R6   610'.92'2 [B]   76-28169
ISBN 0-679-50619-5

Book Design by Arlene Goldberg

MANUFACTURED IN THE UNITED STATES OF AMERICA

For Dr. Paula Seiler,

the beloved physician

Table of Contents

Foreword   ix

Paths of Glory—A Prologue   xi

1. Death Takes a Holiday   1

2. An Ounce of Prevention   35

3. Rebuildable You   67

4. The First Great Victories over Cancer   101

5. The Coming Death of Cancer   135

6. The Way to a Human's Heart   161

7. A Heart for a Heart   189

8. Out of the Mind's Darkness   216

9. Comes the Sexual Revolution   256

10. These Miracle Finders   295

BIBLIOGRAPHY   311

INDEX   321

Foreword

In the course of the past five years, I've traveled tens of thousands of miles and talked with many of the world's greatest medical researchers. I wanted to hear how their discoveries came about and see what kind of people they were.

There are some moments that I can never forget: Watching Dr. Samuel L. Kountz while he gave a father's kidney to his son. Dr. Kountz beamed down at the kidney. "It's got love written on it," he said. Standing alongside Dr. Michael E. DeBakey, the heart surgeon, as he comforted the wife of a dying patient with poignant gentleness. Talking with Dr. Denton A. Cooley, Dr. DeBakey's rival for supremacy in the field of open heart surgery, about their bitter feud.

"Would you let Dr. DeBakey operate on your heart?" I asked Dr. Cooley.

"Yes—if he didn't know it was me," Dr. Cooley declared.

I remember some of the stirring cures I've seen. I'm thinking now of a sixty-five-year-old mailman who was brought into Roswell Park Memorial Institute in Buffalo, New York, with mycosis fungoides, a beastly form of cancer. From his face to his ankles, he was covered with repulsive tumors, sores, swellings, and scabs.

Dr. Edmund Klein tried something new—immunotherapy—on the mailman. By the next morning, some of his worst lesions had vanished. After a month's immunotherapy, not a vestige of the disease could be seen on his body.

"When I look at myself in the mirror," he glowed, "I can hardly believe it's me again."

I recall the cheerfulness of all the doctors, nurses, and patients at Roswell Park.

"We specialize in hope," Dr. Gerald P. Murphy, the director of the big cancer center, stated.

This book specializes in hope, too.

I am deeply grateful to Mrs. Mary Lasker for her interest in my project and her helpfulness. This dynamic woman has done more than any other individual to better the health of America. I'm thankful to Maxwell M. Geffen, one of the most gifted and enterprising of publishers, for his encouragement. The brilliant cancerologist Dr. Isaac Djerassi has given me wise counsel. Dr. George Schreiber, a distinguished New York City surgeon, has made many good suggestions. Walter B. Mahony, Jr., longtime executive editor of *The Reader's Digest*, has been a constant source of intellectual stimulus with his keen, questioning mind. Jess Gorkin, editor of *Parade*, a brave, sensitive editor, has done a lot to widen my medical horizons. Dr. Noel F. Parrish has used a blue pencil on portions of the manuscript with solid judgment.

Thomas J. Rosenberg, who knows hospitals better than almost anyone, has been a reservoir of facts. Ruth Maier of the Albert and Mary Lasker Foundation has been most cooperative, opening countless doors to the great. Robert B. O'Connell of the U.S. Department of Health, Education and Welfare has assisted me hundreds of times in hundreds of ways with unfailing patience, humor, and competence. The same holds true of Huly Bray of the National Institutes of Health. Susan Roberts of the Family Service Association of America, Gilbert F. Martin of the American Medical Association, Theodore Adams of the American Cancer Society, and Suzanne Loebl of the Arthritis Foundation, four of the finest public information experts in the organizational arena, have given generously of their knowledge and resources.

Julian Bach has been a valuable, creative agent, the best there is. Pollie Cluderay has been more than a superb typist. She has been a watchful editor and a loyal, reassuring friend.

Donald Robinson

NEW YORK CITY
July, 1976

Paths of Glory—A Prologue

You needed a lot of courage to be a doctor in prehistoric times. Disease was considered a vengeful act by an angry demon,* and the doctor had to match his magic against the demon's. If the doctor's spells were not powerful enough, the sick person wasn't the only one to suffer. The demon might punish the doctor, too. Yet, from years immemorial, men have gone into the healing professions. There is a painting of a doctor on the rock walls of the Trois Frères cave at Ariège in the French Pyrenees that is at least seventeen thousand years old. The doctor is wearing the formal attire of his profession: an animal skin and a grotesque deer mask with towering, thick antlers.

Disease was there waiting when manlike creatures first emerged from the evolutionary murk. A million years ago, man's apelike ancestor, *Pithecanthropus erectus*, was tortured by cancer. A thigh bone of a *Pithecanthropus erectus* discovered in Java in 1891 bore the grim remnants of a malignant bone tumor. By the time *Homo sapiens*—real man—arrived about 600,000 B.C., hordes of other maladies were rampaging. Evidence exists from early on of the presence in man of tuberculosis of the spine, arthritis, gallstones, serious infections, even migraine. The primitive healers—call them witch doctors, sorcerers, medicine men, priests, or what you will—had a drastic technique for dealing with some of these ailments. They bored a hole in the patient's skull to let out the demon that was causing the trouble.

In 460 B.C., a Greek physician was born who invested the practice of medicine with dignity, logic, and ethics. Hippocrates of Cos developed the first system of diagnosis founded on reason and the careful observation of

---

*Hundreds of thousands of years later, many religions still held to this belief. St. Augustine, who lived from 354 to 430 A.D., decreed that, "All diseases of Christians are to be ascribed to demons."

symptoms. He set forth a code of decent professional conduct that most physicians still embrace.

Hippocrates made medicine into an art. Galen of Pergamum turned medicine into a science. This pushy, conceited genius did some fine research in Rome in the second century A.D. He proved that the arteries carried blood, not air, and he added appreciably to man's knowledge of his brain, nervous system, bones, and blood vessels. He wrote seventeen books on the pulse! Galen also made some bad mistakes. He insisted, for instance, that every woman had two uterine cavities, the right one for a male fetus, and the left for a female. He denied that any connection existed between the arteries and the veins.

Galen could not tolerate disagreement. He was convinced that he had resolved all medical problems and that no more medical research would ever again be necessary. Unfortunately, the medical authorities concurred, and, after Galen's death, all meaningful research into pathology and physiology came to an absolute halt for 1,300 years.

A stormy petrel who went by the name of Paracelsus got the medical procession moving again. His actual name was Theophrastus Bombastus von Hohenheim; he was born in Switzerland in 1493; and he became an itinerant doctor with an international reputation for eccentricity, defiance of authority, and medical skill. Paracelsus refused to accept Galen's words as gospel. On a summer day in 1527, he publicly burned the writings of Galen and other hidbound ancients.

After him, medical men began to think for themselves again.

Andreas Vesalius, a sixteenth-century Belgian anatomist, gave scientific dimensions to the study of human anatomy. He defied the legal ban on dissecting human bodies and wrote a monumental study, *De humani corporis fabrica*, explaining the real structure of the human body. At the same time, a French military surgeon, Ambroise Paré, was laying the foundation for modern surgery. He learned how to stop bleeding by tying a string around a blood vessel. It was far more effective than boiling oil.

In 1868, the English physician William Harvey discovered the circulation of the blood. Forty-five years later, a Dutch draper, Antony van Leeuwenhoek, put his hobby at the service of mankind. Looking through the microscopes he liked to build, he discovered the existence of bacteria, protozoa, and spermatazoa. His "little animals," he called them.

Now medicine was ready to start on the conquest of diseases. Scurvy, which cost the lives of thousands of seamen every year, was the first to surrender. James Lind, a British naval surgeon, found that it was due to a diet deficiency, the lack of vitamin C. He demonstrated in 1747 that sailors could prevent scurvy, or, if need be, cure it, by eating oranges and lemons.

A half century later, the British physician Edward Jenner proved that vaccination could safeguard people against smallpox. In 1816 René Théophile Laënnec, a French physician, invented the stethoscope so he could listen to sounds in his patients' chests.

Pain met its master in America in 1842. A young Georgia physician, Crawford Long, performed a minor operation upon a patient who had been anesthetized with ether. Four years later, John C. Warren cut a tumor out of a patient's jaw in Boston after he had anesthetized him with ether. He had the assistance of a local dentist, William T. G. Morton. Using the ether was Morton's idea.

Rudolf Virchow of Germany, the foremost virologist of the nineteenth century, determined that all cells arose from other cells, not, as most scientists thought, out of some vague invisible "humor." Therefore, to understand a disease, one had to study the cell from which it derived. As Virchow explained it in 1858, disease was simply the life of a cell living under certain abnormal conditions that resulted in an abnormal life for it.

"Disease is life under changed conditions," Virchow wrote.

The French chemist Louis Pasteur discovered that van Leeuwenhoek's "little animals" caused disease. Despite overbearing opposition, he established in 1862 that bacteria produced fermentation and putrefaction. Both could be prevented, he showed, by keeping putrefiable material completely free of bacteria, or by heating the material long enough to kill the microorganisms. Pasteur also developed a vaccine that saved people bitten by mad dogs from contracting rabies, and he did as much for cattle and sheep threatened by anthrax.

A French newspaper once polled its readers, asking, "Who do you think is the greatest Frenchman that ever lived?"

Pasteur came in first. He drew more votes than Napoleon.

Joseph Lister, a British surgeon, introduced antiseptic methods into the operating room in the 1860s. Robert Koch, a German physician, detected the tubercle bacillus in 1882. The German physicist Wilhelm Roentgen discovered the X-ray, one of the best of all diagnostic tools, in 1895. Three years later, Marie Sklodowska, a Pole, and her French husband, Pierre Curie, isolated radium. In 1901, Major Walter Reed, a U.S. Army surgeon, proved once and for always that yellow fever was transmitted by a mosquito.

The medical profession was speeding up its pace now. Chemicals that could cure specific diseases were being tracked down. The vitamin field was opening up. Superb surgical advances were being recorded. Insulin was coming. Medicine was heading toward its greatest age of discovery.

THE MIRACLE FINDERS

1

DEATH TAKES A HOLIDAY

IN THE COURSE OF THE past five thousand years, physicians have prescribed some amazing medications for their unsuspecting patients. Sumerian doctors gave sick people snake skins and turtle shells, ground up in beer. Assyrian and Babylonian doctors, who were internationally known for their medical skill, treated eye trouble in 2000 B.C. with a salve made of frogs' bile and sour milk, carefully preceded by a swig of beer and a sliced onion. In 1553 B.C., Egyptian doctors dispensed lizards' blood, swines' teeth, spider webs, and peppermint in hippopotamus oil. And beer. Chinese physicians administered earthworms, centipedes, and toads' eyelids. Incidentally, the ancient Chinese set aside a special hell—one of 150 individual hells—for pharmacists.

Doctors of the Middle Ages dosed their suffering clientele with everything from mashed jewels to vipers' flesh. As late as the seventeenth century A.D., English pharmacopoeias called for foxes' lungs, crabs' eyes, and moss off a human skull. The formula for Goddard's Pills, which were very popular with King Charles I of England, included "human bones, well dried." These medicines were not cheap. One London apothecary charged thirty shillings a pill in 1633.

Some old-time medicines were not so outlandish. The early Sumerians knew the value of opium as a pain-killer. Hippocrates, the physician-teacher, and his fellow Greeks were aware of some fine medicinal herbs, and the Romans had some good purgatives. By A.D. 1250, the Welsh were using digitalis for heart failure, and the Incas had quinine very soon

1

thereafter. But by and large, the survival of the human race was due more to "T.L.C."—tender loving care—than pharmacological skill.

A few worthwile drugs were developed in the last days of the nineteenth century and the first decades of the twentieth century. Aspirin was introduced in 1899, and the barbiturates in 1903. Dr. Paul Ehrlich, the creative German bacteriologist (he was already a Nobel laureate for his work on immunity), discovered the first chemical cure for a disease in 1909. It was Salvarsan, an arsenic compound that cured early syphilis. The medical profession dubbed it "the Magic Bullet" because it killed the specific germs that caused the syphilis. The first vitamins, A and B, were identified in 1913; insulin, the hormone that mastered diabetes, was isolated in 1921.

Then came the golden age of wonder drugs.

In a comparatively short period, from the 1930s to the late 1960s, medical science discovered the antibiotics, sulfa drugs, cortisone, and a glowing collection of other lifesaving medications. The death rates for dozens of diseases plummeted. In all of recorded time, medical science won its greatest victories.

The year the golden age commenced was 1934. Dr. Gerhard Domagk, a thirty-eight-year-old pharmacologist employed by the German trust I.G. Farbenindustrie to screen chemicals for possible medical applications, found that a dye used to tint cloth a brick-red color seemed to cure streptococcal infections in mice. Domagk's little daughter was dying of a streptococcal infection that she had contracted by pricking her finger with a knitting needle. In desperation, Domagk injected the dye into the child. Her fever dropped at once and she made a splendid recovery. A young Swiss-born scientist, Daniel Bovet, identified the active compound of the dye as sulfanilamide, a white crystalline amide that was deadly to many streptococci and staphylococci.

With the discovery of sulfanilamide and its allied sulfa compounds, pneumonia and a number of other bacterial infections lost much of their threat to humankind.

Dr. Domagk was awarded the Nobel Prize in medicine in 1939, but the German dictator Adolf Hitler forbade him to accept it. The megalomaniacal Nazi Führer had been outraged because the Nobel Peace Prize for 1935 had gone to an anti-Nazi. He had the Gestapo drag Domagk off to prison for a week.

Fleming Discovers Penicillin
—*the First Antibiotic*

Antibiotics were discovered before the sulfa drugs, but for twelve years no one in authority was willing to acknowledge their value. In 1928, a shy forty-seven-year-old Scottish bacteriologist, Alexander Fleming, accidentally left a culture of staphylococci uncovered in his murky laboratory at St. Mary's Hospital in London. One morning, he noticed some mold in the shallow glass dish. Apparently it had drifted in through an open window. He looked more closely and saw that there was a sizable vacant aisle between the staphylococci and the blue-green spotted mold. He brought over his microscope. While he watched, he saw the bacteria disappearing. Something in the mold evidently was killing the bacteria.

It was the classic instance of fortune accommodating a willing mind. "When I saw those bacteria fading away," Fleming said, "I had no suspicion that I had got a clue to the most powerful therapeutic substance yet used to defeat bacterial infections in the human body. The appearance of the culture was such, though, that I knew it should not be neglected."

The mold was identified as *Penicillium notatum*, very much like the mold that grows on stale bread. Fleming cultured it in broth, filtered it, and discovered in the filtrate a miraculous substance that played havoc with bacteria. He named the substance penicillin.

Since Fleming was not a chemist, he could not purify the penicillin himself, and he couldn't get much assistance from anyone else to do it. He correctly predicted that penicillin would be of immense value against venereal disease, but nobody in the upper scientific echelons was much interested. One American university rejected an application for $100 to do research on penicillin. It threatened to discharge a professor who offered to pay for a penicillin investigation out of his own pocket.

The bombs, guns, and torn bodies of World War II made penicillin more appealing to the money-givers. Dr. Howard W. Florey, a forty-two-year-old pathologist from Australia, was funded to do research on penicillin at Oxford University, and he chose Dr. Ernst B. Chain, a twenty-nine-year-old chemist who had fled Nazi Germany, to help him. In the spring of 1940, they were able to extract a tiny morsel of yellowish-brown powder from Fleming's mold—the first purified penicillin. It was a million times more powerful than Fleming's original filtrate.

A forty-three-year-old Oxford policeman was the first human to receive penicillin. He was dying of septicemia; his entire body, his face, his eyes were covered with oozing ulcers. In February 1941, he received an injection of 200 milligrams of penicillin dissolved in water. Every three hours he got another injection, and the next morning he began to mend. For five days, he steadily improved. His temperature fell, his blood count bettered, one eye became practically normal. On the sixth day, no more penicillin was left; the total world supply of the drug had been exhausted. The physicians treating the policeman had to sit back helplessly and let him die. The second patient to receive penicillin was a four-year-old boy who also died. But penicillin then cured eight dying patients in a row.

It proved to be highly effective against a multitude of serious bacterial diseases, among them syphilis, gonorrhea, spinal meningitis, pneumonia, and anthrax, as well as blood poisoning. Later, another great scientist, Selman A. Waksman, was to give the name "antibiotics" (meaning "against life") to chemicals such as penicillin that are produced by fungi and various microorganisms in the soil and that have the ability to destroy or inhibit the growth of other microorganisms. They have turned out to be the best, shrewdest germ-slayers ever furnished to medical science. They are far more subtle and resourceful than the sulfa drugs. They have to be. A natural substance like penicillin is at least two hundred million years old, and it has had to compete with hordes of other species throughout the evolutionary process in order to survive.

Fleming, Florey, and Chain were awarded the Nobel Prize in medicine in 1945 for their work in penicillin, the first antibiotic. Fleming and Florey were knighted, too.

Sir Alexander remained the same unaffected, withdrawing person despite the honors heaped on him. There were never any scientific airs about him. A friend once asked him the best way to treat the common cold.

"A good gulp of whiskey at bedtime," Sir Alexander counseled. "It's not very scientific, but it helps."

He died in 1955. Years afterward, his gallant widow, Lady Fleming, was expelled from her native Greece for stubbornly resisting a military junta that had seized control of the country. She lived to see the dictatorship deposed and freedom restored to the Greeks in 1974. Sir Alexander would have liked that. He could also be obstinate, in the right cause.

Waksman Finds Streptomycin
—Scourge of Many Diseases

Another extraordinary antibiotic soon came out of the soil, the mother lode of these lifesaving microorganisms. It was named streptomycin, and it could do some invaluable things penicillin couldn't do—cure savage forms of tuberculosis, for instance.

One big difference between Alexander Fleming and Selman A. Waksman, the Russian-Jewish immigrant to the United States who discovered streptomycin, is that Dr. Waksman knew from the start what he was looking for. He spent a lifetime hunting for friendly microorganisms that would assault microorganisms hostile to human health.* In the course of this search, he found not one but several splendid antibiotics.

Waksman was eighty-three years old when I talked with him on a November day in his seventeenth-floor apartment overlooking the Yale University campus in New Haven. A little man with grey hair and a bushy white mustache, wearing a brown tweed sports jacket and black slacks, he was brimming with life and warm friendliness. We sat in the big living room surrounded by fine modern paintings. He and his wife had just moved up from Rutgers to be near their only son, Byron, an immunologist on the faculty of Yale Medical School.

Mrs. Waksman, a slim, beautiful woman in her mid-seventies, came in and out of the room, fussing over us. Dr. Waksman looked after her lovingly. "She's been very, very sick," he whispered to me, "but we don't like to think about it."

A student of the Torah, the book of Jewish learning, he had a strong sense of Jewish identity. "As a little boy, I knew every word in the Torah by heart," he bragged.

He was born in Priluki, a little peasant village near Kiev, in 1888. His father, Jacob, was a bit of a ne'er-do-well, and his mother, Fradia, supported the family. Despite the harsh restrictions in czarist Russia against higher education for Jewish boys, he earned a diploma from a gymnasium in Odessa. He wanted to spend his life studying the living processes, he decided.

"I used to go out in the field and watch the peasants plow the land," Dr. Waksman recalled. "I loved the smell of the soil, the crops, the chickens, the cows. I wanted to know what life was. How did it begin? How did it function? What chemical reactions were there?"

He emigrated to the United States in 1910 and went to live with some cousins on their five-acre farm in Metuchen, New Jersey. He milked their cows, fed their chickens, weeded their vegetable garden, and learned English from their children.

His friend Jacob Lipman, the head of the Rutgers College of Agriculture ("He was the first Jew to become dean of a college of agriculture," Waksman boasted), convinced him that he could learn more microbiology at an agricultural college than a medical school, and he entered Rutgers.

---

*It was Louis Pasteur who first observed that some microorganisms were able to destroy microorganisms of a different species, and that medicine might find a therapeutic use for this phenomenon.

Before he graduated in 1915, he discovered a microbe in the soil that he named *Streptomyces griseus*, from the Greek for "white-twisted fungus." He had no inkling yet of its value. He got a Ph.D. in biochemistry from the University of California at Berkeley in 1918 and accepted a teaching and research post at Rutgers paying all of $1,500 a year. He was married now to Deborah Mitnick, a girl from his home town who had come to America to join her brother.

His chief interest was the study of microorganisms in the soil. "Here in the soil a lot of living systems dwelled side by side," he declared. "What did they do to one another? Did they help one another? Did they destroy one another? I was burning to find out."

He was one of the first to explore this territory. As early as 1927, he published a thousand-page textbook on soil microbiology. In 1938, a former student of his, Dr. René Dubos, isolated a chemical from a soil microorganism that killed some bacteria. He named it gramicidin. It was not very useful to medical science, but it changed Dr. Waksman's career. Dubos urged Waksman to look for other chemicals produced by soil microbes that could destroy disease-causing microorganisms.

The recollection of Dubos's advice reminded Dr. Waksman of a story about a famous rabbi. As he recounted it; "The rabbi was asked, 'How did you come to accumulate so much knowledge in a single lifetime?' 'I owe a great deal to my teachers,' the rabbi replied. 'They taught me well. But I owe more to my friends. They encouraged me, they stimulated me. And most of all I owe to my students. They questioned me. They made me realize I didn't know it all.'

"That's how it was with me and René Dubos," Waksman concluded.

He turned from ordinary soil microbes to parasitic, disease-producing microbes, searching for chemicals that could kill man's bacterial enemies. In 1940, he discovered his first antibiotic, actinomycin. It was ultrapowerful, and ultratoxic. It was so toxic that it killed laboratory animals as fast as it killed the disease-producing microbes infecting them. Waksman tried every chemical trick he knew to subdue actinomycin, and none helped. The animals kept on dying.

"There was nothing to do but lay it aside," he nearly moaned. "It was a terrible blow."

In the winter of 1941-1942, when Rutgers wanted to cut down on its expenses, the university's budget cutting almost cost Waksman his job. As one economy measure, a budget expert suggested to the president that he fire Waksman, an obscure microbiologist who was earning $4,620 a year for "playing around with microbes in the soil." That kind of research never repaid the money invested in it, the budget man complained. Only the intervention of Dr. Lipman, his friend from the College of Agriculture, saved Waksman's job.

Since penicillin had proven useless for tuberculosis patients, Waksman decided to go after an antibiotic that could quell tuberculosis germs. It was a mountainous task. He and his students investigated more than ten thousand different soil cultures. Only one thousand of them destroyed bacteria in preliminary tests, and only one hundred showed any promise in later tests. Only ten of these could be isolated. However, one proved to be the antibiotic they were searching for.

They found it on a sick chicken in 1943. A clump of dirt taken from the fowl's throat had a peculiar mold growing on it. Waksman pitted the mold against the steely-coated tubercle bacilli, and it killed them. Coincidentally, the microbe in the mold was of the same *Streptomyces griseus* species he had unearthed in his undergraduate days.

He called the chemical agent in the microbe streptomycin. It was toxic, but not too dangerous to use. It destroyed a wide variety of bacteria, and it appeared to be effective against TB, mankind's ancient, devastating scourge.

When tuberculosis attacks the lungs, people sometimes cough up salty, warm blood. They feel miserably tired. Toward the end they lose weight until they're pseudoskeletons. Death usually comes slowly but inexorably. TB can be even more merciless when it invades the spine, kidneys, liver, lymph glands, or the eyes. Until Waksman's time, medicine had scarcely any methods for treating the disease—bed rest mostly, and some surgery.

On November 20, 1944, physicians at the Mayo Clinic in Rochester, Minnesota, administered streptomycin to a young woman with far-advanced pulmonary tuberculosis. She had undergone stringent surgery on her right lung to no avail, and now her remaining lung was being eaten away.

The streptomycin saved her life.

It literally brought people back from the edge of death. In 1946, Waksman—hailed as the discoverer of streptomycin—received an invitation to lecture in the Soviet Union. Streptomycin was in critically short supply, but Waksman brought a small amount with him. At a dinner in his honor, he met a world-renowned Russian geophysicist who was dying of tuberculosis. He had to leave the table every few minutes to spit blood and was given just six weeks to live. Waksman let him have some streptomycin, and he lived for decades.

Inside of ten years, deaths from all forms of tuberculosis in the United States dropped from forty-two per one hundred thousand to less than ten per one hundred thousand. This decline was not due exclusively to streptomycin. The tuberculosis bacilli developed resistance to the antibiotic, and other drugs had to be combined with it—the drug isoniazid, for example, of which we'll soon hear more. But streptomycin handed tuberculosis its first great defeat.

Dr. Waksman was awarded the Nobel Prize in medicine in 1952 for his contribution to the battle against tuberculosis.

His streptomycin has proven remarkably effective against the plague, many bad infections of the digestive tract, and many respiratory infections and wretched skin disorders. It is also very useful against tubercular meningitis and both syphilis and gonorrhea. Neither penicillin nor streptomycin is effective against any viral infections. No antibiotic is.

Waksman's work with actinomycin was not wasted. Gerhard Domagk, the German pharmacologist whose work led to the discovery of sulfanilamide, reported the isolation of a new form of actinomycin in 1953 that was active against a grim cancer, Hodgkin's disease. Waksman went back to his laboratory, and before a year was up he had isolated another form, actinomycin D, that helped to achieve permanent remissions in most cases of Wilm's tumor, a deadly kidney cancer in children. He also found three more useful antibiotics—neomycin, candicidin, and candidin.

The discovery of streptomycin could have made a millionaire of Waksman. "Listen, after I announced streptomycin to the world, I got offers—you wouldn't believe the offers I got," he said. "People came from the biggest companies in America and said, 'Here's a blank check; just write in how much you want.' I got a telephone call, a serious phone call: 'We're prepared to put $10 million into your account in the bank if you will come and be our research director.' "

"What did you tell them?" I asked.

"I said I wasn't interested."

Merck & Co. and several other drug manufacturers paid sizable royalties for the right to make streptomycin. Waksman turned most of the money over to Rutgers. In the space of a few years, it amounted to more than $15 million. At his suggestion, Rutgers used it to build the Institute of Microbiology. A small portion of the royalties was left for Waksman, and he gave half to his laboratory associates. The remainder he put into a research foundation of his own. One assistant won a lawsuit against him over the credit for the discovery of streptomycin, and its profits. Waksman forever insisted that the verdict was unjust.

He retired from the Rutgers faculty at seventy, but it didn't slow him down noticeably. He wrote three fat volumes on antibiotics and lectured widely in the United States and abroad. He scarcely had time to indulge his hobby, caricatures. He collected thousands of them and more than a thousand books about caricatures. He always hoped to write a book himself one day on the subject.

Mrs. Waksman went out to buy a pumpkin pie, and the three of us ate it together in the kitchen.

I asked what had motivated his research.

"At first it was curiosity, mostly," Dr. Waksman declared. "But then it was the thought of helping sick people. You can't imagine what a pleasure it is to help sick people."

I don't think I've ever met any other man in his eighties who took such delight in life and in studying the miraculous living processes.

He died on August 16, 1973, in Hyannis, Massachusetts. The wife about whose health he worried so much outlived him.

Fleming and Waksman awakened science to the wonders of the antibiotics. Soon, more brave penicillins and streptomycins were found, followed by other staunch antibiotics. Typhus, typhoid fever, amoebic dysentery, and undulant fever were some of the other diseases that were cured.

In the early days, doctors prescribed antibiotics indiscriminately, and patients experienced tragic reactions: swellings, skin eruptions, convulsion, death. For antibiotics are double-edged weapons. Employed recklessly, they can harm faster than they can help. Most physicians seem now to have learned discretion in the use of antibiotics, though.

With the passage of time, some strains of bacteria became resistant to certain antibiotics; they seemed almost to flaunt their immunity. But the antibiotics were not supine about it. Nearly always, when one antibiotic capitulated to invading bacteria, another filled the breech. And medical science has kept on finding new ones.

Conquering TB

Tubercle bacilli are tough little creatures, and wily. They have learned to survive some of medicine's deadliest armaments. But not all.

For a while, Waksman's streptomycin appeared to be the ultimate weapon against TB germs. However, the TB bacilli soon began to develop resistance to the antibiotic. This is not to state that streptomycin lost all its authority over TB germs; it still had a vital role to enact in the treatment of tuberculosis patients. But something more was wanted that could ally itself with streptomycin against the resistant TB microbes. This was the drug isoniazid, and it was fast to come. The credit for its discovery is another matter. I've never seen such a hodgepodge of conflicting claims over the discovery of any drug.

The evidence would seem to indicate that two sets of scientists discovered isoniazid at exactly the same time. Or maybe three. To make matters more complicated, the drug had already been discovered almost forty years before that.

Two Prague chemists, Hans Meyer and Josef Mally, synthesized a new chemical, isonicotinic acid hydrazide, in 1912. (We know it now as isoniazid.) No one saw any medical use for it, and the substance was shoved aside. (One wonders how many other valuable chemicals have been overlooked because of inadequate screening. Is there a cure for cancer sitting idle on some shelf, unrecognized?)

In the late 1940s, scientists at the Nutley, New Jersey, laboratories of Hoffmann-LaRoche Inc., a giant Swiss-owned pharmaceutical manufacturer, started hunting for drugs that might supplement streptomycin in treating TB patients. Dr. Herbert H. Fox, a Hoffmann-LaRoche chemist, put together some compounds called thiosemicarbazones that proved effective in controlling TB in mice but were far too toxic in humans. A neat researcher, Fox retraced his steps and found isoniazid along the way back.

A pair of Hoffman-LaRoche chemotherapists, Drs. Robert Schnitzer and Emanuel Grunberg, decided to test the isoniazid on mice. It completely cured pulmonary TB—by far the most common found in man, and almost the worst—in the mice. Not a lesion was left. But could the drug do that for humans?

Meanwhile, a team of scientists at the E.R. Squibb & Son laboratories in New Brunswick, New Jersey, headed by Dr. Harry Yale, was searching for an antituberculosis drug, and it came up with isoniazid, too. Neither group had any inkling that the drug had been synthesized four decades earlier in Czechoslovakia, nor that some German scientists headed by a Professor Klee were closing in on the same drug.

Isoniazid got its first human trials in 1951 on patients dying of tuberculosis at Sea View Hospital on Staten Island, New York, the world's largest TB hospital. Drs. Irving J. Selikoff and Edward H. Robitzek ran the tests.

I lunched with Dr. Selikoff in his office at Mt. Sinai Hospital in New York City. I found him a very handsome man, stocky, with an imposing head of grey-white hair and strong blue eyes, smartly dressed in a buttoned-down blue shirt with a blue and white striped necktie under his white lab coat. He was pedantic, repetitious, yet very pensive at times.

"I do research for aesthetic reasons," he said. "Scientific knowledge, scientific accuracy, our understanding of the secrets of nature, have an aesthetic appeal. Truth as we develop it can be looked at as an aesthetic achievement. I don't know where aesthetics can be more appreciated than in terms of human health and well-being."

Selikoff was born in New York City in 1915 and graduated from Columbia College and the Royal College of Medicine in Scotland. On his return to the United States, he went into TB research. In 1951, he was an attending physician at Sea View Hospital, working on new surgical techniques for removing diseased portions from the lungs of TB patients.

"It bothered me," he said. "It was illogical for an infectious disease to be treated surgically."

Still, he had misgivings when the Hoffmann-LaRoche scientists brought him isoniazid and a companion drug, iproniazid. It was the same moral quandary that every research-minded physician faces when he has a dangerous new drug to try on sick human beings. No one can foretell exactly what the reactions of human patients will be to an untried drug.

Dr. Selikoff and his colleague, Dr. Robitzek, tried the drugs on themselves first. When this proved to be safe, they went through the roster of all 1,300 patients at Sea View Hospital. They selected the ninety-two "most active, most severe, most unhappy cases, those with the poorest prognosis," who didn't respond to streptomycin, and gave them the isoniazid pills. Every one had advanced tuberculosis in both lungs. Most were walking skeletons who had lost all appetite for food; for living, in fact.

"The worst cases, the most progressive cases, are the ones that teach you the most about the effectiveness of a drug," Dr. Selikoff declared. "You're not going to see much change in an indolent, barely active disease. But when somebody has high fever, loses weight, and is going downhill, you're going to see results pretty fast if the drug is effective."

Selikoff was so tense about the experiment that he stayed at the hospital day and night. His wife, Celia, a rising young sculptress, came to the hospital to help him.

Some patients with 104° fevers were completely normal the next day. All forty-four patients who had high fevers were normal within two weeks. One woman who had tuberculosis of the tongue and larynx suffered with a tongue so swollen that she couldn't eat anymore, and nothing could be done for her. Within three days, the swelling was down so much that she could swallow solid food again. All ninety-two patients gained weight; some went up as much as fifty pounds in three months. Patients who had picked listlessly at their food became voracious eaters, asking for three and four helpings of cereal at breakfast and gobbling down five eggs. One man increased his egg intake to eleven. Their coughing stopped; their X-rays and sputum tests showed amazing improvement.

Of the two drugs they tried, isoniazid was far and away the better in the treatment of tuberculosis. However, iproniazid, or Marsalid, as it was also named, had a great contribution to make in an entirely different type of disease.

Something surprising occurred with many of the Sea View Hospital patients who took Marsalid—they became rapturously happy. Men and women who had been lying in bed dully, apathetically, got up, danced, and sang in a delirium of joy. No one realized the significance of this euphoria at the moment. Later, a sensitive New York psychopharmacologist, Dr. Nathan S. Kline, started to study the Marsalid effect. It led him to a drug for alleviating mental depression that we shall discuss in a later chapter.

While the Hoffmann-LaRoche isoniazid was being tried at Sea View Hospital, Squibb's isoniazid was being tested on tuberculosis cases among poverty-stricken Navajo Indians living on a reservation in Arizona. The findings were equally propitious.

Today, isoniazid—coupled with streptomycin or the new antibiotic Rifampin, and other drugs—can quickly bring tuberculosis under control in 95 percent of all new patients. Once TB patients had to spend years in a sanatorium. Now the average new TB patient can be released from the hospital in a few weeks, three months at the most. The tuberculosis rate in the United States has been dropping at an average rate of 6 percent per year. In 1971, there were 260,000 active cases of TB reported in the United States; in 1974, only 152,000.

Who gets most of the credit for isoniazid? The scientists—Fox (who died, poor chap, running the rapids on the Colorado River in 1973), Schnitzer and Grunberg of Hoffmann-LaRoche and Yale and his Squibb team—or the physicians—Selikoff, Robitzek, and two others who helped test Squibb's isoniazid? In a "joint award," the Lasker Awards judges cited all four physicians as well as the Hoffmann-LaRoche and Squibb organizations, but Selikoff's name headed the announcement that went in the press.

Following his Sea View days (and nights), Dr. Selikoff got into cancer research and helped clinch the evidence linking cigarettes with lung cancer. He became one of the world's leading experts on the environmental causes of cancer. He discovered that asbestos produces a variety of cancers. People who work with asbestos or who live near asbestos plants have an appallingly high incidence of this cancer, he found. Even their children may develop it thirty years afterward as a result of household contamination from dusts brought home from the work place.

Selikoff does his research at Mt. Sinai Hospital in New York. He gets to the hospital at 7:30 A.M. seven days a week. "Sunday is different from Monday only in that there are fewer phone calls," he said.

Work is his idea of fun. "If anything would give me more pleasure than work," he said, "that is what I would do. But nothing does."

Money doesn't interest him at all. "My income is about a third of what I could make in private practice," he declared. "But how many suits of clothes can I wear at a time? How many meals can I eat in a day? I have more money than I can possibly use for the things I want.

"It's my time that I'm jealous of. The only thing that I can't buy is additional years of my life for work."

I asked him if a desire to help people prompted his research.

His voice fell to a whisper. "Perhaps among some scientists this is an overwhelming desire. But with me, there is what has been called 'statistical compassion.' It's a good phrase, statistical compassion. I want people as a whole, in populations, in groups, all of us, to be well."

The Three Heroes of Cortisone

Steroids, unique forms of hormones with a four-ring molecular structure, do salutary things for the sick body that no other kind of drug can possibly do. They can ease the screaming agonies of rheumatoid arthritis as nothing else can do. They can help overcome some devastating forms of cancer. They are the one indispensable drug for preventing rejection after an organ transplant. Without steroids, kidney transplants would not be the routine procedure that they are in many hospitals today.

There is also evil in their nature. Sometimes this evil is indivisible from the good they do, and a patient must accept both if he is to have an endurable life for a while.

Hormones are the chemical messengers of the body and control its functions. They are secreted by glands like the pituitary, the thyroid, the adrenals, the pancreas, and the sex organs. A pair of astute British physiologists, William M. Bayliss and Ernest H. Starling, discovered the key role of hormones in 1902. Nineteen years later, two unflinching Canadians, Frederick G. Banting and Charles H. Best, extracted the insulin hormone from the pancreas and demonstrated its constructive effect on diabetes. Since then, it has probably saved the lives of more than 25 million diabetics.

The first sex hormone was found by a duo of German physiologists, Bernhard Zondek and Selmar Ascheim, in 1927, when they injected the urine of pregnant women into female mice. It promptly roused the mice to sexual heat. This sex hormone proved to be a steroid.

In 1929 came the finding that set medical science on the track of the most thrilling steroid of them all. Two researchers, Dr. Wilbur W. Swingle in Princeton, New Jersey, and Frank Hartman at the University of Buffalo, New York, found that extracts from the adrenal cortex, the outer adrenal gland, injected into animals enabled them to go on living after their adrenal glands had been cut out. This was astonishing. Ordinarily, that operation had a 100 percent mortality rate.

At once a search for hormones in the cortex, or corticosteroids, was launched. The hope was this: The symptoms of Addison's disease, an illness caused by underfunctioning of the adrenal glands, were similar to those that followed removal of the adrenals. Maybe injection of a corticosteroid would help control the symptoms of Addison's disease.

Two men led the pack, Edward C. Kendall in America and Tadeus Reichstein in Switzerland. They raced each other for almost twenty years to see which would be the first to come up with a hormonic remedy for Addison's disease. En route, they did something infinitely more valuable. Simultaneously, they found a drug that eased the tortures of arthritis and more than fifty other diseases: cortisone.

The wreckage done by arthritis is monstrous. There are some 17,000,000 arthritis victims in the United States alone today. One in every five families is affected. At any one time, 3,400,000 people are disabled by it.

Technically, the word "arthritis" means "inflammation of a joint." However, it covers close to one hundred different conditions that torture joints and connective tissues throughout the body. The most agonizing, the most crippling, and the most serious condition is rheumatoid arthritis. It can twist people until their bodies and limbs are distorted pitilessly. Primarily, it invades the joints, but it can beset the lungs, blood vessels, muscles, heart, eyes. About five million Americans suffer from this form of arthritis. And no one yet knows its cause.

No one even knew how to ameliorate the horrible pain of rheumatoid arthritis before cortisone was discovered.

"When an arthritic comes in the front door," the pioneering Canadian physician Sir William Osler said, "I want to go out the back door."

Osteoarthritis is the most widespread form of arthritis. It comes with age from wear and tear on the joints, and those afflicted with it, including ten million Americans, can suffer badly. They may not become crippled, though. Rheumatic fever and gout are serious forms of arthritis, too.

I talked with Dr. Kendall, the American discoverer of cortisone, in his lovely white house on a quiet lane in Princeton, New Jersey. He was eighty-five years old then. A bald, bespectacled little man, quite frail, he lived alone, rather forlornly, cooking his own meals because his wife was institutionalized. It worried him. Suppose he had a heart attack, he fretted. Who would know? But he still drove his own car back and forth to his

Princeton University laboratory five days a week. He worked a full day in the lab, handling the test tubes and chemicals with his own hands.

He was born in South Norwalk, Connecticut, in 1886, and was absorbed in science as early as he could remember. When he was ten years old, he built his own private telephone system between his house and a friend's. He got a Ph.D. in chemistry from Columbia University in 1910 and took a job with a drug company in Detroit. Next, he worked for a hospital in New York City, and in 1914 he joined the staff of the Mayo Clinic in Rochester, Minnesota, as head of its biochemistry section.

He made his first big discovery within a year of his arrival at the Mayo Clinic. He isolated thyroxin, the hormone of the thyroid gland. In 1929, he made another. He isolated glutathione, an important body chemical, in crystalline form and determined its structure.

Late in 1929, Kendall commenced his long, frustrating search for steroids of the adrenal cortex. Initially, he was only interested in examining the chemical implications of the Swingle-Hartman work with adrenal cortex extracts injected into animals. His concern with finding a cure for Addison's disease was casual. And somewhat mercenary.

"A group of physicians at Mayo's was working on Addison's disease, and they wanted me to supply them with an extract of the adrenal gland," he said. "This was right after the 1929 crash, and money was getting very scarce. Salaries were being cut at Mayo's, and lab space was being reduced. It seemed time to pick a subject for research that had clinical applications. If you wanted to keep your job, that is."

By 1938, he had isolated six steroids in the adrenal cortex which he named compounds A, B, C, D, E, and F. Compound E was the one that would become known to the world as cortisone. It was very slow, hard lab work. The adrenal glands of thousands of beef cattle had to be crushed in a wooden press and chopped up in a meat grinder. After that, they had to be chemically treated to get out the tiniest amount of a steroid. From three hundred thousand pounds of the cattle adrenals, Kendall could extract less than two ounces of compound E.

Professor Reichstein and his associates at the Technische Hochschule in Zurich were doing better. They reported that they had already isolated eight separate steroids from the adrenal glands.

Kendall was confronted with a crucial decision. In his words: "Had the time arrived to withdraw from the formidable competition offered by Reichstein's group, or should we continue?"

To make matters tougher, the pharmaceutical concern furnishing Kendall with adrenal glands was getting fed up with his slow progress and was threatening to cut off his supply.

He decided to go ahead with his research. An unwavering man, Edward Kendall!

In 1941, the Allied intelligence services received a top-secret report that the German Luftwaffe was giving adrenal gland extracts to its pilots that enabled them to fly at altitudes of forty thousand feet without difficulty. The report was false, but it stirred Washington to throw its weight behind the Kendall project. With the financial support of the U.S. government, the production of compound A, the most promising of the six hormones, was increased. A sufficient supply of it was turned out to stage human trials.

The tests were a fizzle. Compound A had no effect on Addison's disease.

Some other news was encouraging, however. Lewis H. Sarett, a twenty-six-year-old chemical genius working for Merck & Co., discovered a technique for synthesizing compound E. It meant that compound E could be made from scratch in the laboratory, and Kendall and his assistants would no longer have to wrestle with tons of cattle adrenals. They would eventually have enough compound E to test its effects on human disease.

But on what disease? After the fiasco with compound A, no one had much confidence that compound E would be of any help in Addison's disease. They tried it in cancer, and it did nothing.

"This was our low point," Kendall declared.

The solution came from Dr. Philip S. Hench, the scholarly head of the department of arthritis at the Mayo Clinic. As early as 1929, the thirty-year-old Hench had observed that women with rheumatoid arthritis often were relieved of their agony when they became pregnant. He also noticed that many arthritics felt better when they developed jaundice. He suspected that some glandular secretion was responsible, and he suggested to Kendall that it might be compound E.

The two of them made an odd couple in the Mayo corridors, little Kendall trotting alongside the towering, six-foot four-inch Hench.

"We got along fine," Dr. Kendall said. "Phil Hench knew no chemistry, and I knew no arthritis."

Time almost ran out on them. By 1948, the board of governors of the Mayo Foundation was becoming very upset about Kendall. His investigations of the adrenal cortex had gone on for eighteen years. He was approaching sixty-two years of age and due to retire at sixty-five. Was it possible that anything of value could emerge from his research in three years? Many members of the board doubted it. They recommended that his laboratory be closed. Two of his best assistants were taken away from him. He was very worried, he told me.

One day in August 1948, Dr. Kendall got a message to phone Dr.

Hench. Hench said he had a woman patient, a Mrs. G., at St. Mary's Hospital in Rochester with a racking case of rheumatoid arthritis. She was so crippled that she was practically helpless. She couldn't move her arms and legs without screaming. She was entreating him to try something new on her, anything new, that could ease her pain. Must he tell her that nothing more could be done for her, or could they give her compound E? Could they get enough of it to try it on her?

Kendall promised to get it for her. He was very tense. "I knew that this was the end of the road," he said. "The answer had to be yes or no."

On September 21, Hench started injecting compound E into Mrs. G. On September 23, for the first time in several weeks, she could roll over in bed easily. On September 24, she was able to get out of bed and exercise. She could raise her arms over her head. By October 1, her pain and stiffness were almost completely gone. She went shopping in downtown Rochester for three hours.

"I never felt better in my life," she exulted.

Other patients who were in grisly shape with rheumatoid arthritis were given compound E. They all responded excellently.

Drs. Kendall, Reichstein, and Hench jointly received the Nobel Prize in medicine in 1950 "for their discoveries regarding the hormones of the adrenal cortex, their structure and biological effect." He was quite a researcher, Reichstein. In 1933, he was the first man ever to synthesize vitamin C. Sarett's fine contribution was overlooked by the Nobel Prize committee. Very unfairly, many felt.

It was Dr. Hench who gave compound E the name of cortisone; he derived it from dehydrocorticosterone. Cortisone is not a cure for rheumatoid arthritis, but it does provide blessed relief from its agonizing symptoms. It has also demonstrated its power against Addison's disease, certain kidney diseases, cancer of the breast, many allergic skin diseases, and many inflammatory eye diseases. It operates on a new principle in medicine. It does not kill germs the way antibiotics do. Instead, it produces internal changes in the patient so that his body tissues develop resistance to various kinds of disease, injury, and stress.

Unquestionably, the side effects can be drastic. Protracted use of cortisone can give a patient a grotesque, puffed-up "moon face." It can cause peptic ulcers, diabetes, high blood pressure, cataracts, glaucoma, emotional upsets, and a catastrophic loss of bone calcium. A Long Island, New York, man who underwent a heart transplant dropped in height from five foot eight inches to five foot five and a half in a period of four years as a cortisone immunosuppressant sucked calcium out of his spine.

The beneficial aspects of cortisone are so important that these risks must, sometimes, be run. In some conditions, there is no substitute for it. By the most conservative count, cortisone has saved a million Americans from invalidism.

All three of cortisone's discoverers continued their research work. Before his death in 1965, Dr. Hench demonstrated the helpfulness of another hormone in rheumatoid arthritis cases—ACTH, a secretion of the pituitary gland.

Kendall's Nobel Prize made little impression on the board of governors at Mayo's. He was retired on schedule in 1951. The following year, he moved to the James Forrestal Research Center at Princeton University, and he set out to develop a new form of cortisone. He spent twenty years at it and finally succeeded in combining cortisone with a derivative of vitamin C.

This new form of cortisone was three times as powerful as the regular cortisone and had absolutely no dangerous side effects, Dr. Kendall excitedly told me. He was firmly convinced that he had wrought another, better, chemical miracle.

Tests on human patients were ready to begin, Kendall said, and he was so sure of the outcome that he had prepared an announcement for the press in advance. He let me read it in confidence.

He was fooling himself. The Merck laboratories did the animal testing for him, and his friend, Dr. Sarett, sadly informed me, "Nobody believed in it but him, and the truth is that it didn't live up to what he hoped for."

At eighty-five, Dr. Kendall still went to his laboratory punctually at 8:15 every morning and stayed until four.

"Do you forget the lab at night?" I asked.

"I don't want to," he said.

The one thing that bothered him was that his memory might start to fail. "If you can't carry your work in your mind," he worried, "you have no motivation to keep on going."

His memory seemed excellent to me.

His concept of fun was chess and long walks in the country. He always loved the outdoors. As a younger man, he used to take canoe trips with his three sons down the Flambeau River in Wisconsin. He was married to Rebecca Kenndy in 1915, and he doted on their ten grandchildren and two great-grandchildren.

Talking about his sixty-five years of research, he referred me to a passage in his autobiography, *Cortisone*. It read:

> Some highly intelligent people cannot see why anyone should want to climb mountains; others cannot comprehend the devotion that has overcome

great obstacles to interpret the secrets buried in the ruins of ancient civilizations . . .

But two components of the drive can be understood and are appreciated by almost everyone. These are a love of whatever things are true and a desire to create something. The scientiest hopes to discover a small addition to the accumulated truths of the ages and to create procedures that make this revelation available to all.

He was deeply concerned with helping sick people. I mentioned to him that my doctor had prescribed a cortisone salve to treat a minor little rash on my hand.

"Is it helping you?" he eagerly asked.

"Yes," I assured him.

The Nobel laureate's face lighted up. "Oh, good, good," he happily exclaimed.

Dr. Kendall died in a hospital in Rahway, New Jersey, in May 1972. His friends were at his bedside.

Folkers Versus Pernicious Anemia

A good definition of a vitamin is, "An organic substance, present in tiny amounts in natural foodstuffs, that is essential to normal body functioning and growth." Vitamins are obtained in the diet. Minute quantities of each vitamin work with other chemicals manufacturered in the body to produce the enzymes—pivotal substances that regulate thousands of interrelated bodily processes—that are necessary for metabolism. Lack of any vitamin can cause serious disease. Rickets can come from a shortage of vitamin D. A deficiency of vitamin C can lead to scurvy. A shortage of nicotinic acid—vitamin B_3—can bring on pellagra and its manias.

Some vitamins have an extraordinary ability to rescue gravely ill people from the effects of vitamin-deficiency diseases. One teaspoonful of vitamin B_{12} can save the lives of fifty thousand people. It takes only a fraction of a millionth of an ounce of B_{12} to control a fatal anemia, cure most cases of the tropical killer sprue, and treat other neuralgic diseases.

The isolation of vitamin B_{12} was another collaboration of mind with chance. Dr. Karl Folkers, a chemist with an alert, open mind, happened to be visiting the right university campus at the right time. He recognized the right clue and did the right thing about it.

The beginnings of the B_{12} story date back to 1924, when Dr. George Minot, a thirty-nine-year-old Boston physician, started to investigate pernicious anemia, with its vomiting, diarrhea, and gripping abdominal pain, its desperate panting for oxygen, and its relentless degeneration of the nerves. Six thousand people were dying of pernicious anemia in the United States each year, and tens of thousands more fell ill with it.

Minot and his thirty-two-year-old assistant, Dr. William P. Murphy, found that victims of pernicious anemia could stay alive by eating liver. They won the Nobel Prize in medicine in 1934 for their discovery.

The drawback to their treatment was that pernicious anemia patients had to eat large amounts of liver every day, seven days a week, in order to hold off death. A system of injecting big doses of cooked liver extract was devised, but it was cumbersome. A simpler, better method was needed. Scientists in Europe and the United States started looking for the factor or factors in liver that gave pernicious anemia sufferers their improvement. Dr. Folkers found it.

To talk with him, I flew to Austin, Texas, where he had become professor of chemistry at the University of Texas and director of its new Institute for Biomedical Research. He met me at the airport, a tall, thin man with shell-rimmed glasses. He was sportily dressed in a brown tweed jacket, red striped shirt, red knit tie, and greenish slacks—but he was not a sporty person. He seemed a sober, earnest man, all business. Folkers told me that he was born in Decatur, Illinois, in 1906 and became interested in chemistry as a very young boy. He secured a Ph.D. in chemistry at the University of Wisconsin in 1931, did postdoctoral work at Yale, and accepted a research job with Merck & Co. at its Rahway, New Jersey, laboratories in 1934. He wanted to combine chemistry and medicine by working on vitamins.

His new bosses tried to discourage him. "There'll never be any profit in vitamins," they predicted.

Ultimately, they let him go ahead, and he was first to determine the chemical structure of vitamin B_6, which advances protein metabolism and the operations of the nervous system. Following that, he began his long hunt for the anti-pernicious anemia factor in liver. He suspected it to be one of the B vitamins.

Years went by with little to show for them to the Merck management. The liver is a jumble of thousands of subtle chemicals, most of which are unidentified and highly difficult to detach from one another. Through the use of chromatography, a process for filtering a solution through an absorbent so as to isolate its components, Folkers was able to separate many of these ingredients, but that was as far as he could go. He had no way of telling which of the fractions contained the active compound he was seeking without testing them on animals or human victims of pernicious anemia, and this was practically impossible. No animal contracts pernicious anemia, and the only human on whom a liver ingredient could be tested was a new victim of pernicious anemia not yet receiving liver extract. These were few and far between.

"If you found a patient a month," Dr. Folkers said, "you could count your blessings."

There appeared to be no way out. The pressure on Folkers to quit his research on pernicious anemia grew intense at Merck. He didn't know what to do.

"It's really very difficult to know when to throw in the sponge and when to keep on investigating," he declared.

The celebrated Vannevar Bush, who headed all of America's scientific research for World War II, urged Folkers to continue. "Some people don't give up research on difficult projects soon enough," he counseled, "but some people give up too soon."

Then the dice rolled toward Folkers. On November 5, 1946, he paid a call on Dr. George Briggs of the department of animal husbandry at the University of Maryland. During their conversation, Briggs showed Folkers a contract that had been drawn up in an unsuccessful attempt to secure research funding for Dr. Mary Shorb, who was studying the nutrition of a bacterium, *Lactobacillus lactis lactis* Dorner (LLD). Dr. Briggs had offered Dr. Shorb space in his laboratory after the U.S. Department of Agriculture cut off its backing for her research. So far, all her efforts to obtain financial support for her experiments from foundations and pharmaceutical firms had failed. Briggs merely wanted Folkers to see the kind of a contract they had drafted.

Something attracted Folkers's attention as he glanced at Dr. Shorb's description of her investigations. Her bacteria seemed to flourish when they were fed on liver extracts. Folkers had a hunch that she had fallen on exactly what he needed: a quick way to assay his liver fractions without waiting for human subjects.

He returned to Rahway and early the next morning talked his chief into giving Dr. Shorb a $400 grant to test the liver fractions. It was the best $400 Merck & Co. ever spent. The Shorb bacteria thrived on liver fractions known to be rich in the suspected anti-pernicious anemia factor, and their response was invariably negative to liver fractions without the factor. Now Folkers and his staff, knowing they were on the right track, went searching for a cheaper, more abundant source of the factor than liver. They found it in the fermentation broth used in the production of grisein, a new antibiotic that Merck was testing for Selman Waksman.

On December 11, 1947, the Folkers staff obtained a few bright red crystals that had been concentrated many thousandfold from the grisein broth. They had vitamin B_{12}. Very soon afterward, they got the same red crystals from liver.

"When we assayed it," Dr. Folkers said, "wow, was it active!"

That was his only show of emotion during my visit.

Folkers arranged to give some of the crystals of vitamin B_{12} to Dr. Randolf West of Presbyterian Hospital in New York City, who had been doing the clinical testing on their fractions. They came to three millionths of a gram. You couldn't see them with the naked eye.

Folkers looked at the ampule holding the microsample and said to Dr. Norman Brink, a chemist working with him, "Norm, I'll feel foolish handing Dr. West what looks like an empty vial. Let's put some water or saline in it. At least there'll be something to look at."

They dissolved the crystals in a millimeter of sterile saline, and Folkers delivered the ampule to West. Then Folkers had to wait. It was nearly two months before West could locate one untreated case of pernicious anemia in all of New York City.

On February 16, 1948, Dr. West found a sixty-six-year-old woman with a potentially fatal case of pernicious anemia at Kings County Hospital in Brooklyn. West kept her on a tight regimen for five days, banning all liver, iron vitamins, anything that might cloud the testing of the B_{12}. On February 21, he gave her a single injection of B_{12}.

Inside of five days, an immense surge in the manufacture of her red blood cells was observed. Within six weeks, the woman was entirely normal—all by virtue of that one injection.

Vitamin B_{12}—cyanocobalamin is its full name—does not cure pernicious anemia. The patient has to get a new treatment from time to time. Nevertheless, B_{12} is far more effective than liver extracts, and the patient runs no risk of any toxicity or allergic reaction. B_{12} can also restore normal growth patterns to some poorly nourished children, and it is helpful with some problems arising in pregnancy and old age. New uses for it keep turning up. In June 1974, it was reported that vitamin B_{12} could correct certain inborn errors of metabolism prenatally.

Dr. Folkers got to be vice-president for exploratory research at Merck. In 1963, he surprised everyone by resigning to become a professor of chemistry at Stanford University and head of the Stanford Research Institute. He quit these posts in 1968 to go to the University of Texas at Austin. Since 1957, he has put much of his energy into investigating a new vitamin which he thinks could rank as one of the most important vitamins of all—Q_{10}. Folkers says that it is found in the heart, blood, skin, toes, tissues around the teeth, almost everywhere in the body.

His investigations have convinced Folkers that a deficiency of Q_{10} may be a major cause of heart disease, periodontal disease, which affects the gums and other supportive structures of the teeth, and possibly muscular dystrophy. Big doses of Q_{10} are now being given to hospital patients experimentally as a treatment for cardiovascular disease. Q_{10} is also being given on a trial basis to muscular dystrophy patients and to persons with serious gum trouble.

Folkers has been married since his Yale days to Selma Leona Johnson. They have two children. He is the customarily hard-working scientist who is at his laboratory at 8:00 A.M. and remains until long after dark, six days a week. He does indulge himself with a summer cottage on beautiful Lake Sunapee in New Hampshire, and in twenty-four years, the Folkers have missed only one summer there.

Folkers's work with Q_{10} is scientifically respectable, which is more than one can say for many of the other things going on with vitamins. In the 1970s, the vitamin field was convulsed with controversy. Wild-eyed claims were being made that massive doses of various vitamins could prevent and/or cure anything from cancer to mental illness. Vitamins could even pep up people's sex lives, it was said. A few of these claims had some merit. Dr. Linus Pauling, the Nobel Prize-winning biochemist, had some solid data to support his claim that vitamin C could prevent colds and curtail their miseries. But most of the other assertions—that nicotinic acid relieved schizophrenia and stabilized mental depression, say, or that vitamin E overcame impotence—had little evidence behind them.

All of the testimony wasn't in, though.

Hitchings Tames Gout

Some of the best people have had gout: Alexander the Great, Charlemagne, Francis Bacon, John Milton, Sir Isaac Newton, Johann Wolfgang von Goethe, Charles Darwin. Gout forced King Henry VI of England to postpone his wedding to Margaret of Anjou, and it curdled Martin Luther's disposition.

There is something about gout that makes people snicker. Probably it's because of a widespread impression that gout is caused by riotous living: too much rich food, too much food, too much sex.

Actually, gout derives from a defect in the body chemistry that, most likely, is hereditary. This defect raises the amount of uric acid in the blood and tissues. The uric acid has a tendency to locate in the joints, and the deposits grow there until they create large masses of chalky salts known as tophi. Most commonly, they are found around the big toe and the outside of the ear. The tophi themselves don't hurt, but life is agony when the joints are inflamed.

The pain comes without warning, just before daybreak as a rule, rousing the patient from his sleep like a burning bolt of lightning. Searing, throbbing pain seizes the big toe. If the patient so much as stirs his toe in an effort to ease the torment, a stream of fiery, knifing pains zooms up and down the leg. The least movement, even the reverberations of a far-off automobile, can trigger more torture. This agony can continue ceaselessly for days, maybe weeks.

As are other forms of arthritis, gout is a crippler. It is also a killer. A minimum of 10,000 people used to die in the United States annually from the massive damage that gout wreaked on their kidneys. More than 800,000 people suffer from gout in the United States today. Few die anymore, though.

For many years, physicians had only one drug that helped gout patients, colchicine, an extract of meadow saffron, which reduced inflammation. After that, they got some drugs that increased the excretion of uric acid. But they had nothing that rectified the underlying condition.

Then a pharmaceutical virtuoso, Dr. George H. Hitchings, got into the gout act. Already widely known for his development of drugs that helped in the treatment of leukemia and in making possible kidney transplants, Hitchings now discovered allopurinol, a drug that got at the basic causes of gout and relieved its miseries for most victims.

There are no airs to Dr. Hitchings. He is a no-nonsense speaker, fast and to the point, reciting his achievements in businesslike fashion without a trace of braggadocio.

I spent much of a day with him at the new headquarters of Burroughs Wellcome Co. in Triangle Research Park, North Carolina, a few miles from Durham. Burroughs Wellcome had moved there recently from its long-time location in Tuckahoe, New York.

He turned out to be a tall, thin man with receding grey hair and a bushy mustache who looked every year of his sixty-seven. He smoked incessantly as we talked in his smart, modern office with its towering ceiling made largely of glass and windows that jutted out at stark angles into space.

Hitchings was born in 1905 in the small seaside town of Hoquiam, Washington, the son of a naval architect. He became interested in medical research during his father's long terminal illness, and he got a Ph.D. in biochemistry at Harvard. He taught for a time, and in 1942 joined the Burroughs Wellcome research staff.

"I was the whole biochemistry department," he declared. Now he is vice-president for research of the company and has 250 people on his laboratory staff.

He was fascinated by nucleic acids, those key components of all living cells. At Burroughs Wellcome, he started out to investigate ways of interfering in their biosynthesis. He had an intuitive feeling that this study would bring him to scientifically green pastures. It did.

First, it led him to the discovery of a drug called Daraprim that is a thousand times as effective against malaria as quinine. When it was tested in Africa, it proved so powerful that one milligram protected a man against malaria for a week. Persons living in the tropics had to swallow quinine twice a day to safeguard themselves against malaria. They only had to take Daraprim once a week.

According to Dr. Hitchings, Daraprim prevented malaria, and cured it, by blocking an enzyme essential to the malarial cycle.

The second big Hitchings discovery, 6-mercaptopurine (6-MP), came fast on Daraprim's heels. This is the drug that is widely used today in the treatment of leukemia. Next came Hitchings's development of azathioprine, an immunosuppressant drug used in kidney transplants.

Allopurinol was Hitchings's fourth great discovery. "It grew out of our reflections on 6-MP," he said.

The reasoning was this: The mercaptopurine compound is broken down in the body by an enzyme called xanthine oxydase. This same enzyme converts purines (fundamental components of nucleic acids) into uric acids. If he could interfere with this process, Hitchings theorized, he might have an answer to gout.

He and his staff screened hundreds of purine compounds, hunting for one that would block the chemical activity of xanthine oxydase. They finally came to allopurinol, a purine compound that once had been tried uselessly against cancer. It showed itself to be a potent inhibitor of xanthine oxydase in the test tube.

"From here on out," Dr. Hitchings said, "the development was fairly logical. First, you get a lot of animal toxicology under your belt. You try it on humans as a short-term experiment and watch for whatever might happen. Gradually, you get courage to treat people a little longer, and a little longer. Then you're ready to go."

In 1962, Dr. R. Wayne Rundles, a hematologist, started administering allopurinol to gout patients at Duke University Medical Center in Durham. One of the first patients was a night watchman so crippled by gout that he had had to quit his job. In three days on allopurinol, the level of uric acid in his blood fell to less than half, the agonizing inflammations in the joints subsided, and he went back to work.

Late in 1963, Dr. Rundles published his full findings. He reported that allopurinol did a splendid job of controlling the formation of uric acid and dissolving tophi. It prevented the most dangerous consequences of gout: the stones that destroyed patients' kidneys.

"Almost all patients stop forming kidney stones when under treatment with allopurinol," Dr. Rundles wrote. "Thus, death and, in fact, most complications produced by urate stones, are now preventable."

Dr. Hitchings has developed a number of other useful drugs, among them a powerful new antibacterial, trimethoprim.

He gets to his office promptly at 7:30 A.M. and stays till five or six o'clock, but only for five days a week. He now devotes his weekends to tending the azaleas and camellias in his garden.

While Hitchings was a graduate student at Harvard, he found cheap room and board at the home of a minister with five daughters. He married one of them, Beverly Reimer, in 1933, and they are still together. She is an attractive, serene woman with a talent for languages.

"Beverly is the artistic and literary voice in the family," Hitchings says.

They have two grown children.

"The greatest reward you get from research is seeing a patient who's been benefited by something that comes out of your work," Dr. Hitchings says. "It's a fulfillment of a purpose. It's a confirmation that you were on the right track in your thinking.

Choh Hao Li Fights Dwarfism
—*Isolating HGH*

When red-headed Johnny B. was five, he was merely two feet six inches tall. He had grown only one inch from the time he was two years old. His father had to construct a little ladder for him so he could use the bathroom sink, and the other kindergarten kids at his parochial school in St. Louis toted him around like a baby. In every other aspect, physical and mental, Johnny was on a par with the other children of his age, and a long series of physicians assured his parents that the boy was "just small for his age." His worried parents finally consulted doctors at the Washington University School of Medicine in St. Louis, who diagnosed Johnny as a "hypopituitary dwarf." They said that he suffered from a deficiency in HGH, the human growth hormone that regulates the height children attain. The doctors prescribed regular injections of HGH for Johnny, and he began to grow. By his thirteenth birthday, he was nearly as tall as his seventh-grade classmates.

Ten thousand American children are born every year with HGH deficiencies that condemn them to dwarfism. Some of them can now be helped. Eventually, physicians will be able to help them all. A thirty-odd-year-old contest between a tenacious Chinese biochemist, Choh Hao Li, and the hormones of the pituitary gland is returning admirable rewards.

Dr. Li had more to contend with than the balky hormones of the pituitary gland. He also had to battle the indifference of the scientific bigwigs at the University of California.

I met him in a cocktail lounge at the Waldorf-Astoria Hotel in New York City. He was in New York for a scientific conference. Talk about "the inscrutable Oriental!" Li has more charm, geniality, and joyful humor than one can imagine. He is a very boyish-looking man, tall, with black hair and gold-rimmed glasses.

He was born in 1913 in Canton, China, one of eleven children. His father was a small industrialist with only a high school diploma, and his mother had had no schooling at all (and was brought up with bound feet). But they saw to it that all of their six sons and five daughters got a college education.

An early China memory: "One morning, my mother read in a Chinese newspaper that the sun had a healthy effect on the skin. She went up on the roof and did something heretical. She stripped and took a sunbath. I was only twelve years old. I couldn't understand what she was doing. Suddenly, I realized the importance of sunlight."

He became interested in chemical research as an undergraduate at the University of Nanking. "Pure curiosity," he told me. "I felt that there was something new to find out in nature."

He sailed for the United States in 1935 in hopes of doing graduate work at the University of California at Berkeley. The authorities wouldn't admit him. They said they had never heard of the University of Nanking. But when they saw the results of some of the research he had done in China, they finally accepted him for a six-month probationary period.

"And I've been on probation ever since," Dr. Li wisecracked.

He got his Ph.D. in chemistry in 1938. To support himself, he taught Chinese to Chinese children in Chinatown.

The pituitary is often described as "the master gland"; the ancients called it "the abiding place of the soul." Shielded inside a little saddle of bone in the middle of the skull, the pituitary is no larger than a pea, but it secretes hormones that have immense effects on the vital functions of the body. They control growth, reproduction, lactation, metabolism, and skin coloring. Irregularities in these hormones can lead to cancer, arthritis, and dwarfism, as well as many other critical diseases.

Li commenced his work on the pituitary hormones in 1938 in a makeshift basement laboratory that was scarcely larger than a closet. That was all the authorities would give him. For years, he was strapped for funds. Despite that, he and his coworkers were first to isolate and purify eight of the ten known hormones secreted by the anterior, or front, lobe of the pituitary gland. They were the first to determine the structure of seven of them. Li now has his own Hormone Research Laboratory at the University of California at San Francisco, with a staff of thirty and an entire floor of research space. But it didn't happen easily.

The first victory was the isolation and purification of ICSH. This is the fertility hormone, essential to ovulation and spermatogenesis. The "pill," discussed in a later chapter, is based on it.

Li identified ICSH in 1940, but it took him thirty-one more years to determine its structure.

"You have to be very persistent in this kind of research," he said. "Or stubborn."

By 1944, Li and his colleagues had isolated and purified three more pituitary hormones. In 1953, they isolated and purified ACTH, the pituitary hormone that regulates the adrenal cortex. Injecting ACTH into the body stimulates the cortex to increase the secretion of cortisone. An injection of ACTH can be as effective as cortisone itself with some rheumatoid patients. In 1973 he was able to synthesize ACTH in the laboratory.

Li and his associates first isolated and purified HGH in 1956, and they determined its structure in 1966. "Among the leading achievements of twentieth-century science," it was called, and justifiably so, for the HGH molecule is incredibly complex. Other pituitary hormones consist of thirteen or more amino acids. The HGH molecule has 188 amino acids. To put it another way, water is eighteen times as heavy as hydrogen; cortisone is 400 times as heavy, and ACTH is 500 times as heavy. HGH is 21,000 times as heavy as hydrogen.

HGH can do even more than stimulate growth, Li showed. It can heighten the activities of the sex hormones, improve the production of antibodies against disease, help wounds to heal and broken bones to mend, drop the cholesterol level in the blood, act to develop breast tissue, and increase the milk of nursing mothers. It also affects diabetes, obesity, and gigantism.

The dilemma with it is the same that medical science faced with penicillin, streptomycin, cortisone, and almost every new drug. There is not nearly enough of it available to do the good it is capable of doing. Unlike insulin or ACTH, which can be gotten from animals of other species, HGH must be drawn from human pituitary glands. To help one child afflicted with dwarfism requires the pituitary glands of 150 dead human bodies.

In 1971, Li made a big move toward solving this problem by synthesizing a protein very close to HGH. It has given him confidence that HGH can be synthesized within the next few years and that enough of it will be available to help every child in need of it. And every adult.

Dr. Li used to work all hours and all days. His wife, Sheng-hwai Lu, put her foot down and now he just puts in fifty hours a week at the laboratory. His wife was a student of his while he was a teaching assistant at the University of Nanking. She got a master's degree in agricultural economics and planned to go on for her Ph.D. when their first child interfered. They now have three children: a son who is a surgeon, and two daughters, one an architect and the other a veterinarian.

Outside of reading, mainly nonfiction, Li's chief diversion is his stamp and coin collection. He concentrates on stamps bearing pictures of great art treasures. The Lis bought a beach house sixty-five miles north of San Francisco, where he likes to walk for miles on the white sands.

"But no hobby can equal the fun of looking for something new in nature," he said.

Cotzias Subdues Parkinson's Disease

There is a wonderfully wild and woolly Greek physician, with the mannerisms of a television comic and the exquisite candor of a completely genuine man, who has made life livable again for millions of victims of a misery-streaked disease of the central nervous system. The Greek physician's name is George C. Cotzias. He discovered that the drug L-dopa can control the horrifying symptoms of Parkinson's disease.

This may well be one of the most valuable medical findings of recent times. Certainly, the respected *New England Journal of Medicine* has lauded it as "the most important contribution to medical therapy of a neurological disease in the past fifty years."

A British surgeon, James Parkinson, first described the disease in 1817. It is a progressive malady that destroys the substantia nigra, the deep-seated nerve cells in the brain. A victim's arm begins to tremble involuntarily. His hand begins to shake violently. Gradually, the jerky tremor spreads to the other extremities, to the jaw and to the neck. The victim's back stiffens. His muscles become so rigid that he can walk only with a strange shuffle. The tremor grows so extreme that he becomes bedridden and is unable to shave, wash, or feed himself, even move. His face becomes so frozen that he cannot talk. Saliva drools uncontrollably from the corners of his mouth.

The disease used to mean death or total disablement for most of its victims. A study of 802 cases of parkinsonism was made, covering a period of fifteen years. Twenty-five percent of the victims died or were severely disabled inside of five years. Before the next ten years were done, 80 percent of the patients were dead or severely disabled. Usually, the victims of parkinsonism are in their fifties when the disease appears. Fifty thousand new cases are reported in the United States every year. The total number of cases in America is estimated at 1,500,000.

Brain surgery was the only hope, and a slim one. A brilliant surgical technique to relieve parkinsonism had been developed by Dr. Irving S. Cooper, a young New York surgeon, but there weren't enough trained brain surgeons to do the operation. And not all sufferers could be helped by it. Then Cotzias discovered how to get past the blood-brain barrier with L-dopa.

I heard the dramatic story from him in a torrent of thickly accented words punctuated by his irrepressible jokes, bursting grins, and explosive gestures. We talked in a sunny ground-floor office at the Atomic Energy Commission's Brookhaven National Laboratory in Upton, New York. He invited me to lunch with him there. The menu consisted of Metrecal cookies and coffee.

A small printed sign hung on the wall across from his littered desk. It read, "At every crossing in the road that leads to the future, each progressive spirit is opposed by a thousand men appointed to guard the past."

Cotzias is a heavyset man with bushy grey hair and big ears. He has had a life packed with drama. He was born in Athens in 1918 to a very wealthy, aristocratic family. His father was a politician who rose to be a cabinet minister and Lord Mayor of Athens. While George was in his teens, he told his father that he wanted to be a politician, too.

"Nothing doing," his father said. "You can't have two members of the same family in politics."

George had to think of something else to do with his life. As he tells it, "Not long after that, I entered the hospital for an appendectomy. One day, the chief surgeon kiddingly called me 'Mr. Doctor.' I liked the sound of it so I decided to become a doctor."

He started his medical schooling in Athens. When the Nazis conquered Greece in 1941, his family had to flee for their lives in a rented motorboat. They arrived in the United States virtually penniless.

"Was that your first experience with being broke?" I asked him.

"Yes," he said, "but I can assure you, not the last."

He applied for admission to several American medical schools and was rejected by every one because he couldn't speak English. "My father told me something then that I'll never forget. In life, when you cannot get what you want, try for something better. So I applied to the best medical school of them all, Harvard, and it accepted me."

Cotzias was in and out of trouble during his medical school years, internship, and residency. He almost got fired from Massachusetts General Hospital because he gave advice on contraception to a pregnant woman with a serious cardiac condition.

"But the woman's life was in danger," he protested to his chief. "What would you have done?"

"You stupid bastard," his chief said, "I wouldn't have been caught."

Dr. Means, the chairman of the Harvard department of medicine, told Cotzias's father, "I know he's a black sheep, but go on supporting him. George is difficult. He's crazy, but he has a future. Something good will come from him."

Cotzias spent several years at the Rockefeller Institute doing research on nephrosis, a disease of the kidneys. From there, he went to Brookhaven National Laboratory in 1953 for more research.

Why? "Because no one else offered me a job."

But why for more research? "I don't know why the hell . . . It was the failure, I guess. Everybody tells you that you're no good. Fundamentally, I went to Brookhaven to have another chance. Sheer orneriness."

Dr. Cotzias chose to do his research on manganese. He was perfectly frank with me about the reasons behind his choice. "The easy way to pick a project, the *schlemiel* way," he said, "is to look at the chart of the chemical elements and, acting on impulse, pick one that doesn't have much competition for you. Very few investigators were interested in manganese, so I picked it."

In 1961, the World Health Organization (WHO) asked Cotzias to go to Chile to study chronic manganese poisoning among miners. It is a disease that has virtually the same symptoms as parkinsonism.

Cotzias was confident he could cure the miners, and he failed again. He found lots of manganese, but in the wrong people. Active miners, working daily with the metal, had dangerously high concentrations of manganese in their bodies, but no disease. The sick miners, who had been pensioned off because of manganese poisoning, had all the sad symptoms of the disease but very little manganese in their tissues—only the normal amount. Their bodies had gotten rid of it.

It didn't add up right. Cotzias was forced to conclude that the symptoms of manganese poisoning were not caused by ions of the metal running loose in the body, but rather by some chemical damage done to the brain. However, there was absolutely no evidence of any such damage to the brain.

It was the first dead end on the road to L-dopa, and it begot his first myth. "When something goes wrong in medical research," he confessed, "you must try to find some myth to explain why you went wrong. That's how you keep the spirits up of the people around you, the technicians and nurses whose enthusiasms drop when you have a defeat. It's a way of keeping your own spirits up, too. A form of whistling in the dark. It's a trick that some of us researchers practice whenever we meet defeat, which we continually do."

His myth was predicated on the similarity between parkinsonism and manganese poisoning. If a way could be found to treat Parkinson's disease, it would also work against manganese poisoning, he claimed. As it turned out, there was more truth than myth to his hypothesis.

As soon as Cotzias returned to the United States, he began to research Parkinson's disease.

"I felt that I had to," he said. "I was the guy who promised WHO that he'd get the poison out of the people with manganese disease, and they believed me."

He concentrated on a natural body chemical called dopamine which is vital to normal nerve activity in the central part of the brain. A Viennese pathologist, Dr. O. Hornykiewicz, had performed some autopsies in the late 1950s on the bodies of parkinsonism victims and discovered that their brains were lacking in dopamine.

The logical next step was to compensate for this deficiency. But extra dopamine can't be given to the brain; it can't get through the natural barrier that exists between the bloodstream and the brain cells. So Dr. Hornykiewicz and other physicians gave parkinsonism patients dopa, an amino acid that can cross the blood-brain barrier. Once it arrives inside the brain, the dopa converts into dopamine.

It was a great letdown. The dopa produced short-lived relief from the symptoms, but no more, and the side effects were fierce: intolerable nausea, vomiting, and hypertension to the brink of fainting. The consensus was that dopa was useless.

Reluctantly, Cotzias turned his attention to another chemical deficiency that had been found in the brains of parkinsonism patients. They were lacking in a black pigment called melanin.

"Being utter *schlemiels*," Dr. Cotzias declared, "we decided to increase the patients' supply of melanin by administering the MSH hormone that stimulates the production of melanin in the brain. You know what happened? It made their conditions worse, not better; and it darkened their skin.''

He tried another amino acid, phenylalanine, on parkinsonism victims, and it aggravated their tremors even more.

"At this point of utter defeat," Dr. Cotzias said, "it was tempting to throw up our hands and abandon the whole project."

As a last resort, Cotzias created one more myth: that another trial of dopa might succeed. He hypothesized that the dosages had been too small in the initial experiments. It was necessary to saturate the enzymes in the brain with huge amounts of dopa, he thought, to make them perform at maximum biochemical efficiency.

He launched the new trials in 1966 at the small experimental hospital that the Brookhaven National Laboratory had set up. He began by using D,L-dopa but it harmed the patients' white cells, so he switched to the purer L-dopa. (That's short for levodopa.) He administered it by mouth to twenty-eight patients terribly sick with parkinsonism. They were past help by any other means.

He started them at 300 milligrams a day and raised them gradually to 8,000 milligrams a day. He was very cautious about it.

"I sneaked up on the patients," he said. "I increased the pills just a little bit at a time. That way, I could detect any toxic reactions before they became serious, and it conditioned the patients against side effects."

Dr. Cotzias made his report in February 1969. During a two-year period, ten of the twenty-eight patients showed a dramatic improvement, ten more showed marked improvement, and the other eight demonstrated some improvement.

His report was so sensational that one medical journal refused to publish it. "I was called a crook," Cotzias chortled.

L-dopa has since been proven to be highly effective with about 70 percent of parkinsonism victims. It eliminates most of the tremor and other debilitating symptoms, although there can occasionally be some unpleasant side effects. After many years, the L-dopa can lose its effectiveness with some patients, and the full horror of parkinsonism may recur. But while its effectiveness lasts, it enables the victims of Parkinson's disease to live full, normal lives. And, just as Cotzias promised, it has done as much for people with manganese poisoning.

Cotzias anticipates that something better than L-dopa will be coming along. "I don't consider L-dopa a final solution. It's a mere indication of what's possible," he said.

In the summer of 1975, Dr. Cotzias turned his attention from parkinsonism to cancer. He joined the staff of the Memorial Sloan-Kettering Cancer

Center in New York City to explore the possible effects of L-dopa on cancer. He had a very personal reason for his move. In December 1973, he came down with lung cancer himself. He had to have sections of a lung removed.

It was a harrowing experience. "How did your doctor tell you that you had cancer?" I asked.

"He didn't have to tell me," Dr. Cotzias declared. "The surgeon was a classmate of mine and he couldn't hold his tears back."

"How about your wife?" I said. "Was she told the truth?"

"Yes."

"Did the fact that she was sharing the information give you strength?"

Cotzias's answer was slow in coming, and poignant: "It's a very lonely thing to be very ill."

When last I checked, in the spring of 1976, Cotzias was in fine health with no trace of cancer apparent.

He still gets to the laboratory at 7:15 A.M. and works until 6:00 or 6:30, seven days a week, except when he is teaching at Cornell University Medical College.

"I've been called a masochistically compulsive worker," he said.

Dr. Cotzias is married to Betty Ginos, an American-born girl who grew up in Greece. Their one son, Constantin, wants to be a psychologist. Cotzias has given up gardening and rarely has time now for his motorboat. He loves to play chess, though, when he can find a worthy opponent.

What he likes best is to treat patients.

"I love patients," he said, "and patients really love me despite my very bad manners."

While we sat in his kitchen eating pumpkin pie, Selman Waksman quoted some words of Louis Pasteur: "To him who devotes his life to science, nothing can give more happiness than increasing the number of discoveries, but his cup of joy is full when the results of his studies immediately find practical applications."

Those were his feelings, he said. I feel sure that Fleming, Kendall, Folkers, Cotzias, and most of these others would agree.

2

AN OUNCE OF PREVENTION

MEDICAL MEN ARE A CAUTIOUS lot. Sometimes they insist on discovering the same thing two or three times before they are willing to accept the outcome and set it to work helping their patients. Like the remarkable science of immunology.

Back in the ninth century A.D., Chinese physicians found a way to immunize children against small pox. They scraped dried crusts off the sores of people with mild cases of the disease, crumbled the crusts, and had the children inhale the powder through their nostrils. The idea worked excellently, but naturally got lost in some medical limbo. Several hundred years later, Turkish physicians came up with the same theory. Lady Mary Wortley Montague, wife of the British ambassador to Turkey, had her little son immunized against smallpox in Constantinople in the early years of the eighteenth century. In 1721, she introduced the practice to England, and, of course, the concept got mislaid again.*

Seventy-five years after, a middle-aged country doctor from the west of England convinced the medical world of the value of immunization. As a medical student, Edward Jenner became interested in a notion popular with farmers and milkmaids that catching cowpox, a mild disease prevalent among people handling cattle, somehow safeguarded them against smallpox.

---

*Lady Mary couldn't have been very surprised that the idea came to naught. She had cynically written home to a friend in 1717: "I am Patriot enough to take pains to bring this useful invention in fashion in England, and I should not fail to write to some of our Doctors very particularly about it if I knew any one of 'em that I thought had Virtue enough to destroy such a considerable branch of their Revenue for the good of Mankind. . . ."

"I cannot take that disease," one young woman confidently said to Jenner. "I have had the cowpox."

On May 14, 1796, Jenner put the legend to the test. He got a scraping from a pustule on the arm of a milkmaid ill with cowpox and inoculated it into the arm of an eight-year-old boy. Six weeks later, Jenner took a scraping from inside a pustule on a person seriously sick with smallpox and injected it into that little boy.

The lad didn't contract smallpox. Neither did several other people on whom Jenner tried the same experiment. Every one of them had become immune to smallpox.

Jenner proudly wrote up his findings in 1798, and vaccination against smallpox became the medical vogue. Jenner was knighted and a happy Parliament voted him a grant of £10,000.

The purpose of a vaccination is to stimulate the body to mobilize its defenses against disease. When an antigen—that is, a disease-causing virus, bacterium, or almost any other foreign agent of biological origin—invades the body chemistry, the body's response frequently is to manufacture antibodies against it. These antibodies are extraordinary substances made from proteins in the blood. Each type is carefully designed to recognize and attack a specific antigen. It hunts down the antigen wherever it is in the body and destroys it by uniting with it. Ordinarily, the antibodies remain in the bloodstream thereafter, standing guard against any return of the guilty antigen. It is the reason people who survive some diseases are often immune to them for the remainder of their lives.

Jenner demonstrated that the body's immune system could be artificially alerted *in advance* to produce enough antigens to give immunity against smallpox. After that, a whole armamentarium of vaccines against other diseases was thinkable.

Enders Grows the Polio Virus in a Test Tube

There were times during the long, victorious fight against poliomyelitis when the participating scientists seemed to be as determined to wipe each other out as the disease. It was a vivid episode of dirty medical politics.

Polio has been known for more than three millennia. Mothers have feared it almost more than any other illness because of its appetite for little children. It strikes adults, too. A handsome, athletic, thirty-nine-year-old politician, Franklin D. Roosevelt, was hopelessly crippled by the disease in August 1921. It was known as infantile paralysis then.

Usually, polio is an insignificant viral infection that does little damage. But when it involves the central nervous system, it can become a rampaging horror, starting with a fever, headache, and a cruelly stiff neck and back, and building into partial or total paralysis. In epidemic years, it has done massive harm. As many as ten thousand paralytic cases a year were reported in the United States in the epidemic surges of the 1930s and 1940s. One out of every three victims was left twisted and crippled, with his or her shriveled legs encased in clumsy steel braces.

Karl Landsteiner, an Austrian who later emigrated to America, first isolated the polio virus in 1908. Other scientists tried vainly to find a way to grow it in sufficient quantities so that a vaccine could be developed against the disease. With bacteria, this would have been simple. Bacteria can readily be grown in artificial media in the test tube. However, it seemed that viruses could only be grown in living animals, a highly complicated and expensive system.

In 1948, a generous, self-effacing virologist, Dr. John Franklin Enders—one of the few men in the polio field who did not try continually to cut his colleagues' scientific throats—discovered a brilliant technique for growing the polio virus in a test tube. He was awarded the Nobel Prize for it in 1954. He had already won the fondness and respect of those who knew him.

A laconic Connecticut Yankee, Enders was born in West Hartford in 1897 into a millionaire family. He went to a posh preparatory school and on to Yale, dropping out briefly for duty as a pilot in World War I. After his graduation from Yale in 1920, he started in the real-estate business. He lasted nine months.

"Real estate didn't like me, and I didn't like it," Dr. Enders grinned while we talked in his book-covered office at Children's Hospital in Boston. I found him a bald, stocky man with amazingly big ears. He was wearing a tweedy suit, a gay bow tie, and a cordial smile. He spoke slowly, puffing at a big cigar.

"I'd always had an interest in English literature and teaching, so I went up to Harvard Graduate School and spent several years working toward a Ph.D. in English literature," he said.

That was a detour. His roommate at a Cambridge boarding house introduced him to the inspiring Harvard bacteriologist Dr. Hans Zinsser. Enders was entranced by him. He would visit his laboratory at night and listen to Zinsser talk for hours. It persuaded him to quit English and, at the age of twenty-eight, start after a Ph.D. in bacteriology.

"I had luck," he declared. "It took me only four years to get my Ph.D."

Enders taught at Harvard for seventeen years and moved to Children's Hospital in Boston in 1946. His first research was in tuberculosis bacteria, next in pneumonia. Then he transferred his scientific affections to viruses.

The Australian virologist MacFarlane Burnet had been exploring splendid new methods of growing viruses in chick embryos. Enders followed hard on his trail. He and Thomas H. Weller, a bright young medical student from Michigan, showed that viruses could be continuously cultivated for long periods in chick-embryo cells. They put cowpox viruses in a culture of chick-embryo tissue and kept them growing for months. So long as the chick-embryo cells survived and grew, they found that the virus particles inside of them would multiply.

When Enders moved to Children's Hospital, he enlisted two gifted scientists to work for him. One was Dr. Frederick C. Robbins, a thirty-year-old Alabaman, and the other was Tom Weller, now thirty-one and a full-fledged M.D. Enders and Weller achieved the team's first significant advance in 1948; they discovered a way to grow the mumps virus in a test tube in a stew of chick-embryo fragments mixed with ox blood and other laboratory delectables.

Then Weller tried essentially the same method to grow the chicken pox virus. It had never before been grown in cells cultured outside the body. He didn't use chicken cells, though; he employed bits of human embryonic tissues.

This gave Dr. Enders a big idea. He had in his deep-freeze a tube of polio viruses preserved in frozen mouse brain. He suggested that they try to grow the polio viruses by the same method.

It was an unscriptural thought. The conventional theology among polio researchers was that their virus would grow only in nerve tissue, a very costly and dangerous method, too risky for use in making a vaccine. However, a percipient New York researcher, Dr. Albert B. Sabin, had detected the presence of some polio viruses in the intestinal tract, and Enders had a heretical hunch that they could be made to grow in areas other than the nervous system. Sabin is a name we'll hear a lot more of later in the polio slugfest. He won it. (Two other scientists, Drs. John R. Paul and James D. Trask, of Yale, also found that polio viruses were present in the intestines.)

The Enders heresy became scientific gospel. He and his two young assistants added polio viruses to a test tube containing a concoction of cell nutrients and shreds of human muscle and skin. The polio viruses multiplied like mad. The trio injected these polio viruses into laboratory mice, and the animals got paralyzed.

Enders could hardly believe the outcome.

"We had to prove it three times over before Dr. Enders would accept the fact," Dr. Robbins declared.

Just to prove their point, the trio also grew their polio viruses in human embryonic brain tissue, in foreskin removed from young boys, and in tissue from the human intestine itself.

It was the first major advance in forty years of futile struggle against polio. The trio had proven that polio was not specifically a disease of the nerve tissue; scientists didn't have to contend with brain or spinal-cord tissue anymore in working with the virus. Now scientists could conduct their experiments with the polio virus in a test tube. The road was open to a vaccine.

Drs. Robbins and Weller shared the Nobel Prize in 1954 with Dr. Enders. Robbins moved on to Western Reserve University in Cleveland as a full professor of pediatrics. Weller shifted over to the Harvard School of Public Health as a full professor of tropical public health. Enders stayed at the Boston's Children Hospital to confront measles.

Elsewhere, the infighting got vicious.

The Battle of the Polio Vaccines

It was a barroom brawl with no holds barred, scientific or propaganda. Some of the toughest, most colorful men in the medical world were in the thick of it: Dr. Jonas E. Salk, young and unquenchably ambitious; Albert Sabin, just as ambitious, and equally convinced of his scientific rectitude; Basil O'Connor, flamboyant and the ringmaster of the frenetic polio circus. And others.

More was involved than who would get the glory of developing a universally adopted vaccine against polio. An important doctrinal argument had to be settled: the use of killed versus live polio virus for the vaccine. The accepted approach was to kill the polio viruses, inject them into the body by hypodermic needle, and look to them to stimulate the production of antibodies. The adherents of this line of thought said that it would be safest. Dead viruses couldn't give a child a case of polio by mistake. The opposition wasn't so sanguine. "How can you be sure that all the viruses are dead?" they asked. Besides, dead polio viruses could take months to develop immunity, and the immunity wouldn't last long, they charged. Children would have to be revaccinated annually. By comparison, they stressed, attenuated live viruses—that is, viruses whose paralytic power had been diluted to an infinitesimal fraction of its former self— could be easily administered by mouth, would create much longer-lasting immunity, and would achieve it within a few days. Possibly so, said the backers of the dead-virus technique, but suppose the attenuated viruses were not sufficiently weakened before they were fed to children. What then? It could be wholesale death.

Medical history endorsed both sets of doomsday predictions. In 1935, Dr. Maurice Brodie, a youthful Canadian working at the New York

University College of Medicine, tested a polio vaccine containing killed viruses. The same year, Dr. John A. Kolmer, a Philadelphia researcher, tested a vaccine made from attenuated live viruses. Each vaccine was tried on thousands of children, and each failed miserably. A dozen children developed paralytic polio, and six of them died. The memory of those dead and crippled children cast a shadow over all polio vaccine studies.

The search for a vaccine got new stamina through the efforts of another polio victim. In 1938, President Franklin D. Roosevelt helped organize the National Foundation for Infantile Paralysis to battle the disease, and a sympathetic public rushed to contribute to its annual March of Dimes. Not that everybody applauded F.D.R.'s plan. Despite the fact that the foundation was a private organization, *The New York Times* labeled it "a fairly large experiment in socialized medicine."

In medical research, as in many other fields of intellectual activity, power rests with the checkbook. The National Foundation took in the money, so it became the controlling force in the war on polio. The kingpin was Basil O'Connor, a New York attorney who got to head the organization because he was a friend and law partner of F.D.R. He was a man of great energy, great talent for ballyhoo, and great biases. If he liked you, the scientific sky was the limit for you. If he didn't. . . .

Salk was lucky. O'Connor was very fond of Salk and made a protégé of him. Sabin wasn't as well off. O'Connor didn't like him or his views on polio victims.

Salk was born in New York City in 1914, graduated from the New York University College of Medicine, and went off to the University of Michigan to work on influenza viruses under Dr. Thomas Francis, Jr., a virologist with a lot of political connections. Through Dr. Francis, Salk was appointed director of virus research at the University of Pittsburgh Medical School in 1947, and there he turned his eyes to polio. Along with scientists of three other universities, he participated in a big study which established that polio in the United States was caused by three distinct types of viruses—Brunhilde, Lansing, and Leon. To be effective, it was determined, a vaccine had to protect prople against all three types.

The chances of developing such a vaccine appeared very remote until Enders's great discovery changed all the rules of the game. Suddenly, the only questions were who was going to make the vaccine first? and what kind of vaccine would it be?

The Salk Vaccine
—*A Mass Test Misfires*

Salk was absolutely resolved to win the race. At thirty-five he was slim, dark, and balding, a very intense individual and an almost unbelievably hard worker. Some days he put in twenty-four hours at a stretch. With financial support from the National Foundation, he cultured polio viruses in the kidney tissues of monkeys, killed them with formaldehyde (a technique devised by Dr. Brodie), and made himself a vaccine. He tried it initially on 161 institutionalized children. Early in 1953, he reported to the foundation's pivotal immunization committee that the vaccine seemed effective. O'Connor beat the publicity drums gleefully.

Many of the committee's members were in a hurry to stage a mass field test to prove the vaccine's worth. Dr. Enders, Dr. Sabin, and a group of other members were apprehensive about it, though. They weren't convinced of the safety of the killed-virus vaccine.

"Let us not confuse optimism with achievement," Sabin warned the press.

To be sure, Sabin was not entirely without self-interest. He was busy developing a live-virus vaccine himself.

The Salk adherents, with O'Connor pressing them on, rode roughshod over the Enders-Sabin bloc.

Dr. Thomas Rivers of the Rockefeller Institute conceded that some viruses might be left alive in Salk's vaccine, but he doubted that there would be enough of them to do any harm to anyone. "When it's made right," he remarked, "it doesn't hurt anybody, so what's the difference whether every virus particle is killed or not?"

Sabin pleaded with the committee members not to put all their polio eggs into one basket. He urged them to allot some money for further investigation of the live-virus vaccine, too. O'Connor wouldn't tolerate such split loyalties. By his fiat, the National Foundation committed virtually all of its funds and prestige to Salk and his vaccine.

Starting on April 26, 1954, 1,829,916 children took part in a prodigious test of the Salk vaccine. Some four million doses were administered. (Each kid who completed the series of three injections got a button reading "Polio Pioneer.") Salk's friend, Dr. Francis, was placed in charge of the project.

The results were proclaimed on April 12, 1955, with the full fanfare of a Hollywood movie opening. Dr. Francis, a short, stubby man with a fuzzy little mustache, stepped before an array of sixteen television and newsreel cameras in a colossal salmon-colored lecture hall on the Ann Arbor campus of the University of Michigan. Five hundred hand-picked scientists and physicians were on hand, among others, to cheer his words, plus hordes of media people. It was near chaos as the newsmen battled each other for copies of the Francis report.

Dr. Francis theatrically announced that the field trial had been an epochal success. The Salk vaccine had proven to be 60 percent effective against spinal paralysis and 94 percent effective against bulbar paralysis, although no one knew how long this immunity would continue. Not one child had been harmed by the vaccine. Dr. Salk stated categorically that no live viruses were left in the vaccine.

"It is safe, and you can't get safer than safe," he stated in a tone that allowed no contradiction.

The country was rhapsodic. Church bells rang, factory whistles screamed, cannons fired off salutes. Some cities turned all their traffic lights to red in tribute to Dr. Salk. The man was practically beatified.

Euphoria was short-lived. On April 26, word came from California that five children had fallen ill of paralytic polio a few days after they had received the dead-virus vaccine. A shudder ran through medical circles. More alarming reports started pouring in. Scores of other children were coming down with polio, mostly in California and Idaho, 204 cases in all. Seventy-nine of the cases were among children who had just been given the Salk vaccine. The others had caught it from them. Approximately three out of four cases were paralytic. Eleven children died.

A frightened U.S. Public Health Service ordered a halt to all polio vaccinations while it investigated the case. Vainly, O'Connor protested that "Nothing that has been said affects the safety of the vaccine," but the facts refuted him. The presence of virulent live viruses was conclusively established in batches of vaccine manufactured by one company, Cutter Laboratories of Berkeley, California. Enders and Sabin had been right about the dangers implicit in a killed-virus vaccine.

The Salk vaccine program was resumed later with stricter manufacturing safeguards, and no one can doubt that it cut the incidence of polio measurably in the United States and several foreign nations. But public confidence in killed viruses was weakened. Poor Dr. Salk lost his halo.

The Sabin Vaccine Vanquishes Polio

Now Dr. Sabin's live viruses got their chance. The conflicts over them were just as lacerating. Sabin still bears the emotional scars of battle.

According to Dr. John R. Paul, a fellow virologist, Sabin "possessed not only an uncanny sense for nosing out the fallacies contained in old ideas but also an ability to correct his own mistakes. His was a fierce joy when he turned up a new observation and put it to his own good use.''

He was also vastly egotistic, possessive, and stubborn, Dr. Paul said.

Sabin was born in poverty in 1906 in the city of Bialystok in the Czar's Russia. He emigrated with his family to the United States in 1921.

Why did he become a doctor? ''When I finished high school in 1923, I didn't have any money for college. An uncle of mine, who was a dentist, said he would finance me if I'd study dentistry.'' Then. . . .

After two years at the New York University dental school, Sabin switched to medicine. ''I read Paul De Kruif's *Microbe Hunters* and I felt very romantic about the thought of conquering epidemic diseases.''

That cost him his uncle's support. No dentistry, no money, his uncle barked. Sabin had to work his way through the N.Y.U. medical school as a lab technician.

Several decades later, I talked with him about it in New York City. He was slim, trim, medium-tall, with beautifully groomed white hair, carefully shaped white mustache and sideburns, dressed to a ''T'' in a brownish tweed sports jacket, grey slacks, and a pink shirt. He recited the story of his life intently, as though he were testifying in court.

Once someone knocked on the door of the office in which we were sitting.

''I cannot be interrupted,'' Dr. Sabin called out. ''My flow of thought will be disturbed.''

The intruder went away.

Sabin said that he made his first significant finding while he was still in medical school: a new, speedier system for typing pneumococci. As a young fellow at the Rockefeller Institute, he and Dr. Peter K. Olitsky succeeded in growing polio viruses in a test tube in human nerve tissue. Their method wasn't very practical, but it opened new vistas for other researchers. Sabin also isolated a protozoan parasite at Rockefeller that proved to be dangerous to humans, and a mouse pleuropneumonialike organism that produced the symptoms of rheumatic fever and rheumatoid arthritis in mice.

''I've never been able to be a one-virus virologist,'' he said.

During World War II, Sabin served in the Pacific with the U.S. Army and developed effective vaccines against dengue fever and Japanese B encephalitis. Following the war, he resumed his long-time battle to conquer polio. He and his associates at the University of Cincinnati College of Medicine performed sterile autopsies on every patient who died of polio within a radius of four hundred miles. At the same time, they did autopsies on armies of monkeys. Out of these studies came the observation that brought forth Enders's master stroke. Sabin saw that in human beings the polio virus was present in two places: the intestinal tract and the nervous system, both.

From the outset, Sabin knew that he hadn't a chance of beating out Salk to be first to produce a polio vaccine. It is much easier to kill viruses than to dilute them. He continued, nonetheless.

His immediate goal was to find the best strains of polio virus to use in his vaccine. The viruses had to multiply well in the intestinal tract, but have little or no effect on the central nervous system. Solemnly, he recited his rationale to me.

"It was my conviction that if we could attenuate polio viruses through selection and through experimental modification, we could administer them by the natural portal of entry, namely, the mouth, let them multiply in the intestinal tract, and thereby produce immunity from paralysis."

By the use of 15,000 monkeys (hundreds of chimpanzees, too) and years of work, he was able to dilute three strains of polio virus to a point where they were more than a million times less virulent than their ancestors. But were they safe enough yet? Sabin tested all three strains on himself, his own children, his research associates, and on volunteer prisoners in a Chillicothe, Ohio, penitentiary. The results were excellent: definite immunity to polio, with no dangerous effects.

No one at the National Foundation seemed to care about his progress, though. They were still wedded to the Salk killed-virus vaccine.

"Why the devil don't you throw those strains of yours down the drain?" Dr. Rivers told Sabin early in 1957.

Dr. Sabin almost moaned as he recalled those days. "Oh, there were many heartaches!"

Sabin faced rancorous competition in the life-virus camp, too. Drs. Herald R. Cox and Hilary Koprowski, two scientists employed by Lederle Laboratories, each developed a live-virus vaccine against polio. Each believed unswervingly in his vaccine and angrily abused the other's vaccine. Synchronously, the Lederle public relations machine spewed forth streams of propaganda denouncing Sabin's vaccine. Anything to discredit a rival!

Koprowski's vaccine got the first big test—on 206 humans in Northern Ireland in 1956, and the outcome was incriminating. It was found that Koprowski's attenuated viruses were still a menace. After they entered the human body, they could easily revert to a virulent state. Later, larger-scale tests were run in the Congo and Colombia. They finished both Cox and Koprowski as competitors, if not as propagandists.

The truth is that Sabin outgeneraled them all: Cox, Koprowski, Salk,

Rivers, even O'Connor. He did a consummate job of promoting his vaccine. Since American officialdom wouldn't give his vaccine the right time, he got the Health Ministry of the Soviet Union to adopt it. The Russians checked it for safety and began spooning out his attenuated viruses to children in the spring of 1957. First, 127 children were vaccinated. All turned out well with them, so another 2,000 Russian children got Sabin-type vaccinations. In 1959, 10,000,000 children received Sabin's vaccine in the Soviet Union. In 1960, 70,000,000 people in the Soviet Union were successfully vaccinated with it, and another 30,000,000 in the satellite countries.

I asked Dr. Sabin why the Soviet authorities were so much more susceptible to his vaccine than the Americans.

"Well, I'll tell you," he declared, "before 1954, they used to say in the Soviet Union, 'Under our socialist health system, we don't get polio the way they do in capitalist countries.' Then, all of a sudden, their turn came. They began to have big epidemics—18,000-20,000 paralytic cases a year—and they were frightened. I knew it, and I invited them to Cincinnati to see my experiments."

Sabin traveled extensively inside and outside the Soviet Union, talked to the press, issued statements, took part in countless scientific meetings, pushing his vaccine. He did a real selling stint.

All this time, the National Foundation and the U.S. Public Health Service were still concentrating on the Salk vaccine. For lack of anything better, the Salk vaccine was still being widely used in the United States.

By 1960, the evidence for the Sabin oral vaccine was so compelling that the U.S. Public Health Service had to approve its manufacture. The USPHS was afraid to go any further and order its use, though. It was still playing with the National Foundation. The American Medical Association was as timid. It called for vaccination against polio, but declined to do more about it than deliver pious sermons against disease.

Providentially, a pediatrician in Phoenix, Arizona, Dr. Richard Johns, launched a personal crusade to put over the Sabin vaccine. He convinced the town fathers, the county medical society, the press, and the TV and radio stations to sponsor a Sabin vaccination drive against polio. Vaccine was supplied free, and, one Sunday, hundreds of Phoenix doctors and laymen contributed their services free. Other communities followed suit. Before long, a hundred million Americans had received the oral vaccine safely and effectively.

That wiped out the peril of polio in the United States. Its threat was, for all purposes, soon eliminated everywhere else, too. Sabin had won.

To this day he is soured by the struggle he was put through. He feels that

O'Connor was too much the czar, that the National Foundation had far too much power. No man or organization, public or private, should ever again have such dictatorial control over medical research, he believes. One is hard-pressed to disagree with him on either count.

What are the reactions of a man who created a vaccine that wiped out a major disease?

His answer revealed how deeply he resents the criticism that was heaped on him. "The one thing I had which others didn't was persistence. After I'd completed my research, I didn't sit back like some basic scientists and say, 'Well, I've done my job.' I couldn't sit quietly when I knew that thousands of cases of polio were still occurring. I became involved. All right, so my colleagues called me what they thought was a dirty word. I was a promoter. But the point was that I wasn't happy to see this vaccine available and not being used."

He continued: "Scientists are divided into two categories. There are some first-rate scientists, curiosity-oriented, who really do excellent work but who don't give a damn about humanity. Now, I would not require any scientist to take an oath that he loves humanity before he has the opportunity to do science. If he does good science, he is making a contribution. However, there are other scientists who are just as curiosity-oriented but who are very much concerned that the knowledge they accumulate is used for human welfare. I call them humanist scientists. I'm a humanist scientist. I've always been a mission-oriented scientist. I've never studied a virus for its own sake. I've studied it for what relevance it had to human disease. I've always kept my eye on human problems while other scientists were satisfied to take pot shots at this or that phenomenon."

Dr. Sabin went to Israel in 1970 as president of the renowned Weizmann Institute of Science. His resignation was revealed at the end of 1972. Some said that it was on the grounds of ill health. (He did undergo open-heart surgery in 1972.) Other reports had it that he had antagonized some of the Weizmann staff with his insistence on mission-oriented research. He returned to the United States and research at the National Institutes of Health in Bethesda, Maryland.

He has been working on cancer. In April 1973, he announced to the stentorian blare of N.I.H. publicity trumpets that he had discovered a link between the ordinary herpes simplex virus and nine kinds of human cancer. A year later, he frankly reported that his findings were in error. He couldn't repeat his results.

Sabin has had three wives and two daughters. When I met with him, he was between marriages and enjoying it. "I'm a bachelor, and my biological clock is running backward," he said. "Instead of getting older, I'm getting younger—in spirit, at least. I'm full of beans, just as much as I was thirty years ago.''

Soon afterward, he married a handsome Brazilian divorcee, Heloisa Dunshee De Abranches, a newspaperwoman. They are living in Charleston, South Carolina, where Dr. Sabin is now Distinguished Professor of Biomedicine at the Medical University of South Carolina.

Dr. Salk was also wed again after twenty-seven years of marriage and three children. He made international headlines in 1970 by wedding Francoise Gilot, the former mistress of Pablo Picasso.

Most of Dr. Salk's time and effort go into the Salk Institute, a research establishment he founded in La Jolla, California. He calls himself a "short-term pessimist, but long-term optimist." His vendetta against Dr. Sabin continues. He even wrote an article for the "Op-Ed" page of *The New York Times* in 1973 denouncing the Sabin oral vaccine as unsafe.

"It's not too late to change back" to the Salk vaccine, he urged.

No one paid much attention to his article. Polio was vanquished. Even if Dr. Salk wouldn't admit it, everyone else did.

The Enders Vaccine Attacks Measles

The fight against the childhood scourge, measles, went more easily and decently. This is not surprising when you consider that Dr. Enders was in command.

For more than a thousand years, ever since Rhazes, a physician in Persia, first described the disease in the tenth century A.D., doctors have striven to find a treatment for measles. (Rubeola is another name for it.) Old-time sorcerers prescribed amulets and prayers to the gods. Colonial American physicians recommended bleeding, sweating, drawing plasters, and mustard baths. One tribe of Indians dipped their sick children in water in hopes of rinsing away the measles rash. Another tribe sprinkled their children with ashes.

Most often, measles is a mere nuisance, a joke, a week or two of mild discomfort for a very funny-looking, spotty-faced child. But sometimes it can be a villainous disease that kills children or cripples them mentally. One epidemic in Quito, Ecuador, slaughtered 2,400 children in 1785. Noah Webster reported an epidemic of measles in little Charleston, North Carolina, in 1772 in which "died 800 or 900 children." For sixty-five years, not one case of measles was seen in the Faroe Islands. Then in 1846, measles broke out, and one fourth of the population died of it. In Fiji, an epidemic of measles did to death 40,000 of the 150,000 population. It continually ravaged Black Africa. Every year, it used to destroy at least one quarter of all the babies born in Upper Volta.

According to the textbooks, measles is a highly contagious viral disease whose early symptoms include a burning fever, swollen, reddened eyes, a runny nose, and a hacking cough. White spots crop out inside the mouth. An evil, itchy rash spreads over the child's face, neck, body, arms, and legs.

The disease can do violence in many ways. Sometimes it causes a fatal viral pneumonia; sometimes it sets the stage for a lethal bacterial pneumonia. Sometimes it brews "strep" and "staph" infections. Sometimes it induces encephalitis, an inflammation of the child's brain. Many of these encephalitic children die. About 40 percent suffer lasting brain injury and mental impairment. Some children become totally, permanently deaf.

Dr. Enders first went after measles in the early 1930s and ran up against a brick wall. Encouraged by his success with the polio virus, he returned to measles in 1953. A good-looking thirty-two-year-old pediatrician, Dr. Thomas Peebles, came to work for him, and Enders set him onto measles. Under Enders's guidance, Peebles was able to isolate a measles virus from the blood and throat washings of an eleven-year-old boy, David Edmonston, who was laid up with measles in his prep school infirmary.

Some say that scientists like Enders are great because of their skepticism. Some say it is despite the skepticism. In any event, Enders didn't believe Peebles's report. He looked through the microscope at Peebles's slides and said, "Thomas, I don't see it."

Peebles had to repeat the experiment again, and again, until Enders was convinced.

This time, Enders decided to make the vaccine himself. Naturally, he chose to use live rather than killed viruses. He and his assistants grew twenty-four generations of the Edmonston strain in human kidney tissue and bred it for twenty-eight more generations in human amnion, the membrane that surrounds embryos. They then grew these tamed viruses in fertilized hens' eggs and in chick-embryo cells. By that time the viruses had only a shadow left of their original virulence. Enders tested a vaccine he had made of them on special measles-free monkeys flown in from Java and the Philippines, on himself, and on his laboratory colleagues. It seemed as safe and as effective as he had hoped.

A young pediatrician at Children's Hospital, Dr. Samuel L. Katz, took it from there. He injected the Enders vaccine into eleven little children who were completely susceptible to measles, having never gained immunity through a prior attack. Eight of them developed slight fevers, nine had vague rashes, but inside of a day or two these mild symptoms disappeared, and every child had achieved full immunity to measles.

A demonstration was held at a state school for children on Staten Island, New York. Twenty-three youngsters were vaccinated and twenty-three served as unvaccinated controls. When an epidemic of measles burst loose at the school, seventeen of the twenty-three unvaccinated children became ill, but not one of the vaccinated children got measles, even though they all were permitted to play with the sick kids.

Tens of millions of children have now been inoculated with the Enders vaccine. In 1963, 385,000 cases of measles were reported in the United States. By 1974, that number had shrunk to 22,094. This has pleased Dr. Enders a lot. Nevertheless, he was very disturbed when I last talked with him because the federal government had slashed funds for providing free vaccine to poor children. Enders couldn't understand why a rich country would spend billions of dollars to put a man on the moon but cut back on the few dollars needed to save its children from the risks of measles.

Victories over measles and polio viruses haven't dulled Dr. Enders's scientific thirst. He has now moved against cancer viruses.

I asked him what had led him into a life of medical research.

"It seemed to me as a young man," he said, "that if I were going to spend my life in an academic background, which I wanted to do, that background had to be related to medicine. It had to combine both the intellectual and something that would have tangible value to mankind."

Enders is a very human scientist with his share of superstitions. At the climactic moment in any experiment, he always puts on a banged-up old felt hat (he collects them) for good luck. His chief delight outside of the laboratory is good talk on a large assortment of topics, from science to art to literature and music. He was wed to Sarah Frances Bennett in 1927, and they had two children. She died in 1943, and in 1951 he married Carolyn Bernice Keane. They live simply in Brookline, Massachusetts.

Hilleman Beats a Flu Pandemic to the Punch

When you speak about death in awful, massive doses, you're likely to think of such epidemical horrors as cholera or the plague. Or a world war. Yet influenza can be worse.

Much of the time, flu is a mediocre illness—a few days of misery, that's all. But on occasion, it has been one of history's greatest killers. In 1918 and 1919, it overran most of the world, from the jungles of Africa to the crowded cities of Europe and the United States. The Japanese called it "wrestlers' fever"; the English named it "Flanders grippe"; the Germans spoke of it apprehensively as "Blitz Katarrh"; the Americans knew it as "Spanish influenza." It prostrated practically the whole Swiss army. It exterminated far-off Eskimo villages in Alaska. Twenty-five million people fell ill of it in the United States, and 518,000 of them died. It killed a total of 20,000,000 people throughout the world. That was twice the number of all World War I deaths.

"Had the epidemic continued its mathematical rate of acceleration," A. A. Hoehling wrote in *The Great Epidemic*, "civilization could have disappeared within a few more weeks."

In 1957, a terrible new influenza pandemic—a worldwide epidemic—born in Asia, menaced all of mankind again. Dr. Maurice R. Hilleman, a fast-thinking U.S. Army virologist, a dynamo of a man who works best under intense pressure, defeated that threat. He beat the flu pandemic to the punch.

Hilleman was born in Miles City, Montana, in 1919, the son of a farmer who had to work part-time on the railroad to help make ends meet during the Great Depression and drought of the 1930s. From childhood, the boy was absorbed in the sciences. Graduating from Montana State College, he took a Ph.D. in microbiology and virology at the University of Chicago. He experimented with vaccines for Squibb, then began a ten-year stint on viruses at the Walter Reed Army Institute of Research, the U.S. Army's fine medical establishment in Washington, D.C. In 1950, while at the institute, he discovered the adenoviruses,* a group of viruses responsible for acute respiratory diseases and pneumonia, and prepared a killed-virus vaccine for use against them. He is now employed by Merck & Co. and is vice-president of Merck's research laboratories in West Point, Pennsylvania, and director of virus and cell biology research at the Merck Institute for Therapeutic Research.

We lunched in a private dining room at the laboratories. I found him a tall man, very bald, with penetrating dark eyes, who punctuated his statements on occasion with some colorful profanity.

"I guess I agree with Clarence Darrow," he explained. "Darrow once said that there are so few words that everyone really understands that he was inclined to use them all."

When the Asian flu pandemic broke out in 1957, Hilleman was in charge of the respiratory disease program at the Walter Reed Institute, focusing on influenza. Never could there have been a better example of the right man in the right place at the very right moment.

Ordinarily, flu is a highly contagious disease that seizes the victim within twenty-four to seventy-two hours after he is exposed to its virus.

---

*Drs. Wallace P. Rowe and Robert J. Huebner of the National Institutes of Health discovered the adenoviruses, too, independently of Hilleman. A dispute continues between them as to who merits top credit.

The patient has chills, headaches, pains in the back and legs, an unproductive cough, fever, and a dread sense of anxiety. He is apt to be prostrated for two or three days and to feel absolutely washed out—like "a piece of overcooked macaroni," somebody wrote. But generally, nothing more than that—unless it's the pandemic kind of flu. Then a rapidly fatal pulmonary infection can set in, and the patient may be dead in forty-eight hours from the moment he feels his first chill.

Three types of flu viruses have been identified—A, B, and C. It is the group A viruses that cause the pandemics. Over thirty of these pandemics have been recorded since 1510.

Dr. Hilleman's problem at Walter Reed was to conduct surveillance on influenza and predict when the next pandemic would break out. Flu viruses, especially type A, are tricky foes. As soon as mass immunity to them develops, these viruses form new subtypes against which the population has no natural protection. Minor changes seem to occur in flu viruses every two to three years. Once a decade or so, a major mutation takes place. The new subtypes are spread around the world by travelers, and another epidemic spews up. Or a fearful pandemic.

Surveillance teams with excellent scientists and equipment are on the watch all over the world for the appearance of new flu viruses. Inexplicably, they missed the arrival of the 1957 flu pandemic in Hong Kong. Dr. Hilleman spotted it in the pages of *The New York Times*. There, he saw a small dispatch on the morning of April 17, 1957, reporting that tens of thousands of Chinese mothers were queuing up at Hong Kong dispensaries, carrying babies with glassy stares.

"It means only one thing to me—tens of thousands of children with high fevers," he said. "What else could it be? To me, it was a signal that pandemic influenza had broken out."

He cabled the U.S. Army's 406th Medical General Laboratory in Tokyo, Japan, to get him throat washings from Hong Kong. The first specimens reached his laboratory on May 13. Within five days, Hilleman had isolated a new flu virus. It was a particularly virulent one, called subtype A2. No known vaccine was effective against it.

Hilleman notified the Armed Forces Epidemiological Board, the U.S. Public Health Service, and the World Health Organization that a new pandemic was coming. It threatened to be as bad as the 1918-1919 holocaust, he warned.

Once the virus was isolated, it could be grown in eggs and a vaccine made from it. But could enough vaccine be produced in time to vaccinate millions of people? Hilleman figured that they had only a few months before the pandemic would assault North America.

The big obstacle in the production of flu vaccine is getting fertile eggs in which to culture the viruses. Ordinary eggs are plentiful, but fertile eggs are scarce.

Hilleman telephoned the six major vaccine manufacturers in the United States. "For God's sake, save your roosters," he said.

"Have your suppliers save roosters, too," he added. "Save roosters because there's a new flu virus. I can't prove it now but I think there's going to be a new pandemic."

The drug men saved their roosters, and the fertile eggs came through. In turn, Hilleman supplied the manufacturers with the virus, and they were able to turn out forty-nine million doses of the vaccine in time.

The pandemic was spawned in mainland China in late February. It moved into Hong Kong in April. From Hong Kong, it suffused Taiwan, Borneo, and Australia. By June, it was in East Africa. By July, it was rampaging through the Middle East, had invaded Europe, and jumped the Atlantic. Half the people in the United States were down with the flu. But by December, the pandemic was over. Nearly nineteen thousand people, most of them elderly, had died of it in the United States, and the toll elsewhere was also comparatively low. Hilleman's foresight and quick action had averted a major catastrophe.

In a reflective mood, Dr. Hilleman once wrote, "The practice of science, like the practice of politics, is a game which is best played with one's sights set on the possible and probable."

More characteristically, he remarked to me of his battle with the Asian flu, "Goddamn it, I knew there was no time to waste and we didn't waste any."

In July 1968, the A2 flu virus went berserk in a new disguise in the same old place. Some 500,000 of Hong Kong's 2,500,000 population were seriously sickened, and the virus went marching around the world again. The American actress Tallulah Bankhead died of it. WHO came to Hilleman for assistance, and he helped produce a vaccine to control the disease. Some twenty million people were vaccinated with it in the United States.

Stopping a flu pandemic in its tracks was just a waystop in Hilleman's busy career. In 1963, he developed a live-virus vaccine against mumps that has come to be the standard safeguard for children today.

Mumps is generally considered a minor childhood illness in which a youngster's face balloons up grotesquely and he has some fever, nausea, and aches and pains that soon pass. It can be serious, though. It can cause permanent facial paralysis and bring on impairment of the brain, the ears, eyes, heart, and reproductive organs. Grown men fear catching it mightily because it can set off orchitis, a fiery inflammation of the reproductive glands. Their testicles swell up painfully and may later atrophy. Sterility can ensue. Among women, mumps can cause the ovaries to swell. Primarily, mumps attacks children between the ages of five and fifteen, but it is recorded that a man ninety-nine-and-a-half years old contracted it in 1899.

Killed-virus vaccines have been available against mumps for some years, but their protections are temporary at best. The Hilleman vaccine gives long-lasting immunity. He obtained the virus for it from his five-year-old daughter, Jeryl Lynn.

One night in 1963, a few months after his first wife died of cancer, he was awakened by the child.

"Daddy, my throat hurts," she wailed.

He looked at her. "Oh, my God, you've got mumps, kid," he said.

He had to leave in the morning on an important scientific trip abroad, so he sped to the labs in the middle of the night to get equipment to take a throat washing from the child. It confirmed his diagnosis. The Jeryl Lynn strain of mumps vaccine isolated from this throat washing became the basis for a live-virus vaccine that has since been given to more than eighteen million children. Jeryl's baby sister, Kirsten, was one of the first children to receive it. She cried her eyes out when the needle was injected. Jeryl also wept, in sympathy with her sister.

"Developing a vaccine is nothing but trouble from the day you start," Dr. Hilleman declared. "Learning how to attenuate the virus, finding the culture the virus will grow in, the whole business of getting rid of extraneous viruses, the testing you need to do before you can try the vaccine in man, the computerized field trials you have to run with ten thousand to twenty thousand people—it's problems all the way."

When Merck was first manufacturing the Enders's measles vaccine, an alien leukemia virus was found in it, Hilleman revealed.

"It was a real job getting rid of that one," he said. "We had to scour America for chickens free of the infection.

"Trying to do something to prevent disease in kids is really worth it, though," he said. "I suppose that everybody who's here in the world should try to do something that's useful, and this is my way of doing it. I'm not worth much outside of science. I don't really participate in community affairs or anything like that—too busy—so I try to do my good deeds in science. These philosophical concepts come from childhood. I happen to be a Lutheran, a religion which encourages you to be your brother's keeper. I wouldn't say that I'm religious, but this kind of background was ingrained in me from the time I could talk, and I think it's not at all a bad idea."

Hilleman rarely works in a lab himself anymore. As research director at the Merck laboratories, he oversees other scientists. Usually he is at the lab from eight-thirty in the morning until five-thirty, and spends his evenings reading and writing scientific papers. That's a seven-day-a-week schedule.

He has a second wife, Lorraine Witman. He, his wife, and his two daughters live in a rambling old house in LaFayette Hill, Pennsylvania.

"I don't engage in sports or things like that," he said, "but I do like to be an amateur carpenter, mechanic, electrician, what-have-you. Hell, I did a lot of the rebuilding on my house. It's fun. I'm also very wrapped up in the kids. They both have an interest in medicine, and nothing would please me more than to see them there. Lorraine's a nurse by training, too, you know."

Predictably, the interview ended with an expletive.

Parkman and Meyer Subdue Rubella

An epidemic of rubella—a disease most people call German measles—stalked across the United States in 1964 and 1965. For the tens of thousands of children who fell ill with the virus, there were some sniffles, some swollen glands, a little flu, some malaise, a meek pink rash, and a couple of days' holiday from school. After that, having once contracted the disease, they were almost certain to be immune from it for the rest of their lives.

It was something worse for many thousands of pregnant women. The epidemic brought them the births of an estimated twenty thousand babies with blinding cataracts, defective hearing, abnormal hearts, heads too small for their bodies, and mental retardation. Another thirty thousand babies weren't really born. They ended up in miscarriages or stillbirths.

As a slayer and crippler of unborn children, rubella probably has taken more victims than polio, mumps, ordinary "red" measles (rubeola), chicken pox, and scarlet fever combined. But there is no reason for civilization to endure another rubella epidemic of such dimensions. Two enthusiastic young physicians have developed a vaccine that's fully effective against the disease. They had a cliff-hanging struggle before they were allowed to prove the vaccine's worth, of course. The enemy was their youth. And the myopia of their scientific elders.

Rubella is a totally different disease from the ordinary "red" measles. It primarily mangles the unborn. Back in 1941, Dr. Norman Gregg, an Australian ophthalmologist on duty in the outpatient service of the Royal Alexandra Hospital for Children in Sydney, was impressed by the large number of infants conceived during a rubella epidemic who were born with cataracts. That started the investigators searching. It was found that approximately 50 percent of the babies born to mothers who contract rubella in the first four weeks of their pregnancy are malformed. If the mothers catch rubella in the second or third months, 15-20 percent of the babies are born with defects.

The two doctors who ended this menace are Dr. Paul D. Parkman, a tall, well-built ex-farm boy from central New York State, and Dr. Harry M. Meyer, Jr., a lanky, thin chap, prematurely grey, who hails from a small town in Texas. Both were born in 1932. I saw them together in a stuffy, windowless conference room at the National Institutes of Health in Bethesda, Maryland. Both men were bubbling over with ideas and good humor, in love with mankind and medicine. Parkman was wearing a long white lab coat over a shrieking yellow shirt, blue tie, and blue slacks. Meyer's costume was more restrained. He had on a pale beige shirt and striped brown slacks under his lab coat. Seven pencils stuck up out of his breast pocket.

Parkman chose medicine because of "a certain feeling that you'd be doing good work." It was a hard pull financially.

"My great-grandfather was a very wealthy man with large landholdings," he said, "but he had a problem. He liked fast women and slow horses."

"That is a serious problem," Dr. Meyer interjected.

"So my father was a carpenter. He also worked as a post office clerk and raised chickens and turkeys. Between these three jobs," Parkman recalled, "he somehow managed to scrape together enough coins to send me to medical school. He used to say to me, 'I don't want you to be a carpenter like me. You stick to your books.' "

Parkman studied medicine at Upstate University of New York in Syracuse, did a residency in pediatrics, and was summoned by the Army for military duty. He was assigned to the virology department at Walter Reed Institute. Here he met Dr. Meyer.

Hank Meyer came to research by another route. His father was a horticulturist who taught him curiosity. He also happened to read De Kruif's *Microbe Hunters.* "I can actually remember thinking, Gosh, what could possibly be more exciting than finding something like a rabies vaccine." That headed him toward the University of Arkansas medical school, microbiology, and research.

He talks at a breakneck staccato tempo, and with delicious candor. "You could have asked most of the teachers around medical school to point to the students who looked like they were going somewhere. I don't think you would have found many fingers pointing my way. My medical school record was strictly so-so. If I was interested in something, I worked on it. If I wasn't, I didn't."

An Army internship brought him to Washington, D.C., and the Walter

Reed Institute. "Gosh, I was afraid! I was a country hick. For me to come to a big city like Washington was traumatic. When I saw all those people and all those automobiles, I was very fearful, I really was."

Following his Army duty, Meyer did a pediatrics residency and then joined the N.I.H. research staff. One reason he settled on a career in research, he said, loudly, excitedly, was the futility he felt when he couldn't help a patient. "I'm thinking of a little boy with measles who developed encephalitis. It's a ghastly disease. That kid was in a coma for thirty days, and I couldn't help him at all. You do everything you can for a child, and the best you do, working day after day and night after night, isn't enough. The kid still ends up with permanent brain damage, or dead.

"People like Paul Parkman and me, we say to ourselves, 'Look, if we could find a cure for a disease, we wouldn't be helping just one patient, we'd be helping thousands.' "

Later, Meyer and two other N.I.H. physicians ran trials of the Enders measles vaccine in Africa. "Just think," he said, "three lousy people, with a little help, could save a hundred thousand children from dying of measles because we had a vaccine to use on them!"

Dr. Parkman helped make the first great inroad on the rubella situation while he was serving at the Walter Reed Institute. Together with two other Army physicians, Drs. Malcolm S. Artenstein and Edward L. Buescher, he set forth in February 1961 to isolate the elusive rubella virus. Thousands of Army recruits were sick with rubella, and the Army wanted a vaccine against the disease.

Parkman got the idea that cornered the virus. He read about an English experiment showing that something in nasal washings from patients with colds seemed to interfere with the growth of a poliolike virus called Echo 11. Perhaps, Parkman thought, the same interference phenomenon might work on a rubella washing. He and his two colleagues took some throat washings from rubella patients, made some cultures of them in monkey kidney cells, and added the Echo 11 virus.

"We checked those cultures the next day," Parkman said. "Not a change in them. We checked them the second day and found something strange. It looked as though the Echo 11 virus wasn't growing in the cultures with the rubella in them. So we raced over and looked at them again on the morning of the third day, and this time it was really striking. We could find absolutely no evidence of Echo 11 virus growth in the cultures that had received the rubella throat washings. But in the control cultures—those without rubella throat washings—man, the Echo 11 virus was growing like crazy! In other words, there was a virus in those cultures that was killing the Echo 11."

It was the rubella virus. By mid-June, they had it isolated. Coincidentally, another group of investigators in Boston, led by Dr. Thomas H.
Weller, the Nobel laureate who had collaborated with Enders on his polio
research, reported the isolation of a rubella virus at the same time. It proved
to be the same virus, thereby clinching the Parkman group's findings.

Dr. Parkman quit the Army in 1963 and went to work for the Division of
Biologic Standards at the N.I.H. Hank Meyer was chief of the division's
laboratory of viral immunology, and they decided to work together on a
preventive against rubella. They knew that some of the biggest men in the
medical community—Hilleman, Weller, and Saul Krugman, the distinguished New York pediatrician—were trying to develop a rubella vaccine,
but they resolved to go ahead anyway. Scientific "chutzpah," so to speak.

They tried for a killed-virus vaccine. It would be the quickest, they
thought. Their killed-virus vaccine didn't produce immunity, though, so
they had to commence the long, tedious process of attenuating live rubella
virus. Two years and seventy-seven generations of viruses later, they
finally had a tame virus. They tested it on monkeys and themselves, and it
acted safe.

By late summer of 1965, they were ready for clinical trials. They chose
the Arkansas Children's Colony, a state institution for the mentally
retarded, as the site of their clinical trial, and carefully obtained the written
consent of the parents of every child involved. That done, they applied for
the approval of the all-powerful medical board at the N.I.H.

"You can't just go ahead and stick needles in people's arms," Dr.
Meyer explained. "You have to have your protocol. You have to have your
justification. You have to show what you know and what you hope to gain,
and you have to show all the risks."

The board session was stormy. The grey-headed men around the table
thought that Parkman and Meyer were too young. Furthermore, they didn't
think that either of them was much of a scientific whiz. Most board
decisions were unanimous, but this time the board split right down the
middle. Half of the members were in favor of the plan, half against it. The
decision had to be put off.

Parkman and Meyer were in near-misery. "Here, we'd been working on
this damned project like dogs, day and night, for two years," Dr. Meyer
said, "and we didn't know whether we were going to be permitted to go
ahead or not."

"It was right down to the wire," Dr. Parkman said. "We had our plane
reservations to go, but we didn't have approval. And we knew that if we
didn't get approval, we were out of business."

"Were you both very upset?" I asked.

"We were very hostile," Dr. Meyer said. "We were ready to go over and kill every goddamned one of them."

At the last moment, Dr. James A. Shannon, the N.I.H. director, ruled in their favor, and they made their plane. Sixteen little girls who were completely susceptible to rubella, having never before contracted the disease and become immune, took part in the Arkansas trial. Eight were vaccinated, eight served as controls. For eight taut weeks, Meyer and Parkman took throat swabs every day, blood samples once a week. The samples were encased in dry ice and flown back to Bethesda for analysis.

All eight vaccinated girls developed full immunity to rubella. Not one had any ill effects. Mass trials involving thousands were later held, and the same result recorded.

More than forty-six million doses of the vaccine have been administered since then, and the rubella trend has been consistently downward. In 1972, 25,507 cases of rubella were reported in the United States, 50 percent fewer than the average number in each year between 1967 and 1971. In 1974, just 11,917 cases were reported.

And the immunity conferred upon millions of girls—and potential mothers—protects them from the terrible ravages of rubella among babies born to mothers who contract the disease in early pregnancy.

Some authorities hold that the vaccine should only be administered to susceptible women contemplating pregnancy, but the concensus in medical circles currently is that it should be routinely given to all susceptible children over one year of age.

Incidentally, Parkman and Meyer developed a useful laboratory test which can tell in three hours whether a person is susceptible to rubella. Former tests took three weeks.

The pair now do their research for the U.S. Food and Drug Administration, the Division of Biologic Standards having been transferred from the NIH to the FDA in 1972. Meyer is director, Parkman deputy director. Each likes a reasonable work schedule: 7:30 A.M. to 5:30 or 6:00 in the evening.

Dr. Meyer is married to Barbara Bernheim, an N.I.H. virologist who worked with him in Africa on the measles vaccination campaign. It's a second marriage for both. They have four children between them by their first marriages, and they live actively, gaily, on a sixteen-acre farmette with five riding horses in Waterford, Virginia. For many years, Meyer was an inveterate spelunker, exploring every cavern he could clamber down into. "A period of temporary madness in my life," he concedes. Currently, he hikes up and down the Appalachian Trail, searching for new species of wild orchids, or grows them himself under artificial light.

Dr. Parkman is more restrained in his recreational outlets. He just plays tennis. He and his wife, Emerina Leonardi, live in Kensington, Maryland. They have no children.

"Didn't you ever want to be rich men?" I asked.

"I don't think Paul and I would be in the science game if we were going to starve to death," Dr. Meyer replied. "If we couldn't buy washing machines for our wives, if we couldn't send diapers to the baby services, if we couldn't do at least a few of the things we consider reasonable for professional men in an affluent society, we probably wouldn't be in science, but I'm not interested in making a load of money."

"Hell, I am rich," said Dr. Parkman. "Compared with feeding all those turkeys, I consider myself very rich."

"Is luck a big factor in research?" I inquired.

"Maybe so," Dr. Meyer said, "but only if you've got somebody who's aggressive, who is always searching for other information about his field. God, ideas are the cheapest things in the world! The big thing in scientific discovery is to put the ideas together to accomplish something that wouldn't have been accomplished otherwise. If you're not curious, if you're lazy, if you're just sitting around, good ideas can fall all over you and you'll never capitalize on them."

One comforting bit of news for children about these new vaccines is this: they don't have to be taken individually anymore. Dr. Hilleman has prepared a combination vaccine which permits children to get their measles, mumps, and rubella protection with a single inoculation. Dr. Anatoly A. Smorodintsev, of the Pasteur Institute of Epidemiology and Microbiology in Leningrad, has done as much for Russian youngsters.

"And about time!" Dr. Hilleman growled. "My God, the kids were becoming pincushions."

A Race Against Death with Spinal Meningitis

Take spinal meningitis. "It kills as fast as the plague," Dr. Irving Goldschneider, a pathologist at the University of Connecticut medical school, told me.

It can strike, he said, like this: "Your baby gets a little feverish. She doesn't feel well and she's very sleepy. The pediatrician tells you to bring her in. The baby's throat is a little red, that's all, so he takes a throat culture and just treats her symptomatically—to reduce the fever. A couple of hours later, the baby develops a rash and you can hardly rouse her. Her fever is higher. You phone the pediatrician fearfully. He says, 'I'll meet you in the emergency room.'

"Before you can put down the phone, the baby has a convulsion. You rush to the hospital, but she is DOA—dead on arrival."

Any child who survives meningitis may be left blind, paralyzed, or brain-damaged.

Meningitis is an inflammation of the membrane covering the brain and spinal cord that besets 18,000 children and adults a year in the United States. One wartime epidemic made more than 36,000 ill and killed 6,000. The disease is caused by a wide assortment of bacteria and other microorganisms. The fiercest is a tiny bacterial organism, the meningococcus. There are three important strains of these meningococci. Group A is the kind that starts national epidemics. Group C has done the most damage lately, with a 26 to 29 percent fatality rate among civilians. There is also a group B, but it has never caused a large-scale epidemic.

From the mid-1940s to the early 1960s, meningococcal meningitis was easily kept under control by sulfa drugs. All at once, the sulfa drugs lost their effectiveness. Group C meningitis burst out on several Army and Navy bases in California in the winter of 1962-1963. Every G.I. and sailor at those bases was given sulfa drugs as a prophylaxis, but the disease continued to spread. The medics switched to antibiotics, but more men came down with the disease and died. The Pentagon had to close off Fort Ord in California.

This was another "soap opera" race with death. Thousands of young recruits were passing through crowded Army camps every month. At any moment, a new epidemic of meningitis could erupt.

The Army assigned a combo of three enterprising physicians at the Walter Reed Institute to find a vaccine against the disease. Dr. Malcolm S. Artenstein, the thirty-five-year-old virologist-bacteriologist from Boston who helped to isolate the rubella vaccine, was in charge. The others were Dr. Emil C. Gotschlich, a thirty-one-year-old biochemist born in Thailand of German parents, and Dr. Goldschneider, a twenty-nine-year-old pathologist from Philadelphia.

I talked with Dr. Artenstein in his dingy office at the Walter Reed Institute and found him brawny, informal, full of life and excitement. I met Dr. Gotschlich at Rockefeller University in New York City. He was brawny, too, but owlish and very intense. I saw Dr. Goldschneider in his pathology laboratory at the University of Connecticut Health Center in Farmington. He was slim, quiet, with an acute, probing mind.

How do you defeat a major epidemic-type disease in a desperate hurry, starting from scratch?

The first job was to find an animal to work on. The three injected meningococci into rats, mice, guinea pigs, rabbits, and monkeys. Not one animal got sick. To their dismay, they discovered that no animal outside of man contracts spinal meningitis. Virtually all other animals have antibodies against it.

"The next step was obvious," Dr. Artenstein said. "Somehow we had to see if humans also had antibodies against meningitis."

He arranged for cultures and a sample of the blood of every G.I. who got meningitis anywhere in the Army to be flown instantly to the lab. More than eighteen hundred strains of meningococci were identified in this way. Blood specimens were gathered from fifteen thousand recruits passing through Fort Dix, New Jersey, over a five-month period in 1966, and each specimen was frozen. When seventy of their recruits later developed meningitis, the Army scientists were able to check their original blood samples.

Dr. Goldschneider demonstrated that most people normally have meningococci in their throats but, fortunately, have developed antibodies against them. A sizable number of people fail to produce antibodies, though, and these are always in danger of catching the disease.

Dr. Gotschlich's contribution probably was the biggest. He isolated the specific substance in the meningococcus that stimulated the production of antibodies. It proved to be a polysaccharide, a sugar, in the walls of each meningococcus cell. Through some ingenious chemical juggling, Gotschlich greatly increased the molecular weight of the polysaccharide and made vaccines of it for group C and group A meningitis.

Early in 1968, Dr. Artenstein got authorization to stage a crucial experiment with the group C vaccine at Fort Dix. One foul, rainy afternoon, he addressed three meetings of brand-new recruits. The G.I.s were sitting on their packs, sopping wet, tired, disgusted. Artenstein had to tell them that they were testing a practically untried vaccine.

"We've tried it on ourselves without bad effects," he said, "but I can't in all honesty promise that you may not get some reaction to it."

Most of the G.I.s were tough city kids who had been warned never to volunteer for anything. "Can meningitis kill you?" one asked.

Artenstein had to say yes.

"Can this affect my sex life?" a G.I. demanded. "Will it harm my unborn child?" another inquired.

Here, at least, Artenstein was able to reassure them.

It was a toss-up whether they could get enough volunteers to run the experiment. They barely squeaked through. One hundred and forty-five G.I.s volunteered to take the vaccination.

During the seven weeks of the test, four of the "controls" contracted severe cases of meningitis, but not one vaccinated G.I. fell ill.

That summer, Drs. Gotschlich and Goldschneider returned to civilian life, leaving Dr. Artenstein to continue the Walter Reed work. In 1969, he directed a much larger trial at five Army posts. Some 13,763 soldiers were vaccinated, and the meningitis rate among G.I.s was reduced tenfold. More than a million G.I.s have since been vaccinated, and the incidence of meningitis among all military personnel has been cut by 90 percent.

Promising things also happened with the group C vaccine on the children's front. Dr. Goldschneider joined the faculty of the University of Connecticut medical school and teamed up with Dr. Martha Leopow, a pediatrician, to test the group C vaccine on fifty children between one and nine years of age. Youngsters over the age of two developed antibodies in amounts comparable to those of adults. The younger kids produced slightly less, but more than enough to protect them.

Goldschneider and Leopow planned—in fact, the project was under-way—to run a bigger test, with three thousand children, but the federal government cut off the funds—to save money, it stated. That counted more than children's lives.

The group A vaccine has proven to be equally effective. Seventy thousand people were successfully inoculated with it by WHO in Egypt and the Sudan. In the mid-1970s, WHO was contemplating broad use of the vaccine through the entire "meningitis belt" of Africa, a bloc of black African countries where giant epidemics of group A meningitis occur regularly every year, and thousands die. WHO was confident that the vaccine would end all that.

It was practically ordained that Dr. Gotschlich would go into medicine. His father was an internist, his mother an ophthalmologist. Although they were not Jewish, they fled Germany in 1932, eventually reaching Thailand. Emil went from Thailand to America and to New York University Medical Center to study medicine. Interning at Bellevue Hospital taught him that he preferred test tubes to patients. After he left the Army, he went to Rockefeller University for more work on the meningitis vaccines. He was interested, further, in devising a sure test for detecting gonorrhea. He and his former wife had three children. More than that I can't say of him. Dr. Gotschlich is a very private person.

Dr. Goldschneider worked his way through the University of Pennsylvania medical school as a shoe salesman and short-order cook with his eye always on research. To him, the satisfaction comes "from seeing more deeply than others.

"There are many things I don't know and I never will know," he declared. "But I'd like to know as much as possible about the things that are knowable. If any good comes out of it for mankind, I'm doubly blessed."

He works a six-day-and-night week, at the lab and at home. "The price you pay for research is that you never leave it behind," he said. In odd moments, he sails, paints, and revels in classical records. His wife, Terry, is a former medical technician. They have three small children.

Dr. Artenstein graduated from Tufts University medical school and specialized in internal medicine. The Army called him to active duty in 1959, and he's been at the Walter Reed Institute most of the time since then as an Army officer or civilian researcher. He does research because he enjoys it, he said. That's the only reason. He misses his patients, though. "I like taking care of people," he said. "I like to make people well."

He couldn't be less interested in making money. "I'm no good at business," he said. "As a kid, I invested in a stand at a carnival. Everybody made money but me and my friends. We lost."

He and his tall, attractive wife, Sylvia, have two teen-age children. He is a movie fan, but seldom has time to go. "I always bring home a briefcase full of reports, and spend several hours every night reading them."

"What does a work schedule like yours do to a marriage?" I asked.

He gave me the same sad answer I've heard from dozens of medical researchers. "It's hell," he said.

Still, millions of children and adults are safer because of his endless toil.

Taming the Rh Factor

Until a few years ago, it could be near-murder for a woman with Rh-negative blood to fall in love with any man whose blood was Rh-positive. It meant that some of their children might be born with a luckless condition known as erythroblastosis fetalis—Rh disease. The babies' red blood cells would be ruined by the disease, leaving them gravely anemic, with an accumulation of slaughterous poisons in their blood. Their livers and spleens would swell up grotesquely, and they would die of congestive heart failure. The worst cases would be born dead.

The Rh factor is a substance on the surface of red blood cells. When you have it in your blood, you're called Rh-positive. Those without it are Rh-negatives. Ordinarily, the first child of a positive-negative couple is healthy. But if the first-born baby is an Rh-positive and his mother is Rh-negative, the baby can contaminate her. His blood may leak across the placenta into the mother's blood during the fetal period, or invade the mother's bloodstream through a hemorrhage during delivery. This can literally immunize a mother against her own future babies, with dire results. Her body may produce antibodies that will destroy the red blood cells of any Rh-positive babies she ever conceives.

It is a common event. Some 3,300,000 deliveries occur in the United States each year, and 260,000 end in the birth of an Rh-positive baby to an Rh-negative mother. One out of every ten of those babies is likely to have Rh disease.

Dr. A. William Liley, a jovial, venturesome New Zealand pediatrician, gave Rh babies some hope. He devised a way to diagnose Rh disease in unborn babies by tapping the amniotic fluid in which the fetus floats inside his mother's womb. In the summer of 1963, having diagnosed such a case, Bill Liley skillfully inserted a long needle into the pregnant woman's jutting abdomen, on into the fetus's abdomen, and gave a blood transfusion to the unborn child. He transfused enough healthy blood cells into the fetus to carry it through to a safe birth. All of the baby's blood could then be replaced.

It was an unpredictable technique, though, and some children who underwent it became mentally retarded.

Two separate groups of researchers, working on opposite sides of the Atlantic Ocean, found a better way of handling Rh disease—by preventing it altogether. They had a race to see which would be first. The outcome was, in effect, a draw.

The American group was spearheaded by an Australian, Dr. John G. Gorman, a tall, handsome pathologist with long brown hair curling around his neck, born in 1931. He started out at the University of Melbourne medical school to be a pediatrician but turned to research and blood-banking in the United States. I talked with him in the blood bank he directs high up on the twentieth floor of Columbia-Presbyterian Hospital in New York City.

Gorman and a friend, Dr. Vincent J. Freda, a thirty-two-year-old Columbia-Presbyterian obstetrician, large and boyish, resolved to do something about Rh disease in 1961. Freda had gotten a burning interest in hemolytic disease while he worked under Dr. Alexander Wiener, the man who discovered the Rh factor. The two joined hands with Dr. William Pollack, research director at the Ortho-Research Foundation, a subsidiary of the Johnson and Johnson Company. They had listened to him lecture and fell to talking with him afterward.

A great scientist once said, "Discovery consists of seeing what everybody has seen and thinking what nobody has thought." So it happened here. The three made a search of the scientific literature on Rh disease, and

Gorman was struck with an idea that had been neglected for years. To wit, if you could stop mothers in any way from making Rh antibodies, you could prevent the disease.

"The awful problem was this," Dr. Gorman said. "The antibody mechanism is one of the toughest things to turn off. It's one of the heartiest parts of the body. You practically have to wipe out the patient to prevent him from rejecting a kidney transplant. Blasting people with X-rays, you kill the individual before you kill his antibody factory.

"However, we had an idea that if we gave mothers Rh antibodies ahead of time artificially, their own mechanisms wouldn't bother to make them."

Dr. Pollack manufactured the Rh antibodies out of the blood of a mother whose body was producing large amounts of natural antibodies. He took the serum proteins involved in the immunity process out of her blood and separated from them immunoglobulin G, the small antibody molecule. He made a vaccine of it called RhoGAM that he hoped would stop the antibody factories of pregnant women from going into production.

The three decided to test the vaccine on "pregnant" men rather than pregnant women! "You can mimic a pregnancy situation in men," Dr. Gorman said. "Then, if the vaccine fails and the man gets sensitized to the Rh factor, you won't be doing any harm to unborn babies."

They held the first trial with thirty-six prisoners, each an Rh-negative, at grim Sing Sing Prison in Ossining, New York, in April 1962. All the prisoners were volunteers who got no reward—not even a day's reduction from their sentences—for the risks they ran.

Gorman scrupulously warned the prisoners at a meeting in the Sing Sing lab that they were chancing infectious hepatitis.

"If we get this hepatitis," a prisoner said, "how long will it take before we croak?"

"You'll probably get better," Dr. Gorman declared, "but if you die, it'll be within a week."

"Well, that's all right," the con said.

All thirty-six of the Rh-negative prisoners were given transfusions of Rh-positive blood. Eighteen were given the globulin vaccine; eighteen weren't.

Not one of the men who received the vaccine produced antibodies against the Rh-positive blood. Twelve of the others did.

The first trial of the vaccine with a pregnant woman came in January 1964. She was Katherine Gorman, Dr. Gorman's sister-in-law. Four hundred and forty-four more pregnant women received the vaccine in the following three years. It permanently stopped the manufacture of antibodies in every one without any bad side effects.

Across the Atlantic, a couple of resourceful English physicians, Dr. Ronald Finn and his chief in internal medicine at the University of Liverpool medical school, Dr. Cyril A. Clarke, explored the same idea the same way. They came up with the same globulin vaccine, also tested it on prisoners and pregnant women, and had the same superlative results.

By 1975, the globulin vaccine was acknowledged to be 90 percent effective, and it was being given to 85 percent of all Rh-negative mothers in the United States. In Britain, 75 percent of Rh-negative mothers were getting it. Gorman recommends that the globulin vaccine be administered automatically to every Rh-negative woman within seventy-two hours of her first delivery, abortion, or miscarriage if the child is Rh-positive.

"You've got to get in during the time that the window is open," he insistently declares.

Dr. Gorman has no such problems in his own family. He is Rh-positive and his wife, Dr. Carol Rutgers, is Rh-positive, too. She is a pathologist who used to be one of his residents. They have three little children. He is no compulsive worker. He puts in a normal, easy schedule at the blood bank. He gets most of his fun, he told me, from "taking the children somewhere." And most of his exercise from golf. He adores the game and boasts a handicap of ten.

"Why did I get into this Rh work?" He asked it himself.

"I wanted to do something important," he answered.

Once they could kill and maim at will: polio, measles, rubella, mumps, Asian flu, spinal meningitis, Rh disease. Now men can protect themselves against their forays. Men can also forestall such other executioners as the plague, tuberculosis, yellow fever, typhus, typhoid fever, tetanus, rabies, diphtheria, and brucella.

Someday there may even be a vaccine that will prevent cancer.

3

REBUILDABLE YOU

WHILE GORDON MACKEY, A PHARMACIST, was growing up in the little town of Lampasas, Texas, during the first years of this century, his older brother was stricken by appendicitis. A Dr. A.C. Scott came to town to remove the offending appendix, and he performed the operation in the Mackey dining room. As Gordon recalled it, Dr. Scott boiled enough water for "a hog-killing." Every piece of furniture except the dining table was taken out, and the room scoured. The little boy was astonished that Dr. Scott wasted so much time washing his hands. He scrubbed them three times! To Gordon's mind, any doctor who would fritter away that much time washing his hands could not be very intelligent. Since such a stupid surgeon was officiating, Gordon felt sure that his brother would die. To his amazement, his brother recovered.

With the coming of anesthesia and sterile techniques, surgery had finally become a useful art in the mid-nineteenth century. Once surgeons had to chase fleeing patients up hospital halls and drag them back to their operating tables. Now surgeons could attempt lengthy, complicated procedures in areas of the body they had never penetrated. Infection used to be a more dangerous enemy than the primary disease. Now, most of the time, it could be controlled.

A time of splendid surgery commenced in the operating rooms of Europe and North America. In the latter half of the nineteenth century, the great German surgeon Theodor Billroth did the first successful operation on a stomach. For cancer. He devised a surgical procedure for treating gastric ulcers that is still in use. For his contributions to easing human pain, he was stoned by a Viennese mob.

The Swiss doctor Theodor Kocher streamlined surgery. His clinic was a model of assembly-line efficiency. Every patient arrived in the operating room at the precise instant that Kocher was ready for him.

In seventy crowded years, the indomitable American William Stewart Halsted led a crusade to bring sterile surgical techniques to the United States, revamped surgical education, and did some of history's boldest surgery. Until Halsted came along, many surgeons simply castrated men suffering from strangulated hernias. Halsted developed a surgical procedure that repaired the hernia without risking the patient's sex life. He devised the radical mastectomy, which is the most widely used procedure in cases of breast cancer today.

Early in the twentieth century, Harvey W. Cushing gave major dimensions to neurosurgery. He removed tumors from inside the brain that no one had ever dared to touch. It was Cushing who had the revolutionary idea of taking patients' blood pressure during operations. It saved them from dying of shock.

The scalpel of the Canadian Wilder G. Penfield gave many epileptics good lives. Edward D. Churchill, a Harvard professor like Cushing, demonstrated that a sizable section of a cancerous lung could be cut out of a patient without killing him. In 1901, the Austrian Karl Landsteiner discovered that human blood could be divided into distinctive groups, and that the blood in each group was incompatible with the others. The discovery made blood transfusions feasible. In 1933, the U.S.S.R.'s Sergei Sergeivitch Yukin established the world's first blood bank in Moscow.

All this was the prologue. Since the outbreak of World War II, physicians have learned to do things for the human body that exceed the highest flights of fancy of earlier days. Later in this book you will see what the surgeons can do to help a sick heart. Now you are going to hear about extraordinary things they can do for other parts of the body.

Kolff Invents the Artificial Kidney

There are twenty thousand people in the United States who, by rights, should be dead inasmuch as their diseased kidneys have ceased functioning. There are twenty thousand more in Europe. These forty thousand men, women, and children are alive and active because of an artificial kidney invented by Dr. Willem J. Kolff, a Dutchman with a loathing for Nazis, a tender feeling toward all sick people regardless of their politics, and a rare talent for inventing lifesaving devices.

Kidneys are bean-shaped organs that weigh about a quarter of a pound apiece. If you are normal, you have two of them situated in the small of your back on either side of the spine. Their mission is to remove fluids and waste compounds from the blood and to regulate your body chemistry. Each of your kidneys has a million or so microscopic tufts of blood vessels and membranes called glomeruli which filter more than 425 gallons of blood a day for you, siphoning off impurities in urine.

When the kidneys quit working, poisonous waste products accumulate and the body swells grotesquely. Vomiting, delirium, convulsions, and coma can follow. And death. Fifty-five thousand people die of irreversible kidney failure in the United States each year. According to Kolff, twenty thousand of them could be saved if artificial kidneys were available to them.

I talked with Dr. Kolff on a June day at his laboratories on the campus of the University of Utah, high on a lovely hill overlooking Salt Lake City. He had come to the University of Utah College of Medicine in 1967 with the imposing title of Professor of Surgery, Head of the Division of Artificial Organs, and Director of the Institute of Biomedical Engineering. I found him tall and thin, with sparse white hair and very Dutch blue eyes. He was sixty-one but he looked much older, even in his slacks and blue sports shirt. He was very formal with me.

Kolff was born in Leyden, Holland, in 1912. His father was a doctor he said, so that "for me there was never anything else but being a doctor."

He obtained an M.D. at the University of Leyden in 1938, just in time for war, defeat, and the brutal occupation of the Netherlands by the Nazis. Like most Dutch people, Dutch physicians fought back against the Nazis in every way they could. Kolff used to hide members of the anti-Nazi underground in his small hospital in Kampen.

On one occasion, the head of the Dutch underground was on the run from the Gestapo, and he came to Kolff for help.

"We took a liter of his own blood and fed it to him by stomach tube," Dr. Kolff remembered. "Then we admitted him to the hospital with a diagnosis of gastric bleeding. His teeth were black, he was pale, he was genuinely sick. The Gestapo never caught on to who he was."

In 1944, the Nazi occupation authorities issued a decree enrolling every Dutch doctor in a Nazi medical organization called the *Artsenkamer*. Almost every Dutch doctor promptly wrote a letter to Reichkomissar Artur von Seyss-Inquart stating, "I herewith resign being a physician. Therefore, I am no longer a member of the *Artsenkamer*."

The Nazis reacted violently by arresting virtually all doctors in the Netherlands and putting them in concentration camps. The few left at large—Kolff was one of them—went on resisting.

"We wouldn't sign death certificates," Dr. Kolff said. "We wouldn't sign insurance forms. We wouldn't sign a certificate that a man was too ill to work. The result was that there was a splendid bureaucratic confusion. All these people that couldn't be buried standing around was quite bothersome to the Nazi authorities."

"Were you frightened?" I asked.

"Oh, yes, we were all frightened, but that was no reason not to do it."

After three weeks, the Nazis gave in. They abandoned their *Artsenkamer* organization and let the other physicians out of the concentration camps.

Dr. Kolff started thinking of an artificial kidney in 1938. One of his first patients was a young man slowly dying of renal failure. He was going blind, had horrible headaches, vomited constantly. His mother, a poor peasant woman, her back bent by hard word, came to Kolff dressed in her traditional Sunday black dress with a white lace cap. He had to tell her that her son was going to die. He felt utterly helpless.

If only he could have eliminated twenty grams of urea and other waste products from this young man's blood, Kolff thought, he could have kept him alive. He knew that some researchers had attempted to filter toxic substances from blood and that none of their contraptions had proven practical, but, stubborn Dutchman that he was, Kolff decided to try. Since he could get no support for his experiments, he took the money out of his own meager pocketbook.

He started with a piece of everyday sausage casing—ordinary cellophane—twenty inches long. He poured in 25 cc of blood and added a hefty amount of urea. He fastened the casing to a wooden board and rocked it in a saline bath. The cellophane acted as a filter. After a half hour, the urea had passed out through it, and the blood was normal again.

The theory seemed valid, so Kolff designed a machine the size of a baby carriage consisting of twenty-five feet of permeable cellophane tubing wrapped around a rotating drum whose lower half was immersed in a bath of bloodlike salts and minerals. At one end the tubing could be attached to an artery in the patient's arm, and at the other end to a vein. A small engine rotated the drum. The patient's blood would run into the tubing as the drum revolved, and the impurities would be filtered out through the cellophane into the swirling fluid before the cleansed blood flowed back into the patient.

This cleaning procedure was called dialysis. It sounded fine, but . . .

Fourteen of Kolff's first fifteen patients died. The lone patient who survived might well have recovered without the help of his artificial kidney.

Kolff was not discouraged. "When these patients were brought to me," he said, "they were mostly comatose, practically moribund. I saw them regain their consciousness. I saw them talk to their families. I saw them read the newspapers, write their wills. Even when I lost them, two or three days later, I knew that I had seen a temporary improvement. I was sure that in time I would get one who would be saved."

Patient No. 17 was the one. But first, a moral dilemma had to be resolved. Did Patient No. 17 deserve to have her life saved?

She was Mevrouw Sofia Schafstadt, a sixty-seven-year-old Dutch woman, slim with bobbed grey hair, who had been a vicious Nazi collaborator.

"A lot of my fellow citizens would have liked to strangle this lady with their bare hands," Dr. Kolff said.

Mevrouw Schafstadt was in prison facing prosecution when she fell ill with kidney disease. The prison authorities brought her to Kolff's hospital more dead than alive.

"People begged, 'Let her die,' " Dr. Kolff declared. "But no physician has the right to decide whether a patient is a good guy or not. He must treat every patient who has need of him."

The first day, Kolff dosed Mevrouw Schafstadt with sulfa. Her fever decreased a bit, but her blood urea climbed threateningly, and she didn't pass a drop of urine. She slept and snored weakly. The next day, September 11, 1945, she was hooked up to the artificial kidney. Eighty liters of her blood flowed through the machine in eleven and a half hours. Her blood urea fell, and, most important sign of all, urine began to trickle out of her.

Kolff still remembers her first coherent words. She said that she wanted to divorce her husband.

Mevrouw Schafstadt recovered, and Kolff was confronted with another quandary. The woman faced a death sentence, but Kolff needed to keep her alive to vouch for the effectiveness of his artificial kidney. Reluctantly, he appealed to the Dutch authorities to release her. She might atone for some of her crimes just by staying alive, he pleaded, and the Dutch authorities agreed to let her go free.

The lady was not particularly thankful. Gratitude was never a Nazi strong point.

Initially, the artificial kidney could only be used for short periods, since a large-bore needle had to be inserted into a major blood vessel before each treatment and withdrawn afterward. That played havoc with the patient's blood vessels. In 1960, Dr. Belding Scribner of the University of Washington developed a neat little shunt of Teflon and Silastic that could be left in an artery and a vein in the patient's wrist over a lengthy period of time. It made possible long-term kidney dialysis. Some patients have been kept alive by an artificial kidney for twelve years.

Dr. Kolff emigrated to the United States in 1950. The research horizons were broader there. First, he joined the research staff of the Cleveland Clinic. Seventeen years later, he moved on to Utah.

There was one dreadful drawback to his artificial kidney: the exorbitant expense of treatment with it. The average person required two to three treatments a week in a hospital on an outpatient basis, and his bill could reach $20,000 a year. Who could afford that? Compounding matters was an excruciating shortage of artificial kidneys. Few hospitals had the money to purchase enough of them. They cost more than $10,000 apiece. Not that Kolff got any money for them. He has never taken a penny in royalties for the artificial kidney.

The thought of it still haunts Dr. Kolff. "The miserable fact is that there were selection committees to decide who was going to be treated, and who was not. First, a medical committee had to certify that the patient needed treatment with an artificial kidney. Then you had a lay committee that would ask such questions as, 'Is he married? Is he divorced? Does he have children that go to school? Is he employed? How much does he make? Does he give to the community chest? Does he go to church?' If all the answers were right, then he was considered a good citizen and he might be worthy to be treated with the artificial kidney."

The situation was eased a bit by the development of portable artificial kidneys for use at home. The patients didn't have to pay the astronomic hospital bills. However, the price of the portable machines, around $10,000, was still beyond the means of most people.

It infuriated Kolff that tens of thousands of people with renal failure were being allowed to die although an effective method of treating them was known.

He set out to design an artificial kidney that would be inexpensive enough for anyone to use. He took an ordinary washing machine with a gadget in the center that swished liquids around, and made a perfectly usable artificial kidney out of it. For a total cost of $364, he could send a patient home with his own artificial kidney. It was in vain. The manufacturers of the washing machine wouldn't let Kolff use it. They were afraid that they might be sued by some patient sometime. No humanitarian pleas could budge them.

People continued to die in large numbers for want of an artificial kidney until 1973, when the U.S. Congress authorized the federal government to pay the cost of dialysis for most people in need of it.

The artificial kidney is only one of Dr. Kolff's medical inventions. He has developed an excellent heart-lung machine. He designed the first intra-aortic balloon pump—a long, slender balloon that is inserted in the aorta and helps an ailing heart to pump blood. Lately, Kolff and his staff of biomedical engineers have been working on a whole artificial heart.

Walking through the laboratories with Dr. Kolff, I saw a calf living on one of these artificial hearts. She was mooing contentedly. Kolff and his people have also been experimenting with an artificial eye. A television camera no bigger than a pea reports what it sees to a tiny computer, which gives the proper signals via a pyrolitic carbon button to an array of electrodes in the brain. Totally blind people have been able to distinguish patterns of dancing lights with it.

Getting money for his research has been a continual struggle for Kolff. He becomes quite wrought up about it. "If you're ahead of the field, it's almost impossible to obtain funds. If your ideas are far out, fantastic, very original, the first reaction of the people in charge of research funds in America is negative. Always is. The more original the idea, the less chance there is that it will be supported."

What motivates a mechanically minded physician like him?

"Always, always, it is the needs of patients. I feel a big concern about patients. It hurts me when I see that they suffer."

Dr. Kolff and his wife, Janke, have five children. Three are doctors, a fourth is a hospital architect. Kolff works a businessman's hours, eight to six, five days a week, but he puts in lots of extra hours over the weekend. For recreation, he hikes in the rugged Rockies.

"And I watch birds," he said. "I have a great liking for watching birds."

It is touching to see children during their long, wearying sessions with the artificial kidney. Surprisingly, the children look forward to them eagerly. Because of their maimed kidneys, the youngsters have to adhere to an absolutely tasteless, salt-restricted diet. They can eat anything they want, though, while they are being dialyzed. When I visited Georgetown University Hospital in Washington, D.C., every kid on an artificial kidney was feasting ecstatically on hot dogs, soda pop, and other forbidden foods. Nothing could hurt them since their blood was being cleansed of impurities anyway.

The artificial kidney is only a partial solution, of course. Without it, people with terminal kidney disease would be dead, true, but it means an intensely confined life for the patients, chained, as it were, to their lifesaving apparatus. Some people can't endure it. Ex-U.S. Senator Wayne Morse committed suicide by deliberately refusing dialysis.

For years, kidney patients have prayed for something better: new kidneys that would let them lead more normal lives. Many have now gotten them.

Kidney Transplants
—*Conquering the Rejection Problem*

The first organ to be successfully transplanted from one human body to another was the kidney. Today, a kidney transplant is a routine procedure that can be safely done by a competent surgeon in less than two hours. But it took the pioneers more than half a century to determine the way to do it. A Viennese surgeon, Dr. E. Ullman, did the trailblazing. In 1902, he transplanted a kidney from one dog to another dog. Then he transferred a kidney from a dog to a goat. Soon, the Frenchman Dr. Alexis Carrel was starting kidney transplants in animals. Four years later, Dr. Mathieu Jaboulay, another Frenchman, hooked up kidneys from a dog and a goat to the arms of two human patients. They functioned for an hour. In 1936, Dr. U. Voronoy, a Soviet surgeon, went the whole distance. He removed a kidney from a person who had just died and gave it to a patient critically ill of mercury poisoning. The new kidney went to work for its new owner, turning out small quantities of urine for two days. On the third day, the recipient died, but the doctors knew that a kidney transfer between two humans was surgically plausible.

How long would the body tolerate the presence of a foreign organ, though? It was scientific gospel that the body regarded anything foreign to be harmful and would quickly reject it.

A British zoologist, Peter Brian Medawar, proved that the body's immunological defenses could be overcome. "It is far better to have immunological defenses than not to have them," he argued, "but this does not mean that we are to marvel at them as evidences of a high and wise design."

That was in 1944. Medawar was twenty-nine years old, a gentle six-foot five-inch Goliath who had been doing research on skin grafts for World War II casualties. As he investigated why so many grafts failed to heal, he came to realize that each human body had a distinctive rejection reaction of its own. He recognized that the human body rejected grafts from other bodies because of dissimilarities in their immunological patterns. Through countless experiments on mice, he demonstrated that these immunological mechanisms could be modified. His discoveries were basic to all progress with transplants. He won the Nobel Prize for them in 1960 along with Dr. Frank Macfarlane Burnet of Australia.

Medawar, who secured his doctorate at Oxford, is on the faculty of the University of London. His students idolize him. He never "pulls rank," they say. He washes out his own instruments. When he needs mice, he goes up to the animal room and gets them himself. Medawar and his wife, Jean, live in a two-hundred-year-old house in London and are inveterate opera- and concert-goers. They have four children.

Early in the 1970s, Medawar suffered a serious stroke. He would not yield to it and soon was back in his laboratory with his test tubes and mice.

The first successful kidney transplant between two human beings was performed on June 17, 1950. Forty-four-year-old Mrs. Howard Tucker, the wife of a locomotive engineer, went into the Little Company of Mary Hospital in Evergreen Park, Illinois, in a last effort to push away death. Her sister, mother, and uncle had died of kidney disease, and she was almost dead. Both her kidneys were next to complete failure.

Dr. Richard H. Lawler replaced Mrs. Tucker's left kidney with a kidney from a forty-nine-year-old woman who had just died of cirrhosis of the liver. Mrs. Tucker lived for nearly five years with her new kidney.

But Mrs. Tucker's survival was a fluke. Her transplant succeeded without benefit of immunosuppressant drugs, irradiation, or any other measure for offsetting the body's dislike for alien organs. Scores of other kidney patients still had to die before the transplanters could figure out a means for taming the body's immunological mechanisms.

The kidney transplanters tried huge and small doses of radiation, all kinds of drugs, anything that might break down the patient's immunological ramparts. They had one advantage that the heart transplanters of the next era didn't have, Willem Kolff's artificial kidney. At least they could keep a patient alive until they found a new kidney for him.

Eight attempts at renal transplants from live donors were made in France in 1951, most of them in Paris by a deft urologist named Dr. R. Küss. They all failed. In Boston, a team at Peter Bent Brigham Hospital starring Dr. John P. Merrill did nine transplants in 1951 and 1952. One patient lived a few months; all the others died quickly. Then in 1952, a new approach was tried by Dr. Jean Hamburger at Necker Hospital in Paris.

A sixteen-year-old Parisian boy, Marius R., fell off a scaffolding on which he had been working as a carpenter. He damaged his right kidney so severely that it had to be removed. When the surgeons opened up the lad, they were appalled to find that he had no left kidney. He had been born with only one kidney. On Christmas night, Dr. Hamburger took a kidney from the boy's mother and gave it to him. Perhaps his immunity system would be less resistant to a kidney from a close relative. The new kidney functioned for three weeks.

The Peter Bent Brigham team made the next logical move. If a child were more hospitable to his mother's kidney than a stranger's, a kidney from a twin might do still better—especially one from an identical twin. On the morning of December 23, 1954, the left kidney was taken out of twenty-three-year-old Ronald Herrick and carried into an adjoining operating room where Ron's identical twin brother, Richard, was waiting on an operating table with his abdomen cut open. Dick was dying of kidney disease. An artificial kidney was the only thing that had kept him going. Dr. Joseph E. Murray sewed his new kidney into place, and Dr. Merrill laid out a regimen of drugs and whole body radiation.

Dick made out excellently with his twin's kidney. He fully recovered, married his nurse, and became a father. His twin's kidney gave him eight more years of life.

Merrill and his Peter Bent Brigham teammates did twenty-two successful kidney transplants between identical and fraternal twins. But that solved only a small part of the problem. What could be done for the vast majority of patients who weren't equipped with healthy, agreeable twins? The transplanters got them new kidneys, but they continued to develop the same terrifying symptoms of rejection disease: infections, fever, slackening urine, kidney collapse.

A scientist in Tuckahoe, New York, had some help for them although he didn't know it himself yet. This was Dr. George Hitchings, of Burroughs Wellcome, whose development of allopurinol had done so much to relieve gout and whose discovery of 6-mercaptopurine (6-MP) was to prove so valuable in treating leukemia.

Now 6-MP came to the aid of the transplanters fighting rejection. Two men at Tufts University in Boston, Drs. Robert Schwartz and W. Dameshek, decided that 6-MP might affect the immunity system. They tried it on white rabbits in 1958, and it effectively suppressed their immunological defenses for weeks. A wise young British surgeon (he was twenty-nine years old), Dr. Roy Y. Calne, saw the worth of their experiments. He gave 6-MP to dogs. It also worked for them, the first drug that ever enabled a dog to accept another dog's kidneys.

Dr. Hitchings became very excited about kidney transplants, and he brought out an improved version of 6-MP named azathioprine.

Dr. Calne came to the United States in 1960 for a year's study under Dr. Murray at Peter Bent Brigham Hospital. On the way, he stopped off in Tuckahoe, and Hitchings let him have some of his new azathioprine. Calne tested it on patients who were getting kidneys from non-twin donors, and it proved to be more effective and less toxic than 6-MP. It was the first real immunosuppressant drug.

But, by itself, azathioprine was not enough to protect most transplant patients against rejection. They went on dying right and left. The transplanters grew increasingly discouraged. Were kidney transplants just another passing fad that would be relegated to oblivion like so many other medical innovations before them?

More and more surgeons thought so and stopped doing transplants, both here and abroad.

Out in Denver, Colorado, a skilled surgeon with a knack for juggling drugs wouldn't give up. Dr. Thomas E. Starzl, a tall, handsome Iowan with an M.D. plus Ph.D. in neurophysiology from Northwestern University, became interested in transplants in the late 1950s. He started on one of the most difficult organs of all to shift about: the liver. He originated a new technique for removing livers from animals. The next step, naturally, was trying to switch a liver from one animal to another.

"If I can pull out a liver, I can stick one back," he said.

Starzl did the first successful liver transplant in a dog in 1958. He was thirty-two then. Years more labor in the "dog lab" were necessary before he could attempt the same complicated operation in a human. Meanwhile, he began working on kidneys. He did his first kidney transplant in a human in 1962. By the end of 1963, he had done more than three dozen, and they were amazingly successful. Eighty percent of all the patients in the world today who have survived over ten years with transplanted kidneys got them from Tom Starzl in those two years.

He whipped up a pharmacological cocktail that helped greatly to solve the rejection problem. He added prednisone, a form of cortisone, to the azathioprine that the transplanters had been relying upon. The prednisone was able to reverse the rejection process in most patients. Later, he included a third drug, ALG, antilymphocyte globulin.

Starzl's pharmacological bartending and his persistence helped to restore faith in kidney transplants as an acceptable therapy for people with dying kidneys. His combination drug therapy made kidneys taken from strangers and cadavers almost as useful as kidneys that had come from near-relatives.

A couple of surgeons at the University of California medical school in San Francisco made kidney transplants still more practical. Drs. Folkert O. Belzer and Samuel L. Kountz perfected a revolutionary technique for keeping a kidney alive, healthy, and functioning for seventy-two hours after it had been cut out of the body of a dead person. They flushed the dead man's kidney free of blood and attached it to a perfusion apparatus that had been primed with specially treated cold plasma. With it, a kidney could be flown 10,500 miles from Tokyo to Paris and given safely to a person in need. The world's supply of kidneys for transplant was multiplied.

Some fine advances in tissue matching made kidney transplants safer. Dr. Paul I. Terasaki, a Japanese-American pupil of the famous Peter Medawar, did excellent work here. Dr. Kountz did, too.

I saw a kidney transplanted by Dr. Kountz, now one of the world's foremost kidney transplanters. He's been involved in a thousand transplants.

I met him at 7:00 A.M. in the operating pavilion at Brooklyn's Downstate Medical Center. He had moved east from San Francisco in 1972 to be chief of surgery at two institutions, Downstate and the colossal Kings County Hospital. He was already in his green scrub suit, a good-looking black man, medium-tall, stocky, forty-four years old. There was none of the self-importance to him that so many other big-name surgeons have. I found him a friendly, warm-hearted person, quick to smile, joke, laugh.

The naked man lying on the operating table was a tall, emaciated lawyer, thirty-one years old and the father of three little children. He had been on dialysis for six months and couldn't stand it anymore. He had come up from Washington, D.C., to beg Kountz for help. His own Washington urologist had refused to refer him to Kountz; he thought transplants were too risky. Through the glass walls of the operating room, I could see a huddle of surgeons in the next O.R. slicing into the lawyer's sixty-year-old father. He was giving up his right kidney for his son.

The patient was scarily still, almost completely paralyzed by the curare that the Oriental anesthesiologist had administered. At 8:35 A.M., Kountz started cutting with an electric scalpel. He made a big crescent-shaped incision in the right side of the abdomen. The electric scalpel carved deeper and deeper. The incision became a cavernous hole, eight inches square, six inches or so deep, held apart by dangling metal clamps. An inexperienced scrub nurse kept handing Kountz the wrong instruments, but he never raised his voice to her.

Soon I could see the useless kidney. It looked lifeless.

Dr. Kountz chatted gaily with the resident and the nervous young medical student assisting him. "You shouldn't do surgery unless you love the patient," he declared. "You mustn't love surgery; you must love the patient."

He told them, "A transplant isn't very difficult. The only trouble with it is that it has to be done perfectly."

At ten minutes past nine, the first phase was finished. The lawyer's right kidney was disconnected. The surgical team in the next room wasn't ready, though. The patient had to wait twelve long minutes, his belly open, until his father's kidney was brought in swathed in gauze on a mound of cracked ice.

Kountz studied it carefully. "The most important thing about a transplant is that the donor's kidney is healthy," he said. "This one is nice and firm."

He smiled down at it. "It's a beautiful kidney that's been waiting sixty years to get here. It's got love written on it."

He made a nest for the new kidney in the patient's abdomen. Then he set to sewing it to the blood vessels with infinitesimally small stitches. First to the renal artery, next to the vein. The greyish kidney started to take on a healthy red cast.

Kountz held in his fingers a skimpy little duct of flesh maybe eight or nine inches long. It was the ureter. A drop of urine ran out of it.

"Look," he exclaimed delightedly. "Only two and a half minutes, and the kidney's working."

He sewed the ureter to the bladder. At two minutes past ten, he started closing the incision. I was surprised that he had not removed either one of the patient's own kidneys. The man was left with three kidneys inside him. It's safer that way, Kountz explained.

Several times that day, Kountz visited the intensive-care unit. Both father and son were doing fine. They still were doing fine when I checked a year later.

Few physicians have had to struggle as hard as Dr. Kountz to get a medical education. The son of a moneyless Baptist minister, he was born in 1930 in one of the smallest, poorest towns in Arkansas. It had less than a hundred people in it, all black and all impoverished.

"I think I was twelve or thirteen years old before I saw the face of a white man," Dr. Kountz said.

The town—its name was Lexa—had no doctor. When people fell ill, Reverend Kountz ministered to them as best he could. As a child, Samuel saw many people die for lack of medical care. At the age of eight, he told his grandmother that he was going to be a doctor. His grandmother encouraged him. She had been born a slave, and she wanted him to make much of his life.

He didn't get much book learning as a child. Only one teacher in the church school he attended had received any formal education, and he was seldom present. Samuel knew very little more at his graduation than when he entered. He flunked the entrance examination to Arkansas A & M, an all-black college. However, he talked the president into admitting him, and graduated third in a class of 173. Kountz earned his tuition as a waiter. He was one of the first blacks to win an M.D. at the University of Arkansas medical school. He worked his way through medical school, too, as a waiter; he still can sling hash with the best of them. He did his advance training at California and Stanford.

In 1959, Dr. Kountz was asked to assist at a kidney transplant at Stanford. "It turned all my ideas around," he declared. "Kidney transplants made such good medical sense. I saw at once that I wanted to spend the rest of my life working on them. I wanted to make them surer and safer."

The transplanters now have the technical know-how to transfer kidneys successfully in almost every case, he believes.

Then why aren't a lot more kidney transplants being done?

"We can't get enough kidneys," he said. "Physicians become so emotionally involved with their patients that they can't come to the decision that they're dead. Doctors have a terrible feeling of defeat when they lose a patient. They wait until it's too late for the dead person's kidney to be useful to a living person."

I posed a question to Dr. Kountz that puzzles many people. "Suppose you put the kidney of a fifty-year-old man into a twenty-year-old man. How long will that kidney live?"

"Nobody knows the answer," he stated, "but, probably, the kidney will live a very long time. If you put a kidney from an adult into a child, it gets small. If you take a kidney from a six-month-old baby and put it into a man of forty, it will grow large very fast."

"So a kidney can actually outlive the life it would have had in its original body?"

"Yes, we know that. But it probably can't live indefinitely."

Dr. Kountz starts working at six-thirty every morning. He usually has twenty to thirty surgical patients in the hospital, and he likes to spend a few minutes with each of them. He tells his patients everything. He even lets them see their own charts.

"Will you warn a patient that he has a terminal illness?" I said.

"If he wants to know it, yes. Patients ask you if they want to know something. If they don't want to know, they have unspoken ways of telling you that this is too painful for them to experience. You've got to know how to listen."

Dr. Kountz is married to a beautiful Chicago woman, Grace Yvonne Akin. They live very comfortably on Long Island with their two sons and a daughter. He swims, golfs, and bowls with the children. They all play basketball together.

He has known racial discrimination intimately. He has felt the miserable humiliation of having to ride in the back of buses, of being barred from restaurants, schools, and churches because of his color. He is not bitter about it, but he is determined to do everything he can to help the poor blacks in the ghettos of Brooklyn.

The motivation for his research?

"If I were to answer that honestly, I'd say that it's got nothing to do with fame or what my colleagues think of me. Certainly, it's got nothing to do with money. It's for my own fulfillment. I have to be creative."

The creativity of Medawar, Hamburger, Starzl, Kountz, and the others has helped thousands of kidney patients to lead whole lives again. Not long ago, Dr. Lionel Lobo, an Indian surgeon who is dean of the Christian Medical College in Ludhiana, Punjab, told a San Francisco meeting what his transplant had done for him. He had given up hope, he said. As a physician, he realized how desperate his condition was. He had vomited blood and suffered convulsions so severe that he had bitten off part of his tongue. His intake of food and water was curtailed.

"In summer in India," he said, "you can imagine what it is like to live on just one glassful of water a day."

Now, with his transplanted kidney, he was leading a completely normal existence. He looked like a healthy middle-aged man. And felt like one, he said. He called it a miracle.

We have other wonders to report in the transplant field.

Starzl Transplants Livers for the First Time

On May 5, 1963, Dr. Thomas Starzl felt ready to attempt a liver transplant between humans. For the recipient, there was no alternative. He was William Grigsby, a forty-seven-year-old ex-merchant seaman with lethal cancer of the liver.

The liver is the biggest organ in the body—it can weigh up to four pounds—and it has the longest, toughest list of duties. Sitting over on the right side of the abdomen, it has to produce bile for the digestive system, store vitamins, minerals, and sugars, manufacture vital proteins, and "detoxify" poisons that come into the body. The loss of a liver will cause death in thirty-six hours. No one yet has been able to design any kind of an artificial liver to tide a patient along for a while.

Dr. Starzl and a team of surgeons in Denver obtained a healthy liver from a man who had died of a brain tumor, and they hooked it up to a heart-lung machine to keep it supplied with blood while they worked on Grigsby. Starzl's plan was to build a temporary detour in Grigsby's blood system that would let him cut the liver off from its big artery and three major veins without his bleeding to death. Starzl did it by inserting long plastic tubes into the veins below the liver and linking them to the jugular veins in Grigsby's neck.

Once the blood was diverted, Starzl took out Grigsby's liver. He got the dead man's liver and stitched its blood vessels to Grigsby's while another surgeon sewed its bile duct to Grigsby's small intestines. It required six hours of steady surgery. Before, during, and after the operation, they administered prednisone and azathioprine to hold Grigsby's immune mechanisms in check.

Grigsby lived merely twenty-three days, and every other patient to whom they gave a new liver that year died in short order. Starzl's surgical tactics were brilliant, but he couldn't lick the rejection demons. They were much uglier with the liver than with the kidney.

Dr. Starzl went back to the "dog lab" and more research on immunosuppressants. In 1967, he entered the lists again. He operated on Julie Rodriguez, a one-and-a-half-year-old baby who had a cancerous liver. In this case, he enriched his pharmacological cocktail with ALG.

Julie lived over a year, more than anyone had ever survived with somebody else's liver. In fact, the child probably would have gone on much longer than that, for her liver was functioning well, but the cancer had spread too widely.

I talked with Dr. Starzl in Denver on a snowy January morning. By this time, he had transplanted over seventy human livers. About twenty of the recipients had lived over a year. One had been living nearly five years. (In England, Dr. Calne had a patient with a transplanted liver who had survived even longer.)

Making rounds with Dr. Starzl at the monumental University of Colorado General Hospital, I saw several patients who had received new livers from him. One sixteen-year-old girl with a new liver was due to leave the hospital that afternoon for her home in Montana. She had been next door to death when she was admitted to the hospital two months earlier. Now . . .

"I feel marvelous," she said, "I can't wait to get home."

I saw an adorable little black girl, four-and-a-half years old, in a bright pink dress with bright pink bows in her hair, scampering merrily along the corridor. She'd had her new liver three months. She was the only patient with whom Dr. Starzl, a very terse, no-nonsense type, unbent. He pretended he was trying to steal her doll.

"It's mine," she squealed, and he returned it to her with a big hug.

"How do you feel today, Gerry?" he said. "Does anything hurt you?"

"I feel scrumptious," she said.

I saw a fat man in his thirties, his eyes dull, his face moon-shaped. He had had his new liver four years, and it was acting up. He was very depressed about it. Starzl was concerned. He directed the nurse to modify the fat man's medications.

"What are his chances?" I said.

"Not good. But we won't give up on him."

Liver transplants are still in the experimental stage. Dr. Starzl, who has done more of them than any other surgeon on earth, is categorical about that. But it is self-evident that great progress has been made in recent years. The time will soon be here, Starzl believes, when liver transplants will be as routine as kidney transplants. Patients with cancer or cirrhosis of the liver will get many extra years.

The morning I met Dr. Starzl, he looked like a successful banker in a well-cut grey herringbone suit, blue striped shirt, and dark blue tie. He talked like a banker, too. He never answered with three words when two would do. He said he was born in Le Mars, Iowa, in 1926, his father a newspaperman, his mother a nurse. He never had the slightest doubt that he was going into medicine. He became interested in research in medical school.

"Do you get tense during a transplant operation?" I asked.

"Sometimes."

"Do you carry your worries home when a patient is struggling for his life?"

This was his one show of emotion. His answer was almost wrenched out of him. He almost whispered it. "Yes, I take my worries home. Luckily, I've got a nice wife and a nice family. They can absorb the punishment."

He and his wife, Barbara, have three children. Whenever he gets time, they all go off skiing together.

Although Dr. Starzl is acknowledged to be one of the world's finest surgeons, he derives no particular pleasure from operating. He says that his biggest satisfaction in a transplant comes from defeating the rejection process.

He agrees with his friend Dr. Kountz that research is "a very pure form of individual expression." Research is very much a "creative undertaking" to him, also.

Other transplanters have done important things with other organs. In the fall of 1968, Dr. Fritz Derom, a Belgian surgeon at Ghent University Clinic, put a new lung into Alois Vereecken, a twenty-three-year-old steelworker whose own right lung had been destroyed by silicosis. A year later, Vereecken was still alive. Ghent Clinic surgeons gave a new larynx to sixty-two-year-old Jean-Baptiste Borremans, and he got back his voice. In 1970, transplanters at New York City's Memorial Hospital gave sixteen inches of intestines to a thirty-seven-year-old woman who had lost a big chunk of her lower intestines to cancer. They got them from her sister. They assured the two sisters that a healthy person could get along very readily with only half the normal length of small intestines. In 1971, two Wisconsin children underwent thymus transplantations successfully.

The transplant scoreboard has become very impressive. As of November 1, 1975, it showed 23,305 kidney transplants, 293 heart transplants, 254 liver transplants, 270 bone marrow transplants, 37 lung transplants, and 47 pancreas transplants, as well as several thymus transplants. One person had lived nineteen years with someone else's kidney.

Soviet surgeons have also done some remarkable bone grafting, replacing tumorous bones with bones taken from corpses.

"Bones are not rejected by patients like other organs," Professor Nikolai N. Trapeznikov, deputy director of the Institute of Experimental and Clinical Oncology in Moscow, told me. "Some of our bone grafts have lasted eight and nine years while the patients grew new bone."

The Soviet government has set up special bone banks in its big cities. It has authorized its physicians by law to remove whatever bones they need from any dead individual for use in the bone banks.

So far no one has been able to transplant a human brain, and Dr. Boris Vasilevich Petrovsky, a noted surgeon who is Minister of Health of the Soviet Union, doubts that anybody ever will. "The fact that the brain cannot live more than six minutes without oxygen makes brain transplants impossible. The transplanting of heads in human beings probably will not be possible for two thousand years."

Lacking that, you must admit that the transplanters have done some remarkable reshuffling inside the human body.

Cooper Repairs the Brain

The surgeons may not be able to give you a new head, but they now can do a lot to repair your brain when it gets out of kilter. I watched the greatest, and the most fiercely controversial, brain surgeon alive while he operated on three human brains almost simultaneously. It was at St. Barnabas Hospital for Chronic Diseases, an obscure institution in the Bronx, New York. The surgeon was Dr. Irving S. Cooper.

Two of the patients were lying on operating tables a few feet apart in the main operating room. The third was in a smaller operating room off to one side. Dr. Cooper, tall and rugged with thick blond hair, in a green scrub suit, hurried back and forth from operating room to operating room, and from table to table, with me trailing behind. I looked inside one patient's skull. It was a strange sight. I could see some cerebral fluid bubbling around the brain.

The patient in the smaller operating room was a nineteen-year-old girl named Ruth. She had dystonia musculorum deformans, a ghastly genetic disease which contorts the hands, arms, and legs into grotesque shapes. Ruth's hands were twisted almost inside out, and one of her legs was gruesomely distorted. Before Dr. Cooper devised his operation for this disease, no remedy was known. Children grew up in unending agony, twisted like pretzels. Sometimes their feet bent backward until they touched their heads.

An anesthesiologist injected a "local"—no more than that because Ruth had to stay awake while Cooper probed in her brain. Her head was held absolutely immobile by four steel rods with viselike clamps. An electric drill bit into her shaven skull, and a mist of small particles flew out of the incision. Dr. Cooper called it "dust." He ended with a hole three quarters of an inch in diameter, exposing her grey-colored brain. There was very little blood.

Cooper had a little hook in his left hand and a tiny razor-sharp scalpel in his right hand. With them, he cut away the covering of the brain. He pumped in some air so the X-ray technician could get clearer films—road maps to guide him. He inserted a long, slender cannula, a tube refrigerated by a stream of liquid nitrogen. It could go down to 321° below zero Fahrenheit. This was cryosurgery, an extraordinarily versatile technique that Cooper invented to destroy unwanted tissue.

He advanced the cannula into the brain a microscopic fraction of an inch at a time, searching for the infinitely small section of brain cells that was causing Ruth's dystonia. He found it and attacked it with the liquid nitrogen.

"Ruthy, are you behaving yourself down there?" he joked.

"Yes," she tensely replied. The air that he had put into her brain had given her a throbbing headache.

"Okay," Dr. Cooper said. "See if you can open your left fist."

I watched her slowly, painfully straighten her dreadfully twisted fingers.

"Can you lift your left arm?"

"I'll try."

Inch by inch, she lifted her left arm. "I can, I can," she called out excitedly.

"Touch your nose."

She did.

Dr. Cooper has seen this happen in thousands of operations, but he becomes emotional every time. "That's terrific," he exclaimed. "How long is it since you could bend that elbow?"

"Seven years," she said. She was crying happily. I was crying a little as well.

She could straighten her left leg, too.

That same morning, I watched Cooper successfully operate on an old man with parkinsonism and a middle-aged woman with a spastic condition. During the operation on the epileptic woman, he spent much time exploring the pulvinar, an area of the living brain that had not been operated on before.

Of all the organs in the body, the brain is the most puzzling. Most of it is a vast, uncharted wilderness to medical science. Large sections are unexplored, their purposes unknown. Dr. Cooper has spent his life investigating the functioning of the brain, its diseases, and ways to combat them surgically.

Through the years, he has been heatedly attacked for his research methods, his showmanship, and the publicity he has received. Some medical men are still carrying on vendettas against him. But there is little dispute anymore as to his greatness.

Cooper was born in Atlantic City, New Jersey, in 1922. He chose medicine for the oddest reason of any physician I've met. Between his freshman and sophomore years at college, he had a summer job delivering meat. One day, an old lady customer asked him what career he was planning on.

"I think I'll be a lawyer," he said.

"You're making a big mistake," she said. "You look just like a doctor."

He went home and told his mother that he was going to study medicine. He obtained an M.D. at George Washington University medical school, in Washington, D.C., and a Ph.D. in neurosurgery at the University of Minnesota.

"I was never really driven, as some young men are, by a love of surgery," he said to me. "I never was crazy about tying knots or doing all the tricks that you read about surgeons doing. I was really in love with the brain, and the way to deal with the brain, it seemed to me, was through neurosurgery.

"Neuroanatomy has a lot of fascinations. We know very little about the brain, but what we know is logical. At first, all the things we discovered about it seemed very paradoxical, but eventually we saw that there was great logic to how the brain works."

Feelingly, he added, "You're truly dealing with the soul of man when you're dealing with the brain."

Dr. Cooper's first significant discovery came when he was thirty. It was an operation that helped to control the frightful symptoms of Parkinson's disease in some patients.

For a half century, surgeons had tried to abolish the tremors of Parkinson's disease. They had never been able to do it satisfactorily. Most of their operations ended with the patients partially paralyzed.

Cooper hit on his operation for parkinsonism serendipitously. Joseph Cioppa, a forty-year-old truck driver, came into the neurosurgical clinic at

N.Y.U.-Bellevue Hospital in New York City in October 1952, shaking so badly from parkinsonism that he couldn't even feed himself. He was miserable. He said he would rather have his right side totally paralyzed than go on shaking like a willow in a gale. Cooper, who was teaching at Bellevue, got the case. He started out to do a pedunculotomy, an incision in some motor fibers of the brain. He made an opening about the size of a half dollar in Cioppa's skull, near the ear, and cautiously lifted up the temporal lobe so he could get at the mid-brain. As he was doing this, he accidentally tore a tiny artery in the arachnoid, one of the protective coverings of the brain. Blood poured out.

The bleeding was so heavy that the man's life was in jeopardy. Cooper tensely told his Italian assistant, Dr. Aldo Morello, to go out and tell the family that Joe Cioppa might not survive the next few minutes. However, Cooper was able to stanch the flowing blood with a small silver clip.

By good fortune, Cooper had recently read an article on the torn blood vessel—the anterior choroidal artery. He remembered that it irrigated some important grey matter in the center of the brain, including a section of the thalamus. These areas were related in some manner to the mechanisms of parkinsonism, he knew.

Cooper did some fast, imaginative thinking. Instead of proceeding with the operation, he decided to stop it and see what the results would be of cutting off the blood supply to those areas of the brain. Possibly their destruction would have some effect upon the mechanisms of parkinsonism.

When Cioppa came out of the anesthesia that evening, he wasn't shaking. Cooper couldn't sleep all night waiting to see if the truck driver would be as well off in the morning. He was. His tremors were all gone—his rigidity, too—and he was in no way paralyzed.

Dr. Cooper did the operation fifty-five times in a row successfully. He tried it on parkinsonism patients at Central Islip State Hospital who had been bedridden for years. After his surgery, they got up and walked normally.

Only then did Dr. Cooper report his results. "It was absolute dogma then that nothing could get rid of all the tremor and rigidity of parkinsonism without paralyzing the patient," he declared. "So I wanted the evidence to be incontrovertible."

His fellow neurosurgeons wouldn't accept his reports. Cooper showed them before-and-after movies, but they wouldn't believe them. He brought a patient to a medical meeting, a coal miner who had been 100 percent incapacitated, and had him do push-ups. His colleagues still wouldn't believe him. They maintained that the coal miner had only been suffering from hysteria, and had recovered by the power of suggestion.

"Why do you suppose they wouldn't believe you?" I asked Dr. Cooper.

"There's always been a long history of resistance to innovation in medicine," he said. "But I think there were several other reasons. One is that it went very strongly against dogma that had been laid down by very important men in neurosurgery. Secondly, I was extremely young. I was thirty. I'd never been in New York before. Nobody knew who the hell I was to come along and make this claim. And once it occurred to me that they didn't believe me, I reacted like any young man would. I got mad as hell, and I became very aggressive, maybe too aggressive, in my espousal of the new operation. It was a kind of a vicious circle.

"Another thing. When I reported my results, they got great publicity, which doctors have always had a very hypocritical atittude about. Some of the senior men took a very dim view of seeing my name in *Life* and *Time*. It was something else that they raised hell about."

Then and there, Irving Cooper became known forever in the medical world as a controversial character.

Since blood vessels vary from person to person, the parkinsonism operation was a risky one. The outcome was unpredictable, and the mortality rate sometimes ran as high as 10 percent. Dr. Cooper worked to reduce the hazard. In the course of the next three years, he developed two new techniques for accomplishing the same ends more safely. They were the chemopallidectomy and the chemothalamectomy. In the first, he injected novocaine into the globus pallidus while the patient was awake. If the patient stopped shaking, Cooper knew he was in the correct place and he injected pure alcohol into it. The alcohol destroyed the felonious brain cells that caused the parkinsonism symptoms. Later, he found that he obtained even better results by injecting alcohol into the thalamus. Cooper said that the two operations brought his mortality rate down to 1 percent.

His fellow neurosurgeons criticized him more. Now they denounced him because he had come up with an improvement over his original parkinsonism operation.

"How could your other operation be any good if you're doing something different now?" they carped.

Despite the opposition of the medical establishment, Cooper's operations were soon being done by surgeons all over the United States, Europe, and South America. By the late 1950s, Cooper had performed almost a thousand chemopallidectomies and chemothalamectomies himself, mostly at St. Barnabas.

The technique led to the development of cryosurgery by Cooper, one of the major surgical advances of the century. It was another instance of serendipity in operation. Serendipitous things continually seem to happen to Dr. Cooper.

As he recounted the story to me:

"One Christmas, my wife gave me a gift of a carbon dioxide wine-bottle opener. You know, the kind that ejects the cork by an infusion of carbon dioxide gas. The gadget had a needle in it that looked just like my brain probe. I started playing with it on Christmas morning, squirting the carbon dioxide into my hand. The carbon dioxide made my palm feel numb. Then, as it thawed, the numbness would disappear.

"This might make a very nice tool for me, I thought. I could use the principle of it to freeze very tiny areas of tissue."

Cryosurgery, he was to call this, after the Greek word *kryos*, meaning cold or frost.

He made a probe out of a hollow tube, insulated it like a thermos bottle, and chilled it with liquid nitrogen, a better cooling agent than carbon dioxide. The incredibly cold temperatures at the tip—below minus-300° Fahrenheit—replaced the surgeon's knife in cutting away diseased tissue. He tried it for the first time on a human being in 1961. It was a parkinsonism case, and the cryoprobe did everything he wished.

He wanted it most for dystonia. He didn't dare operate on the brain of a dystonia victim with the ordinary methods.

"In dystonia cases, you're never quite sure how much tissue to destroy for each patient," he explained. "With a cryoprobe, you can reverse the freezing if you've gone too far and thaw out the tissue before it's too late. You can't do that with a knife. You can't reverse the procedure after you've cut into the brain with a scalpel."

Still, he was nervous about the outcome the first time. Most surgeons are when they try a new procedure. A dark-haired little girl, eleven years old, was brought into Dr. Cooper in agony from her dystonia, shaking violently, twisted so horribly that her feet were turned inside out. Her parents wanted Cooper to try his new operation on her and he declined. He didn't know whether he could do her any good. He might do her harm, he warned.

The parents implored him to operate. He hesitated. He advised the parents to go home and think it over.

They telephoned him a week later. They said they couldn't stand seeing the child suffer another day. If Dr. Cooper didn't operate on her, they were going to turn on the gas and kill themselves and their daughter.

Cooper operated on the child. She was out of bed the following morning, her feet straight, her tremor gone. Twelve years later, she was a tall, handsome young woman who walked perfectly normally. She was graduating from college.

Cryosurgery has also proved invaluable for removing cataracts and correcting detached retinas, taking out pituitary glands and prostates, and for several forms of cancer. It provided the most effective treatment for Parkinson's disease until the arrival of the miracle drug L-dopa in 1969. It still remains the best hope for patients who don't respond to L-dopa.

Cooper was in the news again in 1972 with another invention. This time it was a "brain pacemaker,"—to be precise, a cerebellum electrical stimulator. It had tiny platinum electrodes that are implanted on the surface of the cerebellum, a fist-sized part of the brain that regulates movements of the body's voluntary muscles. The electrodes are linked by a miniature radio to a battery on the patient's belt. The battery sends low-voltage electrical stimuli to the brain which relieve the patient's muscle spasticity.

Sixty-one patients suffering from epilepsy, cerebral palsy, and the crippling effects of strokes were fitted out with the brain pacemaker by Cooper. Forty-seven of them were distinctly benefited. One man who had been plagued with uncontrollable epilepsy since he was seven years old became seizure-free. A teen-age boy with cerebral palsy who couldn't move a finger was able to feed himself. He could swim and he was learning to walk.

Dr. Cooper reported the case of an eighteen-year-old epileptic whose frenzied seizures had included several attempts at suicide and physical assaults on his mother. The brain pacemaker kept him free of seizures for years until a wire broke. That day, the boy had thirteen seizures. After repairs were made, the boy became symptom-free again, and he was able to hold down a regular job.

As usual with Cooper, there was loud controversy. Some neurosurgeons didn't believe his claims. They demanded that he conduct controlled tests in which dummy pacemakers were inserted into some patients.

Dr. Cooper flatly refused. "I'm not running an experiment," he said. "I'm treating desperate patients who have come to me for help."

I asked Dr. Cooper, "What does it do to you when your peers insist on challenging the truth of your reports?"

"It tears me apart," he declared. "I think that all new things in medicine should be challenged, but not like this. The facts were all ascertainable here. All anyone had to do was look. It's been an awful ordeal."

He and his first wife, Mary Dan Frost, had three children before she was killed in an accident. He was married again, in 1970, to a stunning Norwegian blonde, Sissel Holm. They have one son. Cooper plays a hard game of tennis, reads constantly, and studies foreign languages. He speaks six of them. He is not much for party-going. He says, "You have to go to bed early if you are going to operate in the morning. You have to train for it; otherwise you're a little shaky."

Cooper is also a very talented writer. His poignant book on surgery, *The*

Victim Is Always the Same, drew critical raves when it was published in 1973.

"I don't think anyone is in medical research solely because they want to help people," he said to me. "Medical men who say that are kidding themselves. If someone says he became a priest solely because he wanted to bring people to God, he's kidding himself. There's always some other cause. The thing that drives me is more artistic than scientific. If I weren't doing surgery, I'd be a composer or a writer."

He analyzed himself for me. "If I have any quality as a researcher, it is an intuitive rather than a scientific one. Many of my discoveries have been serendipitious. A lot of my fellow neurosurgeons have been critical about that, too. When you say, 'Cooper has proven this,' they answer, 'Yes, but he fell into it.' Which is true. But most important discoveries—from penicillin on—have been serendipitous. You have to have the intuition to recognize that you've seen something new and important. And you have to be willing to work at it regardless of the obstacles.

"When I get onto something new and exciting, I can't let go of it. I can't think of anything else. There have been times when I prayed that I could stop thinking about a discovery."

Dr. Cooper's critics are still many. He continues to face them down and find new ways to help dystonics, parkinsonians, epileptics, and other people with malfunctioning brains. Before him, they had little reason for hope.

Rosen Gives Back Hearing to Thousands of the Deaf

To Dr. Samuel Rosen, it's ecstasy to hear a patient say, "I can hear."

Rosen, who was born in 1897, is a chunky man of medium height with a round, cherubic face under a matting of thick white hair. He discovered an ear operation to cure deafness that has been performed close to a million times from Tel Aviv to Tokyo. Today, he is hailed as "the father of stapes surgery," but he had to battle almost as hard as Irving Cooper did against the disbelief and indifference of other ear surgeons. For years, he says, at New York's Mt. Sinai Hospital, he was treated as if he had scarlet fever but it didn't deter him.

"I don't care if God doesn't believe," he told Dr. Eugene R. Snyder, a friend at Mt. Sinai. "I believe."

Now everybody believes.

I talked with Dr. Rosen in the comfortable living room of his Park Avenue apartment. It was filled with exquisite objects d'art he had brought back from his travels. He was youthfully, one might say jubilantly, dressed in a light grey suit, a blue and white checked shirt, and a violent red and black necktie with a matching red handkerchief in his breast pocket. His trim, delightful wife, Helen, served us tea and cookies. The pair were married in 1928. When they go abroad, she assists at his operations.

He was born in the ghetto in Syracuse, New York, the son of Russian-Jewish peddlers. His mother, Lena, earned most of the money that kept the family living by selling crockery on street corners from a baby carriage. She suffered frightful attacks of asthma. Each time the boy heard her painful breathing, he was sure she was going to die. When he was six years old, he went into the sickroom and said to her, "Ma, I'm going to become a doctor so I can cure you."

His four brothers and sisters scrounged the money for his medical education at Syracuse University, and he went on to New York to intern at Mt. Sinai. He chose ear surgery as his specialty, he said, because "it required a meticulousness and precision that surgery in roomier parts of the human body did not demand." As you can imagine, Sam Rosen has always been a meticulous person.

It is impossible to estimate the total number of people in the world afflicted with deafness. The computers gulp at the thought. The best estimate for the United States is that 13,400,000 Americans suffer from a significant loss of hearing. The majority of them—slightly more than half—are deaf because of some disease or an injury that damaged their nerve of hearing. Otologists term this "nerve deafness." However, many of the other deaf people have an absolutely normal auditory nerve. Their trouble is that sound waves cannot get through to the auditory nerve. This condition is known as conduction deafness.

Otosclerosis is a principal cause of this conduction deafness. A bony growth constricts the stapes, the key bone in the hearing process, stopping it from transmitting sound waves to the hearing nerve.

A little course in osteologic anatomy may be in order here. A chain of three small bones—the malleus, incus, and stapes—is located behind the eardrum. These bones pick up sound vibrations and pass them along from one to the other, and on to the fluids of the inner ear which actuate the auditory nerve. That's why you hear sounds. The stapes (the name is the Latin word for "stirrup," which the stapes resembles) is the innermost of the trio of bones, and the tiniest. In fact, it is the smallest bone in the whole body, less than one tenth the size of your little fingernail. In a normal ear, the stapes vibrates just like a tuning fork. In people suffering from otosclerosis, the stapes becomes more rigidly fixed in place, and the patient grows deafer and deafer.

Late in the last century, some French and American surgeons experimented with an operation to cure this condition. It was somewhat akin to the operation that Dr. Rosen devised, but, for some strange reason, otologists abandoned it. Nobody knows why. In 1938, a New York City ear surgeon, Dr. Julius Lempert, developed a new surgical approach. With a Lilliputian dental drill, he cut a hole in the bone encircling the inner ear. He made an artificial window in it that allowed sound waves to detour around the stapes to the auditory nerve. It was a clever operation, called fenestration, but a complicated and lengthy one which had decided drawbacks. It required general anesthesia, it necessitated a two to three-week convalescence, and it often caused permanent dizziness. Still it was the sole known treatment for this type of deafness, and otologists embraced it religiously.

The Rosen operation proved to be far superior. It was much less costly in danger, time, and possible side effects.

Dr. Rosen discovered the operation by accident. "Serendipity" is a favorite word of his, too.

On the morning of April 2, 1952, he was performing a diagnostic test on a forty-three-year-old Midwesterner who was very deaf because of otosclerosis. It was a test he had devised to make sure that the patient really needed the Lempert operation. Occasionally, this condition was misdiagnosed.

A local anesthesia was all that Rosen used. Wearing powerful magnifying glasses, he cut around the man's eardrum, folded it back, and exposed the middle ear with its three little bones. He applied pressure to the top of the stapes. Suddenly, the patient cried out, "I can hear everything, Doc."

This from a man who hadn't heard a normal sound in many years.

"Can you hear what I say now?" Dr. Rosen whispered.

"Sure," the patient said. "You're talking too loud."

Rosen whispered softer yet. "Do you like scrambled eggs?"

"Yes, I like scrambled eggs," the patient answered, "and I like them with bacon."

The man had recovered his hearing. In some way, Rosen's probing had freed his stapes.

After the operation, Rosen was so thrilled that he could barely contain himself. His dilemma was that he didn't know exactly what he had done to the man's stapes. His colleagues claimed that it was just a fluke, but he wouldn't listen to them. He worked on cadavers in the Mt. Sinai morgue and manipulated their stapes to learn to do purposefully what he had done by accident. He experimented on the ears of hundreds of monkeys and dogs. He designed a set of special surgical instruments. He found that the proper amount of pressure applied on the stapes pulsatingly at the right spot and in the right direction could break it loose from the stony tentacles gripping it.

Months later, Rosen tried the operation on another patient, and the patient's hearing was fully restored. It receded following the surgery as the middle ear healed, but within two weeks the hearing had returned.

It was the same old story, though. Rosen's colleagues didn't believe him. He couldn't even get the surgeons in his own hospital to watch him do the operation.

"I begged them to come and see for themselves," Dr. Rosen recalled, gesturing angrily with his eyeglasses. "I implored them to come. Not one came, not one. They all said, 'We don't give a damn what Rosen says. We know it can't work.' "

He suspects that some anti-Semitism may have been involved. He also charges that money was an issue. His operation sharply reduced the value of the fenestration that most ear surgeons were used to doing, a technique that earned them big fees.

Rosen was luckier than Cooper. He was merely held in medical coventry for three years. Finally, word of his successes spread so widely that they could not be denied. In 1955, he was invited to give a paper on stapes mobilization before the august American Laryngological, Rhinological and Otological Society. He reported on twenty-one operations. Stapes mobilization had helped seven out of ten otosclerotics to hear better. Three of the seven had gotten completely normal hearing back. (This record was to mount with the years, and it should be noted that the patients who didn't benefit could still have the fenestration procedure performed on them.)

After 1955, Rosen and his stapes operations were considered to be scientifically respectable.

He has now demonstrated his operation in forty-one foreign countries. When he performed his operation at the Cairo University Medical College, President Gamal Abdel Nasser of Egypt invited him to the presidential palace for a ninety-minute talk.

"I'm very grateful to you for coming here to help my people," President Nasser declared.

"I was surprised that I was invited," Dr. Rosen stated. "I'm Jewish, you realize."

"We're aware of that," President Nasser said. "But your work is above race or country. You doctors are the best diplomats."

During Dr. Rosen's second trip to Israel, Prime Minister David Ben Gurion said, "I'm very glad that you went to the Arab countries to teach them as you taught us. That's very good for everyone."

"You know, I was never trained as a researcher," Dr. Rosen remarked to me. "I'm just a curious guy. I'm curious about people and what makes them tick. Actually, what makes them hear the tick. Or not hear it. I'll go anyplace to find out."

Rosen has gone to some very faraway places to find out what ticks people hear. He and his wife jeeped six hundred miles through the roadless snake-infested jungles of the Sudan to study the hearing traits of a tribe of Mabaans who were living in a Stone Age culture.

Said Dr. Rosen, "We wanted to study a population that had lived for a thousand years quietly, without the insult of noise."

This tribe had never heard anything louder than the roar of a wild animal or the clap of thunder. They had no guns, no radios, no machinery. Rosen found that their hearing as they aged was superior to anything that had ever been recorded for man. He also discovered that their quiet existence and low-fat died saved them from ulcers, coronary heart disease, and hypertension. Their blood pressure was the same at seventy-five years of age as it was at fifteen.

Rosen has made three trips to China. He was very impressed with Chinese medicine.

"I have seen the past, and it works," he told the press.

He has studied the effect of city noises on the health of urban dwellers. It is very harmful, he says. "Each time you hear a sudden noise, your heart beats rapidly, the blood vessels constrict, the pupils dilate, and the stomach, esophagus, and intestines are seized by spasms." He maintains that subway noises, sirens, and rock music are serious health menaces.

"I'm not curious just for the sake of curiosity," Dr. Rosen declared to me. "Whatever I do must benefit people in some way or other."

I remarked, "You're still the little boy who said, 'Mother, I'm going to cure you,' but you're saying it now to all mankind."

"I say it every day," he declared.

He has retired from the daily surgical grind but continues his consultation practice. He does a lot of puttering around their apartment.

"I'm very good with my hands," he boasted.

"But you couldn't fix my zipper," his wife ruefully noted.

The Rosens have two children, a son who is a professor of pediatric research and a daughter who is a magazine editor.

What he does is fun to him.

"It's fun to be truthful," he replied unexpectedly. "It's fun to say you don't know if you don't know. It's fun not to think you're greater than you really would like to think you are. It's fun to pick up a guy and brush him off if he's fallen down. It's fun to cut down a tree that's sick. It's fun to see the sky and the stars. It's fun to walk in the moonlight."

Charnley's Artificial Hip

Both rheumatoid arthritis and osteoarthritis can assault the hip. They can warp and crumble the two bones forming it, the femur and the acetabulum. The slightest pressure on that hip becomes unendurable. The patient is bent over, and all of his ability to walk is stolen from him.

It befell Eugene Ormandy, the veteran conductor of the Philadelphia Orchestra. His hips were attacked so harshly by arthritis that mounting the podium became scourging punishment.

Then he had a man-made hip installed. It let him walk normally again. He could even climb and descend stairs without a vestige of a limp or pain.

"It's like getting a whole new lease on life," Ormandy said.

Men have been making artificial substitutes for parts of their bodies for thousands of years. Wooden legs have been in use since 600 B.C. Metal hands have been attached to people's arms since the sixteenth century. A Boston silversmith by the name of Paul Revere was well known for his high-grade false teeth. But few have invented anything quite as ingenious and pain-relieving as the artificial hip developed by a British orthopedic surgeon named John Charnley. To quote the citation for his 1975 Lasker Award, his mechanical hip has "restored normal living to tens of thousands of patients throughout the world." It is being installed in forty thousand people a year in the United States.

I talked with Mr. Charnley—surgeons are called Mister, not Doctor, in Britain—when he came to New York to receive his Lasker Award. We lunched in the elegant Oak Room of the St. Regis Hotel. I found him a short, light-haired man with very broad shoulders, wearing a conservative charcoal-grey suit, white shirt, and blue necktie. No wild red and black combinations for him. He speaks in a droning monotone, but he gestures often, smashing his right fist against his left palm.

Charnley was born in 1911 in the small town of Bury in Lancashire. His father was a pharmacist.

Why did he select surgery?

"I reckon it's practically the only field where an educated man can use his hands. You can be a sculptor or a painter or a surgeon. My first interest was in dental surgery, but I felt I wanted to do surgery on a bigger scale."

He got his medical education at the University of Manchester shortly before World War II engulfed Europe. Some of his friends stayed out of the army until they could be called up as specialists. It gave them the rank of major. Charnley was too much aware of the threat of Hitler's Germany. "I really thought there was no hope in those days," he said. He joined up early as a captain. He was at Dunkirk, treating the wounded under Nazi bombs during the heroic evacuation of British troops from the Continent. Later, he was posted to Egypt, operating on Tommies wounded at the historic Battle of El Alamein.

He was a general surgeon. "I didn't think anything at all of bones and joints at the time. I thought it was a very unrewarding field. Bones—you just put them straight and waited for God to unite them."

Sir Harry Platt, the medical advisor to the British forces, who was an orthopedic surgeon, saw Charnley's work and had him transferred to orthopedics, to his "complete surprise and slight horror.

"But I found it was really my subject," he declared. "It was mechanical. It offered enormous fields for mechanical development."

Like Willem Kolff of the artificial kidney, Charnley is a mechanically minded physician.

After the war, he studied under Platt at the University of Manchester, then went on to Wrightington Hospital in nearby Wigan. He is director of its Centre for Hip Surgery.

Since arthritis is basic to orthopedics, Charnley's first research was on the stiffening of arthritic knee joints, a very painful condition. In 1948, he discovered a new technique for fusing the knee bones into one solid bone. He did it by cutting off the ends of the bones and putting the fresh ends together under powerful spring-loaded compression.

Naturally, the other orthopedic surgeons were ironclad in their opposition. "People were against the whole idea," Mr. Charnley said. "They thought it was unphysiological."

But it had to be accepted. By his technique, a knee could be successfully fused in four weeks instead of the six months it had previously taken.

The arthritic hip was the prime research target of the orthopedists. It was the most disabling.

The hip is a bulky ball-and-socket joint in which the rounded head of the femur fits tightly. When arthritis ravages the hip joint, the damaged ball of bone at the end of the femur rubs against the roughened surface of the socket and causes agonizing pain. The obvious remedy was an artificial hip. Two of them were developed out of stainless steel in these early years, but neither was reliable, or good. The patients squeaked as they walked.

Charnley set forth to learn why. Replacing the head of the femur with a stainless steel ball was comparatively easy in the average patient. The tough question was how to attach the ball to the femur. In these early artificial hips, the ball was screwed into the femur, and the screw often came undone. Lubrication was another messy problem. No one knew how to prevent destructive friction between the stainless steel ball and the stainless steel socket. The natural body fluids that lubricated normal hips were inadequate in the stainless steel hips.

"Stainless steel wetted by the body fluids just didn't become slippery enough," Charnley discovered. "It squeaked and showed high friction resistance."

A new material was needed that required no lubrication at all. A plastic, no doubt. Charnley made a detailed study of tribology, the science of wear. He read up on the theory of lubrication. He conferred with engineers. He settled on Teflon and used it for the socket of an artificial hip he designed. The hip was a failure. The Teflon wore out rapidly.

Then Lady Luck smiled on Mr. Charnley.

"One day," he said, "a salesman turned up with a sample of high-density polyethylene. I sent him away, telling him we knew that polyethylene was useless. I hadn't heard of high-density polyethylene, but, luckily, my technician had. Behind my back, he told the salesman to leave a sample. We tested its wearing properties, and the results were fantastic." That took care of the socket.

Charnley used dental cement to bond the polyethylene socket to the patient's living bone. He worried that the body might reject the cement, but it didn't.

Clinical tests on the new hip were begun in Wrightington Hospital in November 1972. Patients who had been totally disabled, old people in their late sixties and seventies, were able to walk without crutches two days after the operation. It was thrilling to watch them.

But dangerous complications arose. Almost 10 percent of the patients came down with serious infections. Airborne organisms were getting into the big open wounds needed in hip surgery. Charnley tackled this problem as vigorously, and scientifically, as he had gone after the others. He built a special enclosure around the operating table—a "greenhouse"—and blew clean air down into it from above. That reduced the bacterial count to normal levels. He also designed special air-conditioned clothing for the surgeons. The two precautions lowered the infection rate to an acceptable level.

By 1976, Charnley and his staff had done over nine thousand hip operations with a success score of better than 91 percent.

Ordinarily, it takes Mr. Charnley about an hour and a quarter to implant a new hip. That includes twenty minutes of standing around and doing nothing while waiting for the cement to set. On the two days a week that he operates, Charnley arrives at the hospital at 8:45 A.M. Operating rooms don't start to work in England until a comfortable 9:00 A.M.

Charnley waited until he was forty-six to marry. He and his wife, Jill, have two teen-age children. Neither of the children is heading for medicine.

"I wouldn't press them to be doctors in England today," Charnley said.

He said he is so absorbed in his research that he has let go of all his hobbies. He does the repairs when mechanical things go wrong at home, though.

"I'm not bad at things like that," he conceded.

Charnley said that he went into research "because I was dissatisfied with orthodox teaching." He still is. Now he is trying to develop an entirely new kind of artificial knee. It would give the joy of walking back to tens of thousands more people.

Shinya's Colonoscope Searches Through the Colon

Let us here note some other surgical marvels. The surgeons can save your eyesight by giving you a new cornea. A Russian ophthalmologist, Professor Nils Feodorovich Filatov, conceived the admirable idea of taking human corneas from cadavers and transplanting them into live people. His assistant, Dr. Nadeja Putchkivskaya, is carrying his research further at the Filatov Institute in Odessa. Dr. Charles Kelman, of the Manhattan Eye, Ear and Throat Hospital in New York, has evolved an astute technique for removing cataracts called phaco-emulsification. He makes a tiny incision in the eye with a hollow needle that vibrates forty thousand times a second. It changes the hard matter that forms the cataract into liquid and suctions it out. The patient can go back to work the day after the operation.

We have acupuncture to report on. No question remains that needling is effective as an anesthesia and a pain-reliever for Chinese people.

On his visit to China, Dr. Rosen saw seventeen operations performed for which the only anesthesia was acupuncture. The operations ranged from pulling teeth to the removal of a brain tumor.

"Acupuncture worked in every case I saw," Dr. Rosen declared. "There was no screaming from pain as the patient was operated on. If you saw nothing but the patient's face, you wouldn't think that he was under surgery at all. There was no perspiration. There was no anxiety."

"Even during a serious abdominal operation?" Dr. Rosen was asked.

"Yes."

One hopes that acupuncture will be able to do as much for Occidental patients.

Some of the greatest prodigies are in diagnosis. For example, the nuclear devices. More than one hundred radioisotopes can help to detect diseased hearts, blood clots, cancers, and other conditions.

Ultrasonic frequencies can do many things that X-rays can't do. They can tell the difference between a malignant tumor and a cyst. They can perform echo cardiograms on heart patients. They can locate "internal landmarks" in the brain. They can outline a fetal head to measure the size and shape of an unborn baby.

An adroit Japanese surgeon, Dr. Hiromi Shinya, at Beth Israel Medical Center in New York City, has perfected a masterful technique named colonoscopy that lets him insert a flexible fiber tube equipped with lights and mirrors eight feet up into a patient's intestines painlessly. He can check every section of the colon for tumor, polyps, and inflammations, and the patient doesn't have a shred of discomfort while he is doing it.

A patient with a polyp in his colon usually has to have a major abdominal operation that lays him up for four weeks. I watched Dr. Shinya remove three large polyps from a forty-six-year-old man's colon in his office in thirty-five minutes. He snipped them off with a small wire snare at the end of the colonoscope, a device which he invented. There wasn't a drop of blood, and the patient assured me contentedly that he had felt nothing. He took his wife to a Broadway theater that evening.

The colonoscope is far superior to the rigid proctoscope, which extends only ten inches into the patient.

The use of fiberoptic tubes for medical examinations was pioneered at the University of Michigan in 1957 by a South African, Dr. Basil I. Hirschkowitz. Now fiberoptic instruments are being employed to reach down through the patient's mouth to examine the entire digestive tract. They are being utilized to explore the lungs, the heart, and the kidneys. With these instruments, the surgeons can discover dangerous conditions early enough to cure them. Which really is the name of the game.

4

THE FIRST GREAT
VICTORIES OVER CANCER

DARBY, PENNSYLVANIA, AN UNDISTINGUISHED SUBURB of Philadelphia, on a warm spring morning. I was visiting cancer patients at Mercy Catholic Medical Center. The first was a pleasant, grey-haired woman, fifty-eight years old, with cancer of the pancreas, about as evil a cancer as there is. She had come from Pittsburgh three months before—just skin, bones, and agony. Even morphine couldn't deaden her pain. Her doctors in Pittsburgh had given her eight to ten days to live. They hoped it would be less.

Dr. Isaac Djerassi, a short, dark, boyish man, led me into her room. She was sitting up in an armchair, eating a big slice of birthday cake. She looked in excellent health, her face rounded, her body filled out.

"Hello, sweetheart," Dr. Djerassi grinned. "How are you feeling today?"

Her voice was strong. "Real good, doctor."

Then her eyes turned up at him appealingly. "Do you think, maybe, I can go on feeling this well?"

"Why not?" Dr. Djerassi said.

This Isaac Djerassi—Bulgarian-born, Israeli-trained, and very Americanized—was reputed to do better against childhood leukemia and against many other forms of cancer than any researcher in the United States. He took me on to a chic woman of fifty-five who had arrived at the hospital more dead than alive with lung cancer. Now, two years later, the X-rays showed that her disease was completely gone. Her long white hair had all fallen out as a result of the drugs she had received, but to her surprise and delight, her hair had grown back black. Next was a tall, slender Puerto Rican boy with terrible leukemia who had been sent to the hospital to die. Dr. Djerassi had successfully held his leukemia in check for three years, but the boy was tiring of the struggle. "Let me go home," he pleaded. "I don't give a damn if I die." I listened as Dr. Djerassi urged him to remain in the hospital. Finally, he agreed.

The Saturday before, the hospital had let the boy out overnight to visit his family in Scranton. While he was there, two neighborhood toughs jumped him. One of them got a broken leg, the other a broken arm. Unknown to them and even to the hospital, the gentle Puerto Rican lad was a black belt in karate.

"Tell me, Isaac," I asked Dr. Djerassi, "how can you save all these patients that everybody else has written off for dead?"

He beamed. "Some chemotherapy, some immunotherapy, and some faith."

You can't win them all. Dr. Djerassi sadly spoke of a forty-five-year-old woman who came to him with Hodgkin's disease. He treated her for several months and fully cleared up her condition. She went home happily. Two days later, she came down with hepatitis.

"The poor thing was petrified with fear," Dr. Djerassi said. "She assumed that her cancer had recurred. I assured her that it was only hepatitis, probably due to a blood transfusion. I told her that she had nothing to worry about. But she didn't believe me. She got hold of a gun and killed herself."

An autopsy showed that she hadn't the slightest trace of cancer left.

A wintry evening in New York City. Dr. Edmund Klein, the brilliant Buffalo dermatologist, chunky and bald, had just lectured at Sloan-Kettering Institute for Cancer Research on the magnificent work he was doing in skin cancer. Permanent cures in seven hundred cases! Now we were in a spartan conference room talking about the morality of testing new drugs on dying patients.

"Do you always ask the patients' permission?"

"They are complete partners. There is never any attempt at doing anything without telling them exactly what it is. I point out to them that this not only may not help, but probably will not help. That it may harm, and possibly will. However, the patient usually realizes that there is very little else that can be done for him, and he is definitely willing to try anything new.

"People say, 'Oh, why do you mistreat this poor dying patient?' Actually, you're doing him the biggest favor. Sure, there are some who want to jump out of the window. But I've only known two people who committed suicide. They don't want to die. They don't want to be put out of their misery. It's the family, maybe, that wants to be rid of the problem. It's the nurses who want to get rid of the stinking mess. Not the patient."

Late on a hot summer afternoon in a basement office at Stanford University Hospital in Stanford, California. I was with Dr. Henry S. Kaplan, the radiotherapist who proved that most Hodgkin's disease cases could be cured. He was tall and well built.

"Are you afraid of cancer?" I asked him.

He spoke very slowly. "I guess if I were romanticizing and using language that a scientist wouldn't use, I would say that I have always looked upon my relationship to cancer as a little bit analagous to that of Moby Dick and Captain Ahab. I'm chasing it; I hope it doesn't catch me."

Cancer, the Democratic Killer

Cancer is very democratic. It slaughters the rich, the famous, and the powerful as readily as the poor and the insignificant. It has wasted such notables as King George VI of England; the Duke of Windsor; John Foster Dulles; Democratic Speaker of the House Sam Rayburn and Republican Senator Robert A. Taft; Nobel laureates T.S. Eliot, and Enrico Fermi; Gertrude Stein; Aldous Huxley; Boris Pasternak; Marie Curie; Edward R. Murrow; Fernandel; Walt Disney; and Babe Ruth.

Hippocrates named the disease after the crab whose Greek name is *karkinos*. The crustacean's claws reminded him of the veins that frequently stretch out from malignant tumors.

We first got to know something about the disease in the mid-eighteenth century. Percival Pott, a perceptive British surgeon at St. Bartholomew's Hospital in London, who lived from 1714 to 1788, found the first occupational cancer—chimney sweepers' cancer—in the scrotum of young chimney sweepers. A British pathologist named Thomas Hodgkin (1798-1866) discovered the "morbid alterations of structure" that are now called Hodgkin's disease. For treatment, he proposed "the utmost protection from the inclemencies of and vicissitudes of the weather, to employ iodine externally, and to push the internal use of caustic potash as far as circumstances might render allowable.'' The German pathologist Rudolf Virchow* identified leukemia in 1845. In 1879, two German pathologists, F. H. Hürting and W. Hess, recognized lung cancer; they diagnosed it in Czech uranium miners. In 1895, the German L. Rehn reported that cancer of the bladder was an occupational hazard in the dye industry.

Until recently, cancer was a comparatively rare malady. It merely caused 1.6 percent of the deaths in Paris during 1830. The statistics are infinitely crueler now. In 1975, cancer accounted for almost 17 percent of all deaths in the United States, and the toll was higher in many European countries.

It is estimated that 54,000,000 people who are alive in the United States today will develop cancer, and 36,000,000 of them will die from it. Through the years, cancer is probably going to invade two out of every three American families. Lung cancer is the worst. The statisticians estimated that 93,000 new cases of lung cancer would be reported in 1976, and that 84,000 people will succumb to it. The mortality rate of lung cancer among American men in the early 1970s was 165 percent greater than it was twenty-five years earlier; among American women, it was 182 percent greater. Cancer of the colon and rectum is second to lung cancer in viciousness, with 99,000 new cases expected in the United States in 1976. Some 49,000 Americans will die of it.

It is an eccentric disease, cancer. More than a hundred individual forms of it are known, and sometimes there seems to be no rhyme or reason to their behavior. No one has a good explanation for why the women of Chile have the biggest general cancer rate in the world, with more cancer of the stomach and the uterus than any other women anywhere, yet the lowest rate of skin cancer, cancer of the colon-rectum, and leukemia. No one can tell you why Danish women have the highest rate of breast cancer, and South African men the greatest incidence of cancer of the prostate.

Why, for that matter, do Jews develop so much more cancer of the colon and rectum than Finns or Japanese? Why is cancer of the stomach comparatively rare in South America but very common in Russia? Or look at cancer of the prostate again. Why is it more common among blacks than whites, more common in married men than single men, but, strangely, less common in married men than in widowed and divorced men? No one can say with authority.

Take sex and cancer. Why, one wonders, do Scandinavian prostitutes

---

*Virchow was active in politics as well as medicine. His crusading in behalf of better health care for the German poor infuriated Prince Otto von Bismarck. The Iron Chancellor wanted to fight a duel with him.

get six times as much cervical cancer as other women? Why does cervical cancer occur more often in women who start having sexual intercourse regularly before they are twenty years old than it does among women who wait till later for their lovemaking? Why is cervical cancer uncommon among nuns, rare among virgins? Why is it seldom seen in Jewish women? Is it because Jewish males are circumcised? No one has the full answer.

To this day, no one knows cancer's cause with certainty. The best thinking is that cancer is caused by a number of different viruses, although no firm proof of this theory has been secured.

Yet terrible as cancer is, we are beginning to make headway against it. More than 1,500,000 Americans are alive and well today who have been cured of cancer. Here I'm employing the stringent American Cancer Society definition of the term "cured": no evidence of the disease for a minimum of five years after diagnosis and treatment. In addition, 700,000 other Americans diagnosed and treated for cancer within the last five years are alive and physically well off today.

Most of these cancer victims were saved by conventional methods of surgery and X-ray. But tens of thousands of them were treated by something new—chemotherapy. It is one of the most substantial developments in the whole of medicine.

According to the National Cancer Institute, the federal agency which spearheads the American war on cancer, normal life expectancy has now been achieved in ten different types of cancer by use of chemotherapy.

The N.C.I. says that forty-five drugs are known that can produce complete or partial remissions in a total of twenty-nine different forms of cancer. Of course, some of these drugs are only effective against relatively rare forms of cancer, and some remissions only endure a matter of months. But it is undeniable that some resounding progress has been made.

In 1948, a diagnosis of acute leukemia was a death sentence to any child. Practically 100 percent of all children who came down with leukemia—a cancer of the blood-forming organs that is characterized by uncontrolled production of abnormal white blood cells—were dead inside of a year. Now things have changed. Many children are alive and well today as much as seventeen years after the onslaught of leukemia. Chemotherapy cured them.

Take little Greg Bealer, who became desperately ill with leukemia when he was merely ten years old. "Mommy, I feel like I'm falling to pieces," he sobbed.

I heard about Greg's case at the City of Hope Hospital in Duarte, California. The physicians there warned his horror-stricken mother that her boy might not last the month. A nurse told her not to weep because Greg would "make such a beautiful angel."

"I don't want a beautiful angel," Mrs. Guyneth Bealer cried out. "I want a live devil."

As a last resort, the City of Hope Hospital specialists tested an experimental drug on Greg. In five weeks, Greg was released from the hospital and was leading the life of a normal ten-year-old kid. When I checked on him in mid-1975, Greg hadn't a tinge of leukemia. He was twenty-three years old, a blond giant, six feet three inches tall, weighed 186 pounds, and was graduating from the University of California in Los Angeles. He had just gotten married.

His case is not unique. Dr. C. Gordon Zubrod, the former director of the Divisison of Cancer Treatment at the N.C.I., assured me that "fifty percent of all children who contract leukemia today should be alive and well five years from now."

He went on, "The advances in cancer chemotherapy point to a day that is certainly coming when many forms of cancer will be as curable as pneumonia by means of drugs used in conjunction with surgery or X-irradiation."

Pioneers in Cancer Chemotherapy

The story of cancer research is one of heroism, struggle, and sacrifice. Enormous obstacles have had to be surmounted. Not the least of them was the stubborn opposition of many medical men to the very idea of investigating cancer. To their way of thinking, cancer was a mysterious phenomenon, a plague visited by God upon mankind, and mankind ought not to delve into it.

In 1911, Dr. Francis Peyton Rous, a thirty-two-year-old Baltimore-born physician whose gold-rimmed glasses made him look like a proverbial country doctor, found that a virus could produce cancer in chickens. He proved it by injecting a "cell-free, bacteria-free filtrate" from a cancerous chicken into a healthy chicken. The healthy bird developed cancer—Rous' sarcoma.

Scarcely anyone paid this discovery any attention. Fifty-five years were to go by before Rous was belatedly to win the Nobel Prize in medicine for it.

"In those days," Dr. Rous recalled, "cancer was the disreputable business of crackpots and get-rich-quickers. I used to quake in the night for fear I had made a mistake."

In 1911, a noted Japanese scientist at the University of Tokyo, Professor K. Yamagiwa, with the help of Professor K. Ichikawa, demonstrated that a chemical could cause cancer. He produced cancer in rabbits by rubbing coal tar on the rabbits' ears every day for six months.

Funds for cancer research still remained microscopic or nonexistent. In 1930, Sir Ernest Kennaway and his team at the Royal Cancer Hospital in London synthesized the first known chemical carcinogen—a substance able to produce cancer. They successfully isolated a chemical in coal tar that set off skin cancer. It was 3,4-benzopyrene, a polycyclic aromatic hydrocarbon. But their work had no further impact. The governments of the world could hardly have been less concerned about finding a cure for cancer.

The most rugged resistance was to cancer chemotherapy. The medical establishment was persuaded that cancer could only be treated by surgery and irradiation. Any notion that drugs might cure cancer was regarded as arrant nonsense.

When one of the earliest and most brilliant pioneers in this arena, Dr. Murray J. Shear, started work at the N.C.I. in Bethesda, Maryland, he was expressly forbidden to spend a single moment of his time on cancer chemotherapy.

"It's a waste of effort," his superiors at the N.C.I. declared.

Once a ranking official at the National Institutes of Health asked Dr. Shear what his long-range plans were. Shear submitted a long-term program for research on cancer chemotherapy.

"It's fine as long as nothing happens in seven years," the official said. "In seven years, I retire."

To his credit, Shear pushed on anyway. In the words of the late, great cancerologist, Dr. Sidney Farber, "Murray Shear ran the first program of laboratory chemotherapy research in this country and ran it superbly despite the complete indifference of his chiefs and most of the medical profession."

Shear's tenacity helped to make cancer chemotherapy respectable. Many of the biggest people in cancer chemotherapy today were guided by him: Klein, Djerassi, and the Italian pharmacologist, Silvio Garattini, to mention just three. Incidentally, Shear also did some of the first explorations in the field of immunotherapy.

Decades before most people had awakened to the dangers of air pollution, Dr. Shear went looking for cancer in the air. Back in 1939, he took ordinary soot deposits from the air in St. Louis; Pittsburgh; Charleston, West Virginia; Cambridge, Massachusetts; and the Holland Tunnel in New York City, filtered them until they were as tiny as particles of smoke,

and injected them into mice. The mice promptly developed fatal sarcomas
—cancers of the connective tissue.

As usual, Shear was ahead of his time. No one in authority could face up
to the fearsome fact that pollutants in the air might give people cancer.

Dr. Shear is still a man well worth knowing. Medium tall, bald, with a
thin face and small white mustache, he looks and talks like Arrowsmith. He
has an extraordinary gift for explaining the most complex, technical
subjects in lighthearted, easy-to-understand language. The descendant of a
family of poor Jewish scholars, he was born in New York in 1899 and took
his Ph.D in chemistry at Columbia. He was offered a job in industry at
$7,200 a year but accepted a hospital research post that paid him only
$1,800.

"Shear, I think you're a goddamned fool," his faculty advisor at
Columbia said, "but if that's what you want, go ahead."

He joined the U.S. Public Health Service in 1931 to do research in
cancer. When he retired in 1969, he wasn't content to relax with his wife
and three sons. He started a new job at the Smithsonian Institution.

"I went into science because I was interested in philosophy," he told
me, rather paradoxically, late one night in 1975 as we sat in the study of his
comfortable house in Bethesda. "As a boy of fourteen, I became interested
in knowing more about human beings and their relationships to the cosmos.
Unfortunately, the great figures in philosophy and religion all differed
quite sharply from one another on such matters. The reasoning through
which they arrived at their opinions was subjectively determined, so there
were no criteria for a boy to accept. Ergo, I reached the conclusion that only
valid scientific observations could provide a sound basis on which to build
a philosophy for myself."

"Were you able to create a philosophy for yourself?" I inquired.

"Not yet, but I'm working on it," he said. "Don't forget, I'm still
young. I'm just seventy-six."

The first proof that drugs could affect human cancers came in 1941. Dr.
Charles B. Huggins, a slim forty-year-old researcher born in Halifax, Nova
Scotia, schooled at Harvard, and working at the University of Chicago,
discovered that the female sex hormone, estrogen, retarded the growth of
cancer of the prostate. Twenty-five years later, he would get the Nobel
Prize for his contributions to hormone therapy in cancer of the prostate and
the breast.

World War II brought the next forward stride—the discovery by Dr.
Alfred Gilman and a group of researchers in New Haven that nitrogen
mustard, a chemical relative of the poison gas that wreaked such havoc on

the Western Front in World War I, helped stop cancer. They tested it on seven patients at New Haven Hospital in 1942. Although the drug proved to be very toxic, it produced genuine improvement in a patient with lymphosarcoma—a solid tumor originating in the lymph glands. They had to keep it a military secret, however. In their reports they even had to employ a code name for the nitrogen mustard—"HN2."

A wartime disaster confirmed their findings. On December 3, 1943, Nazi dive bombers sank an American Liberty ship, the *John E. Harvey*, with a hundred tons of nitrogen mustard gas aboard her, during an air raid on the harbor at Bari, Italy. Many American sailors who lived through the bomb blasts and the burning oil that covered the water died later of mustard gas poisoning. Keen scientists of the U.S. Army's Chemical Warfare Service analyzed samples of the victims' tissues. They found that the mustard gas had affected their bone marrow and lymphatic systems, suggesting that the mustard gas could be of value against cancer of the tissues that form white blood cells.

Shortly after World War II, chemistry won mankind's first success against leukemia, the worst of all child-killers. Dr. Sidney Farber was the hero here. A gentle person, tall and slender, with deepset, thoughtful eyes, he suffered a serious case of cancer himself and two crushing heart attacks before the final one that took his life. On each occasion, he hastened back to his crusade against cancer the moment he could get out of bed.

I chatted with Dr. Farber for hours in his smartly furnished office high up in Boston Children's Hospital, where he headed research for more than twenty years. A bird carved of Italian marble sat on his desk.

"It's a symbol of hope," he whispered. "It's always looking up, up, up, always up."

Farber was born in 1903 in Buffalo, New York. His father was a jeweler of moderate means who worshiped education. He didn't have much of it himself, but he wanted his son to have a lot. The boy decided to be a doctor when he was eleven years old. It was during a bad epidemic of diphtheria and scarlet fever.

He said to me, "I was deeply disturbed by seeing all those little white caskets leaving the houses, with tiny victims of diphtheria and scarlet fever in them. Ever since, working with children and wanting to help them have been natural to me."

At Harvard medical school, Dr. Farber said, "Our professors told us that cancer had always been with us and always would be with us. It was passed over as a problem that would never be solved." In spite of that, he went into cancer research. He became a pathologist and joined the staff of the Boston Children's Hospital. He taught at Harvard medical school, too.

It was Dr. Shear who got him to concentrate on cancer chemotherapy. They were walking together in Lafayette Park, opposite the White House in Washington, one morning near V.J. Day.

"There are plenty of people in the field already," Farber argued.

"The ones you hear about most are not to be trusted," Shear said. "They are promoters and self-servers. We need honest people for research in cancer chemotherapy."

Farber had to agree.

In 1946, a team of scientists at Lederle Laboratories directed by an Indian chemist, Dr. Yellapragada SubbaRow, synthesized folic acid, a member of the vitamin B group that is essential to the growth of a wide variety of organisms ranging from bacteria to man. Dr. SubbaRow was an old friend of Dr. Farber from Harvard medical school, and he brought the folic acid to him. Farber tested it on mice with leukemia. He found that it did the wrong thing. It accelerated the mice's leukemia.

This gave pathologist Farber an idea. If folic acid aggravated acute leukemia, a folic acid antagonist might inhibit it.

Dr. Farber explained his theory to me. "Perhaps the leukemia cell looking for nourishment could be tricked into absorbing the antagonist because it was chemically similar to the vitamin. Once absorbed, the antagonist would provide no nourishment, and the leukemia cell would starve."

He asked the Lederle scientists to develop a folic acid antagonist. They came up with several. Farber successfully tested one, pteroyltiglutamic acid, on mice. Optimistically then, he tried it on a nine-year-old girl very sick with acute leukemia. To his despair, the drug didn't ease the child's disease. It made her condition worse.

Farber hurried back to SubbaRow at his laboratory in Pearl River, New York. "We need something more powerful," he said.

SubbaRow and his staff created a new folic acid antagonist called aminopterin that seemed to be much stronger. After testing it on mice, Farber took the plunge. In November 1947, he gave it to sixteen children who were crucially ill with acute leukemia.

For the first time, a form of drug therapy produced a complete remission in acute leukemia, albeit a temporary one. Ten of the sixteen dying youngsters were restored to a completely normal state of health for a short period.

An improved version of the drug that was less toxic was brought out by Dr. SubbaRow in 1948. He called it methotrexate, and it has since proved to be a major weapon against many forms of cancer. It was the last drug that SubbaRow developed for Farber. SubbaRow died of a heart attack in August 1948. He was scarcely fifty years of age.

Now Dr. Farber went forward and demonstrated that chemotherapy could cure a cancer permanently. The enemy here was Wilm's tumor, a savage cancer of the kidney. Although comparatively rare, Wilm's tumor accounts for 20 percent of all the malignant growths in children. It is usually present as a painless abdominal mass that is discovered by the mother while she is bathing her child. Occasionally, it is accompanied by some pain and blood in the urine. Uncontrolled, it can spread to the child's lungs, liver, brain, and skeleton.

Dr. Farber teamed up with the Nobel Prize winner Dr. Selman A. Waksman, the discoverer of streptomycin, to battle Wilm's tumor. In the spring of 1954, Waksman brought Farber his antibiotic actinomycin D. Tests showed it to be "the most powerful anticancer agent by weight that we'd known till that time," Dr. Farber said. The drug was extremely toxic, though.

Farber devised a neat method of using relatively low dosages of the actinomycin D in conjunction with a small amount of radiation that, to all intents and purposes, eliminated the fatal consequences of Wilm's tumor. The antibiotic and the radiation reinforced each other to wipe out the spreading cancer without perilous side effects. The technique achieved permanent remissions in 89 percent of the cases.

It was rough sledding for Dr. Farber at the Boston Children's Hospital at the start. The clinicians splenetically opposed his research. As a pathologist, he had no right to treat patients with dangerous drugs, they claimed. They said he was "a backroom boy" who should stick to his microscope and frozen sections. Farber held to his guns and finally obtained backing for his experiments. He even got a fine tall building erected at Boston Children's Hospital just for child cancer patients. He named it the Jimmy Fund Building after a little boy who came to him dying of cancer of the lymph nodes. Farber cured him with chemotherapy.

I found the Jimmy Fund Building an enchanting place with a small, delightful merry-go-round in the lobby, charming Walt Disney drawings on the walls, and children riding gaily up and down the corridors on tricycles. You would never think that all the kids there have cancer. It might be very depressing if you didn't recall that some of the world's best researchers are at work there seeking new ways to treat cancer.

As the years moved on, Dr. Farber won the Lasker Award for Clinical Research and many other medical honors. He became the commanding figure in world cancer research. When Congress wanted an expert opinion on cancer, its leaders invariably turned to Sidney Farber, and, more often than not, his views were written into federal law. A tough in-fighter, he was as effective at national politics as he was in medical politics, and it is hard to say which breed is more combative.

Most medical authorities esteem Sidney Farber today as "the father of cancer chemotherapy." And justifiably so. He was the first person to prove that drugs could cure cancer where knives and X-rays alone were of no avail. For more than two decades, he led cancer researchers carefully, cautiously, but unswervingly forward.

Dr. Farber was married to Norma C. Holzman in 1928, and they had four children. Mrs. Farber has had two good careers, one as a concert singer and the other as a widely published poet. Outside of work, Farber said to me, his idea of fun was "music, reading, a rare movie, and no television." He was a very conservative dresser; his colleagues used to call him "Four-button Sid."

Early in the spring of 1973, Sidney Farber died, as he expected he would, of his third heart attack. When I heard the radio bulletin carrying the news of his death, I couldn't help remembering something he had said. "How fortunate to be young at a time when progress in medical science was so rapid."

A Growing Arsenal of Anticancer Drugs

Dr. Djerassi described to me a tense medical meeting he attended at Boston City Hospital one Wednesday evening in 1954 at which the most powerful big-name physician on the staff laid down the law to the young residents and interns.

"All these drugs for cancer chemotherapy," he said, "I want you to throw them out of the window."

Dr. Farber, who was present, couldn't keep quiet. He rose out of his seat and said to the young doctors in his calm, dignified manner; "Maybe you shouldn't throw them out of the window just yet."

By 1960, the "big shot" physician had changed his tune. "These damned drugs, they're the best things that've ever happened to cancer patients," he told a hospital conference.

Chemotherapy has not replaced surgery and X-rays as the prime weapon against cancer. Most conscientious physicians feel that surgery is still the best way to treat cancer in cases where the malignant tumors can be completely excised. Irradiation is considered a highly valuable tool against certain other cancers, particularly inoperable ones. It is vastly useful in destroying some cancer cells that the surgical scalpel may have missed. But chemotherapy can do some things better than either surgery or irradiation. It can get remissions where surgery and irradiation are of no avail—in leukemia, for instance. It can cure some cancer conditions that are too far gone to be helped by surgery or irradiation. And, of course, drugs are widely used to supplement the scalpel and the X-ray.

To be effective, a drug must seek out the wild-acting cancer cells wherever they are located in the body and kill them or stop them from reproducing. To cure, it has to get every last one of them. Slaying 999,999 out of 1,000,000 cancer cells is not enough. One microscopic cancer cell that is left behind can multiply until it is again a big, rampaging cancer.

Two New Yorkers, Drs. Jacob Furth and Julius Kahn, proved this back in 1937. They took a single malignant cell from a leukemic mouse and transplanted it to a healthy mouse. In eighteen and a half days, the healthy mouse was dead of leukemia. For years, no one saw much significance to their experiments. Then in the 1960s, some depressing calculations were made at the Southern Research Institute. They showed that a solitary leukemia cell that reproduced inside a human body every four days could create a condition of acute leukemia in exactly 164 days. That is to say, the patient would have more than a thousand billion leukemia cells at large in his body. The report demonstrated the need for "total kill" of cancer cells, right down to the last cancer cell wherever it might be lurking.

Five principal types of cancer drugs have been developed. They are: 1) alkylating agents, quick-acting, highly reactive compounds that are often called "cell poisons" because they destroy many species of cancer cells; 2) antimetabolites, such as methotrexate, which structurally resemble the nutrients every cell needs in order to grow. They sneak inside the cancer cell through mistaken identity and prevent them from growing; 3) antibiotics, which can kill some cancer cells; 4) hormones, which can prevent certain cancer cells from multiplying; and 5) alkaloids from plants.

Dr. George H. Hitchings, of Burroughs Wellcome Co., the persistent biochemist who developed the drug that helped end the miseries of gout, spent ten years looking for antimetabolites that would interfere with the metabolism of nucleic acids. He was one of the first to theorize that cancer cells might have unusually critical requirements for these nucleic acids.

"I had a hunch that nucleic acids would be highly important to cells," he told me the morning I saw him at the Burroughs Wellcome laboratories in Triangle Research Park, North Carolina. "I was fascinated with them."

He was ten years ahead of the scientific field. No one knew much then about DNA (deoxyribonucleic acid) or RNA (ribonucleic acid), the two varieties of nucleic acids. No one had any notion that they were the two most important substances in life. It was not until 1953 that Francis H.C. Crick and James D. Watson figured out the structure of DNA, a discovery that has become the cornerstone of scientific research into all genetic replication.

DNA has been lovingly called "the mother molecule in the heart of living cells." Crick and Watson described it as a double helix, somewhat like two long, interlaced, spiral stairways. The "cross rungs" of these DNA "stairways" carry the genetic message that fixes our heredity patterns. The RNA has a very different job. It makes our private enzymes and other proteins.

Dr. Hitchings set out to synthesize molecular modifications from "pieces" of the DNA and RNA.

"Had you any idea where you were going?" I asked.

"Well, we had some idea because we felt that most parasitic things, including tumors, had to replicate DNA rapidly in order to survive in the hostile environment of a host. If we could stop the DNA from growing, we figured the cancer cells would be unable to reproduce."

He focused on the fundamental parts of DNA and RNA known as purines and pyrimidines. With a few enzymes as his tools, he jockeyed molecules back and forth, hoping to find something that would prevent nucleic acids from multiplying. In 1948, he picked up a lead that the compound diaminopurine might do the trick. It led him to synthesize a new compound that he called 6-mercaptopurine (6-MP). It seemed to choke off the lifelines of nucleic acids, and he tried it on transplantable tumors in mice with excellent results.

Would it do as much for leukemia in children? Hitchings sent it to Dr. Joseph H. Burchenal, a gutsy investigator at Sloan-Kettering Institute for Cancer Research in New York City, to test. Dr. Burchenal gave the 6-MP to children dying of leukemia. These were children at the end of the road. They were resistant to methotrexate.

The 6-MP produced complete remissions of their leukemia for periods ranging from six months to three years. True, all had relapses and died, but for a time they were absolutely normal. They went back to school. They even played baseball.

It was joy to Hitchings when the results were tallied in 1953. "There is nothing more thrilling than to see kids benefit from something you thought up," he declared.

The 6-MP is constantly used now against acute leukemia in children. For some reason, it is much less effective in adults with leukemia.

A third great antimetabolite came on fast. In 1954, a Philadelphian, Dr. Robert J. Ruttman, was making a laboratory study of uracil, another pyrimidine. He noticed that the uracil was taken up by tumor tissues in greater amounts than by normal tissues. His report caught the imagination of a thoughtful thirty-four-year-old biochemist at the University of Wisconsin, Dr. Charles Heidelberger. He got an idea for synthesizing a special compound that looked and acted like ordinary uracil but had a poisonous fluorine atom hidden inside each of its molecules instead of an innocuous hydrogen atom.

Dr. Heidelberger brought the concept to the Hoffmann-LaRoche pharmaceutical company in New Jersey. Hoffman-LaRoche assigned a fifty-four-year-old chemist, Dr. Robert Duschinsky, to work on it. Duschinsky was a short Viennese with a penchant for crazy skiing, hazardous mountain climbing, and driving a Mercedes roadster on curving roads at breakneck speeds. He succeeded in synthesizing a counterfeit uracil in less than a year, an incredible feat. Hoffmann-LaRoche called it 5-Fluorouracil, 5-FU for short.

The 5-FU quickly showed that it could dupe cancer cells. It is now employed against advanced solid tumors of the colon, rectum, stomach, and breast. It is applied externally to skin cancers.

Another auspicious antimetabolite was discovered in the U.S.S.R. Dr. Salomon Hiller, of the Soviet Institute for Organic Synthesis, reported in 1973 that a drug, Ftorafur, was 65 percent effective against breast cancer, 55-60 percent effective in controlling intestinal cancers. And it was "absolutely nontoxic," he said.

Antimetabolites are not all. A fine variety of other types of anticancer drugs has been developed. Two different drugs were made from the alkaloid portions of the humble periwinkle plant—vincristine and vinblastine. They are being effectively utilized against acute leukemia, choriocarcinoma, Hodgkin's disease, and other cancers. A valuable antileukemia drug was fashioned out of serum taken from the blood of healthy guinea pigs. Dr. John G. Kidd, of Cornell University, discovered in 1953 that the guinea pig serum was effective against leukemia in mice, and a colleague at Cornell, Dr. John D. Broome, put eight arduous years into trying to find out why. He learned that the active element in the serum was the enzyme L-asparaginase, which deprived the leukemia cells of the L-asparagine they needed to survive. In 1963, Dr. Georges Mathé, the most eminent of French cancer researchers, discovered that a new Italian antibiotic, daunomycin, had a strong anticancer punch. A broad assortment of hormones was also found to be helpful against certain forms of cancer.

The search goes on. It is an unbelievably difficult one. In one year, the National Cancer Institute spent $75 million testing 30,800 natural and synthetic chemicals as possible agents against cancer. Just 4 of the 30,800 had enough promise to be accepted for human experimentation.

Chemotherapy Scores the First Total Cure of a Solid Tumor

We tend to forget that it requires a special breed of bravery to do clinical research on disease. A patient may be only days away from death, beyond all hope of rescue by any known remedy, but if you hasten the patient's going even one day by trying a new, unproven treatment, you can be accused of near-murder. Your career can be ruined.

On October 20, 1955, Dr. Min Chiu Li, a thirty-nine-year-old physician at the National Cancer Institute, was conscious of this risk as he looked down at Peggy Longoria, a pretty woman with glorious copper-hued hair, in the Clinical Center of the National Institutes of Health in Bethesda, Maryland. Mrs. Longoria, twenty-four years old and the mother of a two-year-old daughter, was dying of choriocarcinoma—a cancer in the womb. It had metastasized—that is to say, the cancer had spread—and a tumor had perforated her right lung. She was hemorrhaging. No treatment was known that was effective against her disease.

Dr. Li recalled that moment. "I was facing a dying woman. I was forced to consider an unprecedented methodology of treatment. If I didn't do anything, this woman would surely die in a short while. If I did something, this woman might also die, but if she died, I'd get the blame. I'd get my head chopped off. Yet if my imagination was correct, there might be some hope for her to get well. What was I do do?"

He decided to try the new treatment on her. "I was ready to risk my reputation and my career."

Li was up against a rare but grisly kind of cancer. Choriocarcinoma comes in two forms. Gestational choriocarcinoma originates in the placenta during pregnancy and eats its way through the wall of the uterus into the veins. It spreads rapidly to the pelvic structure, to the lungs, the brain, liver, and almost every tissue of the body. Nongestational choriocarcinoma starts in the sexual glands of both sexes and quickly spreads everywhere, too. Both cancers secrete a hormone called chorionic gonadotropin. Each type is equally virulent. Untreated, each kills 90 percent of its victims within a year.

Peggy Longoria had gestational choriocarcinoma. She had been operated on for it twice, including a full hysterectomy. Each time, the choriocarcinoma had recurred, and now it had spread to the lungs.

"If I have to die," she told her husband, Bob, "I want to die at home with my baby and you."

He insisted that she go into the N.I.H. hospital and let the N.C.I. researchers try to save her. It was very late in her game, though. Ten days after she entered the hospital, the tumor gnawed through her lung. Blood was pouring out of her faster than it could be restored by transfusions.

More surgery was out of the question. "She'll die on the operating table," a chest surgeon warned.

Li was counting on the drug methotrexate to save Mrs. Longoria. He had in mind some pioneering research by his chief, Dr. Roy Hertz, which indicated that a folic acid antagonist like methotrexate could affect the condition of female genital organs in animals. Li also remembered a mysterious thing that happened while he was in training in New York at Sloan-Kettering. A woman patient who had a cancer known as a malignant melanoma, for some reason, secreted chorionic gonadotropin hormones. She was given some methotrexate. Although it did not cure her cancer, it stopped the secretion of the chorionic gonadotropin hormones.

It was a long shot. Methotrexate had never been successfully employed against a solid tumor. It could be toxic. But Dr. Hertz and his colleagues in the N.C.I. endocrinology section agreed with Dr. Li that it should be tried.

There wasn't time to administer the methotrexate orally or intramuscularly. It had to get right into Mrs. Longoria's bloodstream if she was to survive the day. But no one knew what amount of the drug to give her intravenously so that it would have an immediate effect. Methotrexate had never before been administered to a patient that way.

The usual dose in leukemia was 2.5 milligrams of methotrexate by mouth. Li chose to give Mrs. Longoria four times as much, intravenously, in a single dose. It was a large dose and very dangerous.

"I couldn't sleep the whole night," he told me.

Peggy Longoria was still alive the next morning. Late that afternoon, Li tested her urine for the presence of chorionic gonadotropin hormones. (Dr. Hertz had devised a sensitive test for gestational choriocarcinoma by measuring the amount of chorionic gonadotropin hormones in the urine.) The level of Peggy Longoria's hormones had dropped noticeably.

Li "went for broke." He increased the dosage of methotrexate to 50 milligrams. Three days later, Mrs. Longoria's hormone count was down to zero. It was nearly unbelievable.

Working under Hertz's supervision, Li continued the methotrexate regimen. In three months, Mrs. Longoria was completely rehabilitated. Not a sign of a tumor remained anywhere. Twenty years later, Peggy Longoria was still in excellent health, with no evidence of the disease.

It was the first time a solid tumor had been totally cured by chemotherapy.

Some choriocarcinoma patients developed a resistance to methotrexate, and Dr. Li later found a fine substitute for it, actinomycin D. Together, the two drugs can cure 90 percent of all victims of gestational choriocarcinoma if they are treated early enough—within four months of the onset of the tumor. Seventy percent of the patients whose disease has metastasized can be cured by drugs. Now, women afflicted with this cancer can have normal pregnancies.

In 1958, Li conceived a technique of treatment for choriocarcinoma of the testicles with combinations of drugs. As yet, it has only a 25 percent cure rate, though. What made it noteworthy is that it was the first demonstration of the value of combination drug therapy—the use of several drugs simultaneously—against cancer that is all the medical vogue today.

Drs. Li and Hertz both received Lasker Awards in 1972 for their achievements against gestational choriocarcinoma.

The two men could hardly have had more different backgrounds. Min Chiu Li was born in Tekhing, a little town near Canton. His parents were missionary-teachers.

"Are you a religious man?" I asked him on the rainy May afternoon I talked with him in his cramped office at Nassau Hospital in Mineola, Long Island.

"I was a very religious man until I came to the United States," he said.

I found him an intense man with almost no sense of humor. Like many other researchers, he complains bitterly that his contributions are not sufficiently honored.

He got his M.D. in Mukden, Manchuria, and came to the United States in 1947 on a church scholarship, in part to get away from the advancing Chinese Communists. He had to leave his young wife and two small children behind. He didn't see them for eight years, until the Communists finally let them out of China to join him.

He became interested in choriocarcinoma because it is ten times as common in China as it is in the Western world. He left the N.C.I. for Sloan-Kettering in 1958, and was promptly farmed out to Kings County Hospital, a mammoth municipal institution in Brooklyn, to set up a cancer research program. He was miserably frustrated there.

"It was impossible to do disciplined clinical research," he said. "People held on to their patients as their own property. It's the American tradition. The physician here feels he owns the patient."

In 1963 Li moved to Nassau Hospital, a medium-sized community hospital, where he became director of medical research and head of the cancer service. He has been working overtime recently on a test for diagnosing cancer of the ovary.

Dr. Li and his wife, Rebecca, live with their three children in a modern ranch house with wide grounds in Old Westbury, Long Island. There, whenever he has the time, he enjoys gardening. He is delighted that Mrs. Li is "an ordinary housewife" who is very supportive when he gets home in the evening.

"It's very important for a scientist to have peace of mind after a day in the laboratory," he said.

He likes to travel, but he'll spend no more than two or three days in any city. "It makes me nervous to stay in one place too long."

Dr. Hertz was born in Cleveland in 1919, fifth of seven sons of a Polish-Jewish immigrant. He got a Ph.D. in physiology at the University of Wisconsin. Jobs were Depression-scarce, so he took an M.D., too. He supported himself financially "by scratching around and by marrying a young lady who managed to stay employed." He started his hormone research at the N.C.I. in 1946. In addition to his work on choriocarcinoma at the N.C.I., he helped to develop drugs that are getting one-year remissions for 30 percent of patients with cancer of the adrenal glands. In 1969, he left the N.C.I. to do research on population control at Rockefeller University. He moved in 1972 to head the endocrinology department at New York College of Medicine in Valhalla, New York, and was talking of a new move and a new career when I saw him in the summer of 1973.

Hertz loves caring for patients. Frequently, he quotes from Maimonides's Oath of a Physician: "I shall never see before me in a patient other than a mirror of myself."

I spoke with him in his pleasant laboratory at Valhalla, a short, slim, white-haired man with rimless glasses in the usual white lab coat. I found him as intense a person as Dr. Li. He doesn't chat; he lectures.

Hertz was widowed in 1962 and remarried to the widow of a former classmate. He resides in South Salem, New York, "where my hobby is watching my wife, Toby, garden." And doing a lot of gardening himself.

The motivation for Li's research stemmed from his missionary rearing. "I was brought up with the concept that we live for other people's benefit," he declared. Hertz has different views: "I would say that the primary motivation of most medical scientists is the desire for acknowledgement of their accomplishments by their peers."

Both men fell upon their discoveries accidentally. Hertz was surprised to see that the female sex hormones of chicks in his laboratory needed folic acid to be metabolized. Similarly, Li was amazed to find his woman cancer patient excreting chorionic gonadotropin hormones in her urine. Both men knew what to do about it, and did it.

The sad facet to the choriocarcinoma work is a twenty-year feud between Drs. Li and Hertz over who merits the credit. When I spoke with him, Li was not disposed to share a shred of the credit. "It was my idea," he said. "I designed the model and Dr. Hertz utilized my model to expand it. Dr. Hertz made his main contribution by having confidence in me and supporting my work."

Hertz maintains that Dr. Li was merely one member of a large scientific team which he headed. "I am not particularly interested in any kind of controversy regarding anyone's participation in various phases of the work," he said coolly. "I will simply stand on the record."

I checked the record. It shows that virtually every important paper published on this program was signed by both men.

Actually, there is enough honor for each of them. Chemotherapy won its first full-sized victory over cancer here.

Klein Finds a Cure for Skin Cancer

Every year, three hundred thousand new cases of malignant skin cancer occur in the United States, mainly among thoughtless sun-worshipers who overdo their exposure to the sun. Most of these cancers are easily handled by surgery, but some of them get out of hand through patient neglect or a doctor's misdiagnosis. Horrible lesions cover large portions of the face and body. Portions of the nose and other features are eaten away, leaving revolting holes in the face. Surgery is ineffective then.

As Dr. Edmund Klein put it, "You'd practically have to skin the patients alive to rid them of their cancers."

As a result, four thousand people a year have been dying of skin cancer in America alone.

Dr. Klein has found a way to end this ceaseless toll. He is curing skin cancers with a simple salve.

The first time I saw Dr. Klein was on that winter evening in New York City as he lectured on his skin cancer work to a group of distinguished researchers at Sloan-Kettering. He showed a long series of before-and-after pictures of men and women with mutilated, cancerous faces and bodies who had been completely cured. The Sloan-Kettering men were very impressed. Afterward, I talked with him for hours in an empty conference room at Sloan-Kettering. He proved to be a delightfully informal, effusive chap, full of good humor, warmth, and wisecracks in English and Yiddish.

He was born in Vienna in 1921, the son of a very poor rabbi. "How did you happen to get interested in being a doctor?" I inquired.

"I didn't want to be a rabbi."

"To escape theology, you went into medicine?"

"Well, not necessarily. I don't think you can practice medicine without practicing theology."

All of his family, save his sister and him, were exterminated by the Nazis. He escaped to Canada, supported himself at medical school as a laboratory assistant, and trained under Dr. Farber at Children's Hospital in Boston. He preferred research to private practice.

"Didn't you want to be rich?"

"Sure, I wanted to be rich, but I thought there were other things that were more important."

"Such as?"

"Such as doing things for people."

In 1961, he joined the dermatology department of Roswell Park Memorial Institute in Buffalo, New York, one of the country's leading cancer research hospitals. He wanted to investigate skin cancer.

The only way chemotherapy was then used in skin cancer was internally. If surgery and radiation didn't help, the patient was given drugs orally or by injection. Once in a while, the drugs helped a little.

Dr. Klein had a better idea. "We had a patient in Buffalo who was getting 5-FU by vein. A number of his lesions seemed to respond reasonably well, but one lesion on the tip of his finger continued to grow. It occurred to me that if I took 5-FU in a much higher concentration than one could dare take internally and put it directly on the lesion, it might give us effects that we could not see otherwise."

He put the 5-FU in a cream base, made a paste of it, and applied it to the patient's finger.

"I expected it to act the same as sulphuric acid. I thought it would make a hole in the finger. It didn't. It destroyed the tumor, but it didn't hurt the finger a bit. I didn't believe it. Nor did anybody else. The tumor just melted away. It was incredible."

That was late in 1961.

Klein repeated the experiment with another patient, and it turned out as well. No one would believe him when he first published on it in April 1962.

"Everybody was terribly skeptical. All my requests for research grants were turned down. The N.C.I. said it couldn't possibly be done, and I had to agree with them. I wouldn't believe it either if I sat on the committee and somebody said, 'You smear on a cream and the tumor goes away.' I'd also say that the guy's crazy."

Happily for Klein, his work was easy to confirm. Within eighteen months, two medical papers appeared reporting similar results. At last count, Klein had cured 1,000 patients with 210,000 precancerous and cancerous lesions on their skin. He is getting complete, permanent remissions in 95 percent of all cases of widespread skin cancer. The technique is employed all over the world.

I had lunch at an elegant New York restaurant with Dr. Klein and a patient whom he cured of a hideous case of skin cancer. He was Alfred Rosenthal, a wealthy, retired New Jersey textile manufacturer, short, stocky, and brimming with energy. He looked and acted ten years younger than his seventy-six.

Rosenthal liked sunbathing too much. In 1965, he developed a lesion on his face that wouldn't heal. A physician misdiagnosed it as eczema. By the time a biopsy identified it, the cancer was on a rampage. In the course of the next four years, Rosenthal was operated on more than two hundred times. Tumors were cut out, recurred, and spread. He had to have two big skin grafts to cover holes in his face.

In 1969, Rosenthal read a magazine article about Dr. Klein and flew up to Buffalo. Klein started treating him with 5-FU. Inside of a few weeks, he had the skin cancer under control. Since then, Rosenthal has only undergone two minor surgical procedures on isolated lesions.

"Dr. Klein gave me back my face," Rosenthal said to me. "I idolize him."

In 1972, Dr. Klein received a Lasker Award for his discovery of a cure for skin cancer.

Klein, who is vice-chairman of the dermatology department at Rosewell Park, works around the clock. He gets to the hospital at 7:00 A.M. and usually stays until 1:00 in the morning, seven days a week. His only hobby is solving differential equations. His pretty wife, Martha, used to be an X-ray technician. They have two boys and three girls, and every one of them wishes to be a doctor.

For twenty-one years, Dr. Klein has had a Damon-and-Pythias relationship with Dr. Djerassi. They talk three or four times a day by long-distance phone between Buffalo and Philadelphia. The friendship has led to some very promising discoveries on the latest frontier in cancer research—immunology. But that story comes later in this book.

Dr. Klein takes much better care of his patients than he does of himself. Despite all the scientific reports on the dangers of cigarette smoking, he puffs on a cigarette incessantly.

"Why do you smoke so much?" I asked him.

"Because I'm a shmuck," he confessed, using a dirty Yiddish word for "fool."

"May I quote you as saying that?"

"You can say that I said I'm a shmuck," he pleaded, "but please don't say that I smoke."

Truth will out.

Isaac Djerassi Subdues Childhood Leukemia

Isaac Djerassi has no use for clinicians who temporize with cancer. He doses his leukemia patients with drugs at two hundred times their normal strength. Yet instead of dying in toxic turmoil, most of these leukemia victims are being cured. He doses other cancer patients with drugs at a thousand times their normal potency, and most of them are being helped.

Dr. Djerassi is more than a daring medical genius. He is a physician with a heart. To many research clinicians, patients are merely statistics. Not to Dr. Djerassi. He spends endless hours with all the cancer patients who come into his hospital, comforting them, helping them to understand and cope emotionally with their disease. They worship him. As Stewart Alsop, the writer, said, Djerassi's patients have a "religious faith in his curative powers."

"You know something," Dr. Djerassi said to me. "I cry when a patient dies."

Before Djerassi decided to move to Mercy Catholic Medical Center on the outskirts of Philadelphia in 1969, he told the heads of the hospital, "I'll only come if you promise me one thing—that you'll take all my patients whether they have money or not, whether they have insurance or not. You'll only collect what the Blue Cross pays. When the Blue Cross is finished, you'll continue giving the same care regardless of whether the patient can pay or not."

The hospital consented. Djerassi's patients stay in the hospital as long as they need to and they never have to pay the bills out of their own pockets. Djerassi himself doesn't charge any patient a penny for his services beyond the insurance benefits.

He is a nonstop talker, and a candid one. I listened to a monologue by him for seven hours in his messy office and enjoyed every minute. A microscope sat on his desk amid disorderly piles of medical reports, correspondence, and newspaper clippings. He was wearing a blue blazer, grey slacks, and a gay red tie. No lab coat. He smoked Kent cigarettes incessantly. Outside the open door, I could see a blonde woman lying on a stretcher, giving blood and getting it back. Her blood was feeding into an exotic machine invented by Djerassi for the purpose of filtering out white cells from the blood of a normal donor for transfer to a leukemic patient—in this case, the woman's sister. The machine could collect up to one hundred billion white cells in five hours.

Djerassi was born in Sofia, the capital of Bulgaria, in 1925, the son of a wealthy Jewish merchant. He was always first in his class, he said. His English is good although accented.

"One thing I was absolutely sure of. I wanted to make big discoveries that would be very helpful to people, and become very famous."

"Why?"

"That's how I felt as a child. You wanted to know and I'm telling you."

The Nazis acted to ship all Bulgarian Jews to extermination camps in Poland in 1943. Djerassi and his family were sent to a small provincial town in preparation for the move to the gas ovens. Their lives were saved when large numbers of the Bulgarian people protested openly, angrily, against the deportations. The Nazis backed down. After the war, Djerassi entered medical school. In 1948, a month from graduation, he dropped out to fight against the Arabs in Israel's War of Independence. The war ended before he could get there, and he had to spend two more years in an Israeli medical school before he could get his M.D.

Hematology and pediatrics were his first interests, then cancer. In 1954, he went to Boston to learn American research methods from Dr. Farber at Children's Hospital. He was paid $1,000 a year by Farber plus room and board.

"Some board," he winced. "I lost twelve pounds in the first three months."

He already had an ingrained disrespect for medical dogmas, medical bureaucrats, and the medical establishment in general.

His immediate boss was Dr. Klein. Their long friendship and scientific collaboration began with an investigation into platelets, one of the three main components of blood. The red blood cells give us life and energy; white cells combat infections; and platelets supply the clotting power that keeps us from bleeding to death. Klein and Djerassi had a theory that dry platelets could be transfused into leukemic patients to halt the hemorrhages that so often kill them.

They worked like Trojans. Djerassi's chic Bulgarian wife, Tika, whom he met and married in Israel, used to sit in the laboratory with them until three in the morning, shaking test tubes. It was the only way she got to see her husband.

There was no such thing as it could not be done. Djerassi recalls, "We need more blood? Okay, we go to the fire station around the corner, we drag out a couple of firemen, we take them to a close-by bar, we buy them beers, we bring them in, we bleed them. Anything works as far as we are concerned."

The results of the experiments with platelets looked splendid—for a while. But when they announced them in 1956, it developed that they had made some serious mistakes.

"We went too quick, too fast, and we did harm," Djerassi said.

They were berated on all sides. "Ed Klein and I became very undesirable people in hematology," Djerassi declared.

Disheartened, Klein switched to dermatology. Djerassi stuck to his work with platelets. He began all over again, using fresh platelets now. By the early 1960s, he had proven his point. Platelets were halting hemorrhages in leukemic children. By the mid-1960s, platelet transfusions were an acknowledged modality of treatment in cancer and other diseases. Djerassi received a Lasker Award for this in 1972. Thousands of patients have now had this kind of blood transfusion.

Djerassi moved to the Children's Hospital in Philadelphia in 1960. He vowed that he would never work on leukemia again. His reasons are revelatory.

"At that time, our leukemia patients were just living a year, or a year and a half. They were dying a very uncomfortable death. It was a very discouraging thing. You go through that often and you break down.

"My platelets? The main reason I was transfusing platelets was for the comfort of the patient so he wouldn't have his nose bleeding and blood spilling all over his face. It didn't make any difference to his survival really, because there was no way of treating the leukemia itself then."

His new chief in Philadelphia insisted that Djerassi treat leukemia patients, however. Luckily so. It started him searching for a leukemia cure.

He focused on the drug methotrexate because it seemed to have such biochemical vigor and versatility. He took ten leukemia patients who had developed resistance to methotrexate and had suffered bad relapses. Despite the risks of fatal toxicity, he put each of the patients on a methotrexate regimen again, but he gave it to them in vastly bigger amounts—twenty to thirty times the normal daily dosage—and he administered it in a different fashion, by dripping it continuously into the patient's bloodstream.

The rationale he gave me was vivid. "After you've killed off a couple of generations of leukemia cells with methotrexate, the surviving leukemia cells are tough. They have a thicker membrane, let's call it, around them, so the methotrexate does not get inside them anymore. I figure if I give a higher concentration of the methotrexate and keep the methotrexate there for a long while by continuously dripping it, there is more of a chance that I will get the methotrexate inside those leukemia cells. Basically, it's like making a pickle. You take a cucumber or something and you dip it in salt water. The salt is not going to go right into the cucumber. You have to leave it sit there in order to saturate it. That's what I wanted to do—to pickle the leukemia cells in methotrexate.''

His pickling procedure proved out. All ten of his leukemia patients had remissions. Djerassi wasn't satisfied, though. The risk of toxicity in taking such large doses of methotrexate on a daily basis was too great.

As usual, he went the unorthodox route. He didn't reduce the dosage. He gave even bigger doses of methotrexate, but less frequently.

"I decided you've got to give the methotrexate on a hit-and-run basis. You've got to give an awful lot of it—a hundred to two hundred times the normal dose—but only for one day or at the most two days. After that, you don't give the patient any for three to four weeks. Then you can give him the same big dose again. That way, you get an effect that is many times more than if you'd given the same amount in divided doses through the whole period.''

The N.C.I., highly impressed, gave this system the apt name of "pulse therapy.''

To protect his patients against the unholy side effects implicit in such huge doses, Dr. Djerassi developed a special "rescue" technique—for rescue of the patient from toxicity. He followed up each methotrexate treatment with another drug, Citrovorum Factor, which contained a direct antidote to the side effects of methotrexate. He also gave heavy transfusions of platelets.

Djerassi tried his system first on twenty-five near-death leukemic children in 1964. He was able to report in 1967 that 80 percent of them were alive after thirty months.

"Thirty months for eighty percent of the patients was an awful lot," he bragged to me. "This was at a time when everybody was losing them after a year. Maybe they had ten percent surviving for two years.''

In the spring of 1973, Djerassi was able to boast some more. Seventy percent of the leukemic children had passed the crucial five-year survival line!

Since he switched to Mercy Catholic Medical Center in 1969, Dr. Djerassi has been applying his "pulse" system to several other forms of advanced cancer. He has attacked terminal lung cancer with doses of methotrexate a thousand times bigger than the usual. All of ten patients so treated were living after a year. Under ordinary circumstances nine of the ten should have been dead. According to the authoritative magazine *Medical World News*, he has made "sensational progress" with both childhood lymphosarcoma and reticulum cell sarcoma, two gruesome cancers that had been unresponsive to conventional methotrexate treatment. More than half of his patients here were fully cured and off treatment after six years. He has obtained optimistic results with cancer of the pancreas and breast cancer, too.

The Djerassi regimen has even been effective against osteogenic sarcoma, a hopeless cancer that starts in the bones. Early in 1971, Dr. Djerassi flew up to Boston, where he is a consultant to the Children's Hospital. A physician on the staff grabbed him.

"Isaac, you won't believe it."

"What?"

"Dr. Farber told us to give your methotrexate to a patient with osteogenic sarcoma."

Djerassi, who says he tends to be a bit paranoic, broke in furiously. "Is that where I told you to use it? I told you to use it in lymphosarcoma. So now don't tell me that it doesn't work in osteogenic sarcoma. Nothing works in osteogenic sarcoma."

"Isaac, don't get so excited," the doctor soothed him. "It worked. It's incredible. This patient had his chest full of masses of tumors, all over the place. They're all gone."

It was a gag, Djerassi thought, until he looked at the X-rays. It was true. The tumors were entirely gone. The patient was still alive a year later with no evidence of tumor.

The Djerassi method got an official seal of medical approval when Senator Edward M. Kennedy's twelve-year-old son, Edward Jr., had his leg amputated for bone cancer in 1973. After the operation, the boy was put on the Djerassi methotrexate regimen to prevent a recurrence of the disease. At the close of 1975, the lad was doing fine.

Djerassi is a seven-day-a-week worker, from nine in the morning till seven in the evening at the hospital. He returns home to a gracious brownstone in Philadelphia, has dinner, spends some time with his nineteen-year-old son and fourteen-year-old daughter, and goes back to work at ten until one or two in the morning.

His son, Rami, does not wish to be a doctor. He told his father, "If I become a doctor, I would always have to compete with you."

What does Djerassi do for fun? "I used to be a champion dancer in Bulgaria, a real jitterbug. Now the only thing I take time out for is old friends."

One medical matter maddens Dr. Djerassi. "The leaders in the cancer field don't want to try out new methods," he charges.

"Why?"

"Because they're jealous. This is called medical politics. That's what it's called. The price is paid by the guy who chokes in his bed and is not given the opportunity to be treated."

It brought to mind something Dr. Min Chiu Li had said. "A sound investigator must also be a politician."

Djerassi is no slouch at politicking (as witness his long list of research grants), but American medical politicians can play very rough.

Among other medical men who have made gains against cancer, Dr. Donald Pinkel of St. Jude's Children's Hospital in Memphis, Tennessee, has obtained a 50 percent cure of acute children's leukemia by combining multiple drug treatment with radiation. Dr. Emil Frei III, who now heads the Sidney Farber Cancer Center in Boston, has gotten excellent results with combination therapy against Hodgkin's disease and leukemia. Early in 1976, Dr. Gianni Bonadonna of the Instituto Nazionale Tumori in Milan, Italy, electrified the medical world with a report that a new form of combination chemotherapy he had developed was having near-miraculous effects on women with breast cancer. As a rule, 55 percent of women with breast cancer who have serious lymph node involvement die within five years of surgery. But not Dr. Bonadonna's patients. He started a large group of breast cancer patients with extensive lymph node involvement on three drugs—cyclophosphamide, methotrexate and 5-FU—immediately after surgery. More than two years later, 95 percent of them were alive and thriving, cancer-clean!

N.C.I. officials were enthusiastic. "This is the kind of stuff dreams are made of," Dr. Frank J. Rauscher, the N.C.I. director, told me.

Although he has made no major discovery himself, Dr. Joe Burchenal, now director of clinical investigation at New York's Memorial Hospital, has stimulated leukemia research on many continents. A businesslike man, of medium height and bald, born in 1912, Burchenal aided in the research in East Africa that led to the cure for Burkitt's lymphoma. He was called in to treat Senator Robert A. Taft for cancer in 1953. It was much too late. Taft's cancer was everywhere. And Taft realized that it was.

"Bob Taft was the bravest man I ever saw," Dr. Burchenal told me. "He knew the jig was up but he didn't flinch."

Two decades later, "Mr. Republican" might have been saved by the advances made in cancer therapy.

But don't be misled. When you think of the remarkable gains that have been recorded, remember that chemotherapy still is more promise than performance in most forms of cancer. Remember that a long, sad lag invariably occurs between the discovery of a new cure for a disease and its use with patients.

This is especially so in cancer. Dr. Seymour Perry, special assistant to the director of the NIH, remarked to me one day: "I go to medical meetings in big community hospitals and I'm appalled to see how slowly information obtained in clinical research reaches physicians around the country. For example, when I talk about the great progress that has been made in Hodgkin's disease, I find that many doctors have never heard of it. Some doctors let a year go by without treating a patient for Hodgkin's. Well, a tumor doesn't stand still."

Advances in Cancer Surgery

Surgery and radiation are the preferred modes of treatment in most forms of cancer. The big advances in these two fields were made long ago. However, some interesting things have been done by interesting people in recent times.

Dr. Charles Kennedy of Grace Hospital in Detroit did the first hemicorporectomy. He cut a cancer victim in half to rid him of his rectal cancer in February 1960.

The seventy-four-year-old man had undergone surgery in vain for his cancer. He was in agony, and nothing more could be done for him with conventional surgery. In a last effort to ease his torture, Dr. Kennedy cut through the old man's spine between the third and fourth lumbar vertebrae. He did both a colostomy and an ileostomy to handle all his excretions. The operation lasted thirteen hours. When it was over the upper half of the old man was alive and cancer-clear. The pain-encrusted lower half was thrown away.

The old man lived eleven days before his heart collapsed. It proved that the operation was practical, and twenty months later the same procedure was performed at the University of Minnesota medical school on a twenty-nine-year-old patient with cancer. This man lived for years. Since then, the operation has been successfully performed many times. One man who had the operation at Memorial Hospital in New York can drive a car and earn his own living.

A surgical team at Memorial headed by Drs. Joseph Fortner and Edward J. Beattie, Jr., has devised an imaginative way to repair cancerous livers. They completely cut off blood from the liver and keep it alive by perfusing it with an ice-chilled solution of lactate and heparin. They can cut out tumorous lesions without blood blocking their view. They can even operate on blood vessels inside the liver. Some of their livers have gone 147 minutes without blood. It's real bench surgery.

The most original development has been the cryosurgery created, as we have seen, by Dr. Irving S. Cooper. This novel technique is used to destroy cells with supercold liquids. After employing it first to freeze portions of the brain in Parkinson's disease, Cooper tried his cryoprobes on some advanced rectal cancers in the mid-sixties. They worked. The frozen cancer cells died off and the tumors disappeared or dwindled. Cryosurgery is also used in recurrent cancers of the rectum. Miserable people who cannot eat sitting down, ride in automobiles, or lie on their backs because of their pain are enabled to live normally for a time.

Today, cryosurgery is routine in many other cancer situations. It is curatively used for some skin cancers, and palliatively for many internal cancers where surgery and radiation are impossible. It is ultravaluable for eliminating pain and stopping bleeding.

Surgeons at Memorial Hospital told me of a man in his forties with a melanoma of the neck—a cancer stemming from a black mole—that had spread. His pain was uncontrollable. He had even become a morphine addict, but it didn't help. "We froze the melanoma," the surgeons said, "and black ink came running out of it as if we'd exploded the cells. You'd have supposed an octopus had secreted it. We froze right up into the nerve channels from which his agony had proceeded."

The man was pain-free after the operation. He went off morphine, returned to Detroit, became a breadwinner once more. He died six months later, but he never had pain again.

A variation of the freezing technique was announced by Dr. Arthur W. Weaver, of Wayne State University, Detroit, in 1973. He has found a way to remove cancerous bones and superfreeze them in liquid nitrogen to destroy the cancer. Then he grafts them back into the patients. They look as good as new.

Kaplan Beats Hodgkin's Disease with Massive X-Rays

The finest advance with radiation has been in Hodgkin's disease. Ten years or so ago, most doctors thought this disease virtually untreatable and fatal. Today, 80 percent of its victims can be saved in the early stages of the disease by the audacious radiology of Dr. Henry Kaplan of Stanford University Hospital in California. Even many patients in the later stages can hope for cures.

Hodgkin's disease strikes eight thousand people in the United States a year, ordinarily between the ages of twenty-one and thirty-five, and kills five thousand of them. It is a cancer of the blood-forming tissues, the lymphoid system, and is too spread-out for surgery. "You'd be nitpicking," says Dr. Kaplan. "You'd be berry-picking, plucking something here and plucking something there." For a long time it was thought to be too widespread for X-rays, too. Then in the 1920s, a Swiss radiotherapist, Dr. René Gilbert, tried high doses of X-rays on the affected areas, and smaller doses on nearby areas to which the disease was likely to spread. The results were excellent, but Gilbert was a voice in the wilderness. Hardly anybody listened to him. Two Canadian radiotherapists, Dr. Gordon Richards and his disciple, Dr. M. Vera Peters, carried the Gilbert work forward. Their results were impressive, but they had only old-fashioned X-ray machines at their disposal. Kaplan showed what could be done against Hodgkin's with massive X-ray power.

I saw him in his tasteful little office at Stanford University Hospital. He was on time to the second for our 4:30 P.M. appointment. He talked very carefully, pedagogically, as we discussed causes, including his reasons for being interested in the disease.

"Cancer is not only a phenomenon with a tremendous impact on people, with implications of tragedy for families," he said. "On a strictly intellectual level, it is also one of the most fascinating problems in human biology. Although cancers differ enormously among themselves, they are fundamentally disturbances of the basic growth controls of the cells of the body. We come very close to the most essential concepts in biology when we seek to understand these fundamental growth-control mechanisms."

He was born in Chicago in 1918. Like so many other great medical researchers, the death of a relative turned him to medicine. In Kaplan's case, it was his dentist-father, dead of lung cancer at the age of forty-five.

"I felt a very personal challenge because of my father—the feeling that cancer struck him down while he was a very young man."

After he graduated from Chicago's Rush Medical College, Kaplan taught radiology at Yale and did some significant research on the role of viruses in causing cancer. When he moved to Stanford as chairman of the radiology department in 1948, he heard that some of its physicists were developing "a new kind of gadget called a linear accelerator" which would put out a colossal 5,000,000 volts of energy. Kaplan saw that it could open up new aggressive techniques of radiotherapy, the sort that Vera Peters had been crusading for. He went to the physicists and persuaded them to adapt their gadget to medical purposes. The first, the LA-I, was completed in 1956. It was a mammoth apparatus with a six-foot vacuum tube that could accelerate electrons almost to the speed of light and hurl them against a target of gold or tungsten to make deep, penetrating X-rays. It could deliver a fantastic 100 rads a minute. That was four times as many as any conventional X-ray machine.

Kaplan recalls the first patient he treated with the new accelerator, a seven-month-old baby with retinal blastoma—cancer of the eyes. The first eye had already been taken out, and now the second was in jeopardy. "It never dawned on us that this very rare cancer would be the first to come in for treatment. We had to improvise. I had to go down to the garage and borrow a heavy-duty jack to position a big block of lead just opposite the baby's eye. We drilled a hole in the block of lead so that the right aperture could be created for the X-rays to go into the back part of his eye without hitting the lens farther forward. Well, that baby is now sixteen years old, has approximately 20-20 vision, and is the leader of his class in high school."

He had good success with the LA-I against testicular cancer, ovarian cancer, and cancer of the prostate. After that, he attacked Hodgkin's.

"The prevailing thought at that time," Dr. Kaplan declared, "was that Hodgkin's was incurable. You were supposed to treat it palliatively because you couldn't cure it anyway. People were using low doses against it with the thought that they'd have to treat the patient again anyway, so they might as well preserve his tissues as long as possible."

Kaplan felt that the disease could be cured in the early stages, when the tumors were localized, if the X-rays were used aggressively enough. You had to eradicate every last tumor cell.

In 1956, a forty-one-year-old woman was admitted to Stanford Hospital with Stage II Hodgkin's. (The disease is divided into four main categories, from Stage I, when it is restricted to one area, to Stage IV, when it has spread into the bones, bone marrow, or lungs.) The woman had tumors in her neck and in the region behind her breastbone. Kaplan put 3,000 rads—an unprecedented amount—into the two tumorous areas and the adjacent lymph nodes. The tumors vanished. Twenty years later, the woman was totally free of cancer.

Even at 3,000 rads, though, the disease recurred in 10 percent of the patients. Warily, gradually, Kaplan raised the dosage higher. He found that the problem of recurrence in the treated area was inversely related to dose. The higher the dose, the less the chance of recurrence. At 4,000 rads, the recurrence rate fell to 1 to 2 percent.

"This was almost as good as a written guarantee that there would be no recurrence," Dr. Kaplan said.

Cassandras had wailed that the immense dosage of radiation would desperately sicken the patients. It didn't.

The radiotherapists' work was aided with the development of a sterling new diagnostic tool, the lymphangiogram. In 1962, a British surgeon, John B. Kinmonth, and a Norwegian physician, Dr. Arne Kaare Engerset, devised the technique. It permitted X-ray pictures of the lymph nodes, even those deep in the abdomen and pelvic regions, where doctors couldn't feel tumors with their fingers.

Next, Kaplan went at Stage III Hodgkin's, which involves lymph nodes all over the body. Radiotherapists were merely giving palliative doses of 1,500 rads for it. The most they hoped was to ease its pain and stop the fiendish itching. Now and then, if they were lucky, they were able to reduce the tumors a little.

Kaplan resolved to smite every lymph node with high-dosage radiation. According to him, "At the time, this was essentially an unthinkable concept." He was warned that all that radiation might destroy the bone marrow, that it might produce terminal anemia, that it might kill vast numbers of white cells and leave the body prey to deadly infection.

He had to try. Patients with Stage III Hodgkin's hadn't a chance otherwise. Together with Dr. Saul Rosenberg, he ran the first randomized trials ever conducted in Hodgkin's disease. He separated Stage III patients into two groups. One group received the customary 1,500-rad dosage. The remainder was given 4,000 rads to every lymph node in the trunk and neck over a four-week period.

To Kaplan's joy, "This very radical treatment proved remarkably well tolerated. We didn't kill patients. They weren't nearly as sick as we thought they might be. Blood counts didn't go down as far as we feared. We didn't have the episodes of infection, sepsis, and bleeding that one would have feared."

The trials opened a new chapter in the treatment of late-stage Hodgkin's. Kaplan not only got remissions, but cures. He told me, "Some of those patients we treated ten and more years ago are still alive and have never had a relapse."

He was not yet satisfied. In 1968, he and Dr. Rosenberg added chemotherapy to their arsenal. They took fifty of their sickest patients— men and women in Stage III B—treated them first with a 4,000-rad dosage, then gave them a combination of drugs known as MOPP (for nitrogen mustard, vincristine, procarbazine, and prednisone). Four years later, forty-four of the fifty hadn't a sign of Hodgkin's.

Dr. Kaplan expects still better results when a new 30,000,000-volt linear accelerator goes into operation at Stanford.

He is a typically hard medical worker. He is at the hospital from 8:00 A.M. until 7:00 P.M., six days a week, and works at home four or five nights until 1:00 A.M. He and his wife, Leah, who is a psychiatric social worker, dote on classical music indoors and skiing outdoors. They have two children.

He believes devoutly in the importance of chance in research. "I don't think there is a scientist alive who's honest with himself and others who would deny that chance has played a part in his work," he said to me. "When that fortuitous thing does happen, you have to realize that you've stumbled on it. You must never discourage it."

The first victories over cancer had been gained. The war was far from being won, but a small group of spunky scientists had shown that the disease that most frightens mankind could be beaten.

Now the war grew more intense.

5

THE COMING DEATH OF CANCER

DR. ISAAC DJERASSI IS NOT the kind of physician who stifles his feelings. He wore a mile-wide grin as we walked down a corridor at the Mercy Catholic Medical Center on the outskirts of Philadelphia. We had just come from the bedside of a patient with a brain tumor who was doing very well on the Djerassi brand of chemotherapy.

"That guy is going to pull through. I bet he does," Dr. Djerassi gloated.

He went on happily. "The day is coming, I'm sure of it, when most of cancer will be just a bad memory."

"What makes you so sure?"

"Because we're hitting cancer from all sides now. We're finding new cures, we're developing tests for detecting it really early, and we're finally discovering some of its likely causes. Damn it all, we're going to lick cancer. I'm positive of it."

Chemotherapy Defeats Burkitt's Lymphoma

The British surgeon Denis P. Burkitt is responsible for three victories in man's war on cancer. First, he discovered a deadly form of cancer in African children that no one had reported before. It is named after him, Burkitt's lymphoma. Second, he found it could be cured quickly and permanently. On top of that, his work led to the detection of the first human virus that seems almost certainly to cause cancer.

"He is unique," Dr. George Klein, the eminent Swedish cancerologist, said of Burkitt. "He has climbed Kilimanjaro. He does it every day. His whole life consists of climbing Kilimanjaros."

Mr. Burkitt is one of the most attractive scientists I've met. He is a genuinely humble man.

"I was never an unusually clever chap. I was bad at everything at school," he told me. "Anything that I've been able to do has been because of opportunities that have come my way. It's not that I'm a chap with any undue aptitudes. I just say that by the grace of God I have done what I have."

He is a tall man with a very military carriage, born in 1911, spare, his white hair thinning. I scarcely noticed that he had lost an eye in a childhood accident. He speaks very loudly. I interviewed him first at an East Side restaurant in New York City on a rainy day in November 1972. Everyone in the restaurant could hear him describe the more squalid facets of cancer in stentorian tones. After lunch, we talked away the afternoon in the elegant offices of the Albert and Mary Lasker Foundation overlooking the United Nations. (Burkitt had come to the United States to receive a Lasker Award.) It was a very graphic interview. Once he squatted on the floor to demonstrate how some Africans move their bowels.

He is a simple, pious man. "I was born in Enniskillen in the north of Ireland from very wonderful parents whom I dearly, dearly loved."

His grandfather was an itinerant Presbyterian minister, living on a pittance, who rode around his parish on horseback, carrying a revolver for protection against footpads. His father was a civil engineer, but spent much of his spare time watching birds. He was named one of the seven persons who have done most for British ornithology. Burkitt is very proud of that.

As a youth, Burkitt did not want to be a doctor. But "I was led to seek God's will for my life," he said. "I prayed and it was quite overwhelmingly borne in on me that I should be a doctor." He graduated from Dublin University medical school and went to Edinburgh for advanced surgical training. When he got there, he couldn't afford the $6 a week for room and board. He searched out a boarding house providing them for $4. He served through World War II as a British Army surgeon in Kenya, Somalia, and Ceylon. After demobilization, he joined the Colonial Service and was assigned to a small town in Uganda. He had the help of one assistant to run a one-hundred-bed hospital, and handle malaria and sleeping sickness control, all school health problems, and every other aspect of medical care for a population of 275,000. He performed more than six hundred operations a year.

In 1948, the Colonial Service switched him to Mulago Hospital in the Ugandan capital, Kampala.

"If anybody had said to me in those days that I'd do research, I would have just laughed because I never had any training in research. I never had any training in laboratory work. I hadn't worked in a laboratory for one day in the whole of my life.

"I really got interested in cancer as a hobby. What happened was that we'd been operating on the tumors which now bear my name, but we'd never really investigated them. Then the time came when I realized that these jaw tumors we were operating on were only half of a tumor. . . ."

One day, early in 1957, Burkitt was requested to examine a seven-year-old African boy named Africa who had large swellings on both sides of his upper and lower jaws. Burkitt was puzzled.

"They just didn't fit in with any textbook description of malignancy."

He photographed the swellings and held the child under observation. Some weeks later, Burkitt saw another child with the same kind of swollen jaw. In the following months, he saw many more, and he made photographs of each one. He noticed something strange about them. Every time he saw a jaw tumor, he was certain to find another tumor in the child's kidney, liver, ovary, testicles, eye, or somewhere else in the body. Obviously, this tumor was a multiple malignancy. It grew at incredible speed, practically doubling in size every forty-eight hours. A child with the tumor was practically sure to die within a few months. Surgery was useless.

The tumor proved to be a lymphoma—a tumor originating in the lymphoid tissues. Burkitt showed his photographs to A.G. Oettlé, director of the Cancer Research Unit of the South African Institute for Medical Research. To Burkitt's surprise, Oettlé said, "This tumor doesn't occur in South Africa."

Where does it occur? Burkitt wondered. "If they don't get it in South Africa and we get it here, it must stop somewhere. If only we could learn where it stops. . . !"

He set forth to find out. Untrained though he was in research techniques, he handled his project wisely. "It was like a geographical biopsy," he declared. "When a surgeon cuts a bit of a lesion to give to the pathologist, he cuts the edge wide so he can give the pathologist a bit of normal tissue and a bit of tumor. I decided to do the same thing."

He obtained his first research grant, all of $42, and had a thousand leaflets with pictures of the mysterious tumor printed. He mailed them to almost every government and mission hospital in Africa, inquiring whether they had seen the tumor in their localities. Many of them had. Their replies showed that the tumor was widespread in a belt across tropical Africa.

In October 1961, Burkitt bought a battered old Ford station wagon and embarked upon a ten-thousand-mile safari through Africa with the tumor as his quarry. Two medical missionaries went with him. Both were good doctors. More to the point, they knew how to make emergency repairs to a broken-down automobile. None had much money, so they slept in government rest houses and made meals out of tea and biscuits.

The three visited fifty-seven hospitals in nine countries in ten weeks. At each, they showed pictures of the tumor to the doctors. They found out something no one had ever known before. This was the most common cancer in children in tropical Africa! It was more common in some areas than the sum total of all other cancers of tropical African children.

Burkitt remarked to me, "It is not often that you can describe a new tumor and at the same time can say that it is the commonest tumor."

The tumor occurred in children between the ages of two and fourteen. Ages four to seven were the most dangerous.

The biggest discovery emerging from the trek was that the incidence of the lymphoma was directly related to altitude and temperature. Near the Equator, few tumors were reported anywhere at an altitude higher than 5,000 feet. In Nyasaland, none occurred above 3,000 feet; in Mozambique, and Natal, none above 1,000 feet. The tumor was most prevalent in the hot, moist southern areas where the rainfall is sixty to one hundred inches a year; it was almost unknown in the northern regions where the climate is dry.

One look at Burkitt's tumor map suggested that the incidence of the tumor was approximately the same as the incidence of yellow fever and several other insect-transmitted diseases. It was a galvanic thought. It suggested that the tumor might be caused by a mosquito-borne virus, as yellow fever is.

Burkitt lectured about his findings in London at the Bland-Sutton Institute. A forty-year-old virologist at the institute, Dr. Michael Anthony Epstein, happened to be at the lecture. Burkitt's news was "hot coals" to him, and he raced up at the conclusion of the lecture.

"We'll provide all the expenses," he said. "Can you send us tumors from Africa?"

"Fine," Burkitt agreed.

A stream of biopsy specimens in glass thermos jars started by air mail to the institute in London. For three years, Tony Epstein worked on them. In 1964, he and his associate, Dr. Yvonne Barr, detected a large number of a herpes-type virus in tumor tissue under an electron microscope. Two urologists, a married couple at Children's Hospital in Philadelphia, Drs. Werner and Gertrude Henle, exposed cells from healthy people to some of these Epstein-Barr (EB) viruses taken from Burkitt's lymphoma patients. The healthy cells were transformed into cancerous cells. The Henles also found antibodies to the EB virus in Burkitt's lymphoma patients. Although the proof is not all in, the evidence strongly indicates that the EB virus causes Burkitt's lymphoma. It is the closest medical science has so far gotten to identifying a viral villain in human cancer.

Coincidentally, the Henles discovered that the same EB virus causes infectious mononucleosis.

It is now known that Burkitt's lymphoma occurs, albeit very rarely, everywhere in the world. Burkitt has, therefore, modified his views as to the reason for its high prevalence in places like tropical Africa and New Guinea. His theory now is that every person carries the EB virus at some time in his life, but it causes cancer only in regions where malaria is hyperendemic. The malaria acts as an immunosuppressant and lets the cancer loose, he believes.

Most scientists find cures for diseases because they are expert in their spheres. Burkitt found the right treatment for his lymphoma because he knew so little about it. It was another case of medical fortune rewarding a receptive mind. In January 1960, Dr. Joe Burchenal and a team of Sloan-Kettering scientists came into Kampala on a trip through East Africa to test new anticancer drugs. Burkitt told Burchenal about his lymphoma, and Burchenal suggested chemotherapy for it. He gave Burkitt a supply of methotrexate.

"It would hardly be an exaggeration to say that I found myself the most ignorant cancer chemotherapist in the world," Mr. Burkitt told me. "I did all the wrong things."

His wrong things turned out to be right. He was instructed to give the methotrexate in very large, frequent doses. He didn't. "I had so many other things to do as well as treating patients with this tumor, and I had to wait such a long time to get my blood counts back, that I treated my patients very badly. I gave them what in the United States people would have laughed at as a ridiculously small, ineffective, and inefficient therapy regime."

As luck would have it, this is a very sensitive tumor, and small doses are all that it requires. Burkitt treated a five-year-old boy named Kibakola with a few small doses of methotrexate. The horrible tumor he had on his jaw disappeared. Ten years later, it was still gone. A seven-year-old girl named Namusisi had one treatment of a three-course schedule of methotrexate, and her tumor vanished. Eight years later, it was still gone.

Today, chemotherapists in Africa are achieving total, permanent remissions of Burkitt's lymphoma in most of their cases.

Mr. Burkitt left the Colonial Service in 1964 to join the staff of the Medical Research Council in London. He has been principally concerned since then with a controversial thesis advanced by a Royal Navy doctor, Surgeon Captain T.I. Cleave, that a number of the worse diseases of Western man, among them cancer of the colon and rectum, coronary heart disease, diabetes, and diverticulosis, are largely due to the lack of roughage in people's diet. Cleave maintains, and Burkitt agrees, that these diseases are rare in countries where people eat carbohydrate foods in their natural state, but are rife in the Western world where carbohydrate foods are refined and the roughage removed from them.

They point out that cancer of the colon and rectum seldom occur in Africa, where the people eat a lot of roughage, but kill close to fifty thousand people a year in the United States, where white bread and other refined foods are popular. Burkitt feels it has to do with the amount of time that food takes to pass through the digestive system. "A long hold-up in the bowel" allows carcinogetic substances to form, he claims.

"There is no country in the world on a high-fiber diet which gets coronary heart disease," Burkitt goes on to say, "and there is no community that changed from a high- to a low-fiber diet for long enough which didn't subsequently get a high incidence of coronary heart disease." He devoutly urges that white bread be banned.

Both Cleave and Burkitt have been sternly criticized for "their far-fetched theory," but they are completely persuaded of its validity.

Burkitt and his wife, Olive, a former nurse, live out in the English countryside, near Shiplake, forty miles west of London. "I'm a wife-made man," he loves to say. "She is the greatest gift I have ever been given. We celebrated out twenty-ninth wedding anniversary this year, and I think I can say we find it harder to part from each other than we did when we were first married."

The Burkitts are religious people. He said, "In the morning, I make the tea. I give my wife a long kiss while the kettle is cooking. Then we both, on our own, spend about half an hour in quiet prayer and study of the Bible before we start the day."

They have three daughters.

He made no pretenses to me about his motivations. "I didn't ever set out to do research. It was a hobby, just as somebody might have a hobby in botany or birds. It eventually made my life more interesting if I tried to find out the reasons for things."

Mr. Burkitt watches his pennies very carefully. He hates to spend more than $3 for a meal, and he always turns off the lights when he leaves a room. He was shocked to hear of the multithousand-dollar fees some American surgeons demand. While he was in the Colonial Service, he was allowed to do some private surgery. The highest fee he ever charged for the most difficult operation was $100, and he only asked that much four or five times in his career. He normally leaves home at eight in the morning and returns at six. Unlike most other world-famous medical scientists, he objects to a frenetic work schedule.

"Somebody one time said, 'Beware of the barrenness of a busy life,' and there is something in it," he said to me.

The Search for Viruses in Human Cancer

"Cherchez le virus" are the watchwords of many cancer researchers today. They feel sure that viruses will prove to be the prime villains on the cancer stage. There is testimony to bear them out.

Not that skeptics haven't abounded. A high-level scientific committee was appointed in the late 1930s to draft a research program for the newly founded National Cancer Institute. It ruled that mammalian cancer could not possibly be infectious. Therefore, it decreed, viruses and all other microorganisms should be disregarded forever as etiological, or causative, agents for cancer.

Evidence linking viruses to solid cancer tumors in animals goes back to 1911, when Dr. Peyton Rous made his great discovery that a virus caused tumors of the connective tissues. Twenty-two years later, Dr. Richard E. Shope of the Rockefeller Institute fortified the case against viruses by taking a virus from a wild, cancerous rabbit and producing cancer with it in domestic rabbits. In 1940, Dr. Ludwik Gross, a fine researcher at the Bronx Veterans Administration Hospital in New York City, did something no one had ever been able to do—that is, find a viral cause for soft tumors in animals. He produced leukemia in newborn mice by injecting them with cell-free extracts taken out of a leukemic mouse. In 1951, Dr. Gross also induced leukemia in healthy adult mice with a virus he had gotten from leukemic mice. In 1952, Dr. Maurice R. Hilleman demonstrated at the Merck Sharp & Dohme laboratories that a virus labeled the SV 40, which was harmless in its natural host, the monkey, was violently carcinogenic when he injected it into newborn hamsters. In 1957, two scientists at the National Cancer Institute, Drs. Sarah Stewart and Bernice Eddy, isolated a "polyoma virus" that produced more than twenty different kinds of tumors in several different kinds of animals. In 1964, Dr. Arthur Jarrett, a British dermatologist, showed that cats could infect each other with cancer. Dr. Robert J. Heubner, the N.C.I. virologist, went him one better. He induced leukemia in healthy cats merely by inoculating them with drops of saliva from a leukemic cat.

A minimum of 110 individual types of viruses that cause cancer in animals were known by 1974.

What good does it do for us?

There are two principal reasons for seeking the cause of a disease. One is to help find a cure for it. The other, which may be far more important, is to develop a means of preventing the disease. This is what has occurred with one form of animal cancer, and the implications are boundless for humans as well as animals. For the first time, a vaccine has been produced that can prevent a naturally occurring cancer.

The cancer is Marek's disease, grimly described as "a debilitating, neoplastic condition of chickens of all ages characterized by the development of lymphoid tumors throughout the chicken's body, particularly in the nerves, skin, muscles, and internal organs." Its death rate is very high. Fifty percent of a flock can develop paralysis and die within four to five months. The disease used to cost American poultry growers $200 million a year. It was eradicated by Dr. Ben R. Burmester, a quiet, self-effacing physiologist-pathologist who is the world's top authority on a variety of poultry diseases.

Tall, white-haired, and spectacled now, with the look of a schoolmaster, Burmester was born in 1910 on a poultry ranch in Petaluma, California. His father was a German peasant who emigrated to the United States and started one of the country's first poultry farms. The boy was guided into the sciences by a professor during his undergraduate days at the University of California. He took his Ph.D in physiology at California, went back to school years later, and became a Doctor of Veterinary Medicine. He is director of the U.S. Department of Agriculture's Poultry Research Laboratory in East Lansing, Michigan.

For decades, scientists had searched for a weapon against Marek's and other leukemic diseases in poultry. In 1965, a team of USDA researchers under Dr. Burmester set out to track the virus they thought was responsible for the disease. Their biggest difficulty was finding a medium in which to grow the suspected virus. By accident, they tried some duck egg cells, and they worked. They were able to isolate the viral culprit in 1967. It proved to be a highly infectious herpes virus, the same genre that causes Burkitt's lymphoma.

It was a very mystifying virus. As Dr. Burmester explained it to me, "No one could figure out how this cancer spread from chicken to chicken. We couldn't find one virus particle in the body of a cancerous chicken where there should have been billions. What happened to them? We discovered that the cancer viruses grow in the cells of the feather follicles. The surface cells of the feather follicles are shed as the feathers grow out. They dry up and float about in the air with the viruses still alive inside them. Then they are breathed in by the other chickens through the mouth and nose. In essence, the cancer is spread by the respiratory route, just like TB or the flu."

A British team under Dr. Peter Biggs isolated the herpes virus at Houghton, England, at the same time as the Burmester people did. The two groups vied to see which would be first to turn out an effective vaccine from an attenuated herpes virus. The Biggs team came in ahead, but its vaccine wasn't satisfactory.

The Burmester people tried a different gambit, and the dice rolled their way. One of Burmester's scientists, Dr. Richard L. Witter, happened to examine a turkey's blood and found a strange new virus in it. It obviously was related to the Marek's virus, but it didn't cause Marek's in turkeys. Burmester wasted no time. See if the turkey virus causes Marek's disease in chickens, he directed.

As he recounted the story, "Lo and behold, it didn't. The next question was: If it didn't cause Marek's in chickens, would it prevent it?"

They grew the turkey virus in the same duck-cell culture, inoculated chickens with it, and the chickens became solidly immune to the cancer for the rest of their lives.

It was the same "stalking horse" technique that Edward Jenner employed so successfully against smallpox.

Today, virtually every chicken grown commercially in the United States—and in all other advanced nations—is inoculated with the Burmester vaccine against Marek's disease at a cost of less than one cent per dose. None ever gets the cancer.

I talked with Dr. Burmester in East Lansing by telephone. He told me that he met his scientist-wife, Mary Alice, while they were both students at the University of California. Until her recent retirement, she was a professor of biology at Michigan State University.

He gets most of his fun from remodeling their summer cottage on Bass Lake. About his motives, he was very subdued. "You'd like to discover something significant. That's part of the motivation. I suppose the other part is that it's your job and you want to do well at it."

Dr. Hilleman, who isolated a cancer virus himself, was not so subdued when he spoke to me of Dr. Burmester's work. He knew it well, for his company manufactures the vaccine.

"You can sit around and talk about oncogenes and theories and why vaccines won't work and so forth, but I want to tell you that them damn chickens are staying alive. To me, this dwarfs everything in the cancer field for the past twenty years.

"This vaccine gets inside the chicken, produces an infection with its attenuated virus, and that infection stays for the rest of the life of the chicken. A virulent cancer virus can get inside the chicken, sure, but the virulent virus cannot express itself as a tumor anymore.''

The hope now is that human beings can someday be given the same protection that chickens get.

First, however, it has to be conclusively proven, once and for all, that viruses also cause human cancer. Then each culpable virus has to be identified.

Dr. Leon Dmchowski of the M.D. Anderson Hospital and Tumor Institute in Houston, Texas, made the opening stride here in 1957. He did a biopsy on a fifteen-year-old girl with leukemia and discovered some strange particles in her lymph node tissues. He thought they looked like viruses. In 1959, he noted several other instances of particles that looked like viruses.

The poor fellow quickly learned that a virus hunt is one of the more precarious activities in cancer research. Almost any time anyone claims to have discovered a cancer virus, dozens of other scientists stand poised with verbal bludgeons to attack the claim and the claimant. The rivalries are very intense on this front, as Dmchowski found. He was assailed for everything but treason.

He didn't retreat. The particles were definitely C-type viruses, he reported.

I talked with him at the Anderson Hospital in 1972. He was a jovial man, stocky, with very black hair, boasting a very multinational background. He was born in 1909 in what was a part of Austria but became a part of Poland and is presently a part of Russia. He secured an M.D. and a Ph.D. at the University of Vienna and spent years doing research in England before he came to the United States.

He told me that he had just isolated particles of C-type viruses from cells he had extracted from the tumor of a five-year-old boy with Burkitt's lymphoma. The particles, he said, were identical in appearance to those known to induce leukemia in every species of animal from monkeys to mice.

The discoveries of the role of viruses in Burkitt's lymphoma followed hard on the original work by Dr. Dmchowski. Since then, considerably more documentation has accumulated. Dr. Dan Moore of the Institute for Medical Research in Camden, New Jersey, and Dr. Sol Spiegelman of Columbia University reported in 1971 that they had detected a B-type particle in the milk of Parsi women in Bombay. They were ''certain'' that it was ''a human breast cancer virus.''

In November 1972, an N.C.I. representative presented a box containing thirteen suspected cancer viruses to the U.S.S.R. Academy of Medical

Sciences at an impressive ceremony in Moscow. The greatest cancer specialist in the Soviet Union, Dr. Nikolai N. Blokhin, reciprocated by giving the N.C.I. man twelve species of Russian viruses to take home with him.

A year later, the N.C.I. sorrowfully informed me that the Soviet viruses would not grow in the Washington environs. The Russians weren't talking about the behavior of their American viruses.

There is, it must be said, a radically different concept of the virus's role in cancer that has won wide currency. It was advanced by Dr. Robert Joseph Huebner, one of America's most prominent and unorthodox virologists.

Dr. Huebner heads the Viral Carcinogenesis Branch at the N.C.I. He is a big man, ruddy-faced, with baggy eye pouches. Born in 1914, oldest of nine children, he started law school but decided that he preferred medicine. He got an M.D. at St. Louis University in 1942 and went to work for the National Institution of Health in 1944.

I saw him in his gloomy office at the N.C.I. He told me that he decided on a career in research during his senior year at medical school. He was not overly burdened with modesty.

"I found that if I concentrated on anything, I could learn more about it than almost anybody else."

He proved to be an excellent medical detective. In 1946, he was sent to New York City to investigate an epidemic of a strange new disease that looked like Rocky Mountain spotted fever. He tracked down the guilty rickettsia that caused it and named the disease rickettsiapox. He helped discover the adenoviruses that cause conjunctivitis and other unpleasantnesses. In the 1950s, he switched his attentions to cancer.

He started his research with a conventional view of cancer viruses. But "I had to take my head off and screw it on in a 180-degree different direction."

He and his staff checked the antigens in every animal they could lay their hands on: mice, monkeys, cats, snakes, hamsters, chickens, guinea pigs, rats, swine. In every one of these animals that had cancer, Huebner or his colleagues found evidence of RNA C-particles.

It convinced Huebner that most, perhaps all, cancer is caused by an RNA C-type virus.

He maintained, "This cancer virus is definitely not the same kind of a bug that causes such well-known infections as measles, polio, or the common cold. It isn't spread horizontally—that is, from person to person, or from an animal, or a toilet seat. You don't catch it."

Huebner's intriguing concept is that the C-type particle is a noninfectious virus that has become a normal part of all living cells. He thinks that we transmit it vertically to our offspring the same as a gene that gives you red hair or blue eyes. Usually, it lies quiescent in the cell, but sometimes it runs riot, he says. It is triggered by other viruses, by chemical carcinogens, or radiological carcinogens. Then, cancer!

In brief, Huebner declares, you can inherit from your parents a specific group of genes—known as oncogenes—that are potential cancer causers.

"What we're looking for now," Dr. Huebner said, "is a way of preventing these oncogenes from getting out of hand."

Huebner is one more twelve-hour-a-day, seven-day-a-week worker because "work is a lot of fun." He was married to Grace Berdine Hoffman for more than thirty years; they had nine children. A rare man among scientists, Huebner has a keen business sense. He bought a broken-down 154-acre farm in Maryland for a few thousand dollars and made a fortune out of it breeding prize Black Angus cattle.

Huebner can even make scientific capital out of business setbacks. A few years ago, a valuable Black Angus heifer died of lymphosarcoma. "It was a hard loss," he declared, "but it was one of the best breaks I've had." He recouped a hundred pounds of cancerous tissue from the carcass for his researchers.

The critics of Huebner's heretical concept of the cancer virus are myriad, but so are those who see its merits. Certainly, it has stirred up intellectual ferment in the cancer laboratories.

Immunotherapy
—The Promising Anticancer Weapon

You've heard in earlier sections of this book of the portentous cures that chemotherapy has attained with some cancer patients, the salutary affects of high-dosage radiation and surgery, the promising research into viruses. Now you are going to hear about the most threatening enemy that cancer has—the human immune system, and the scientists who have enlisted its aid for the anticancer crusade. It could be the ally physicians have dreamed of: a way for the body to help cure its own cancers, or prevent them.

Immunity is the remarkable ability of the body to build a specific, long-lasting immunity against a foreign substance to which it is exposed. Take the mumps vaccine. When a child is inoculated with a vaccine made of attenuated mumps viruses, he comes down with a small case of the mumps, but speedily recovers as the body unleashes an irresistible attack on the viruses. Then, for many years afterward, his body has an impregnable defense against the mumps virus. Immunity also explains why the body rejects transplanted organs and skin grafts. It is the body's protection against all foreign invaders.

The immune system in every normal person is constantly at war with cancer. "I think malignancies are continually arising in the body," Dr. Robert A. Good, the great authority on immunology, declares "Nearly always they are recognized by the immune system as foreign and are knocked out. But every once in a while, a malignancy manages to escape the surveillance system and—bang—you've got cancer."

"The question is not how come we develop so much cancer," Dr. Edmund Klein, who has pioneered in cancer immunotherapy as well as chemotherapy, says. "The question is how come we develop so little cancer."

The big push is to spur the body's immune system to do more against cancer—much more. To wipe out cancer altogether, maybe. There are many who are convinced that the immune system will eventually help to defeat all forms of cancer. They have some early triumphs to point to.

Dr. Good has for many years led the immunological forces. When I interviewed him in the spring of 1973, he had just taken over as president of the Sloan-Kettering Institute for Cancer Research and director of research at the entire Memorial Sloan-Kettering Cancer Center. I saw him in his smart modern office at 7:15 A.M. That was very late for him. His day at the office starts at 4:30 A.M. A tall, shambling bear of a man with long grey-black hair, Good dresses very informally. That morning, he was wearing a black turtleneck sweater with a grey sweatshirt over it. "I've never been persuaded that a necktie has any real function except to get in the way," he stated. I found him a good-humored man with a warming smile, and more than a touch of the actor. He used his low, musical voice theatrically, with a wide range of highly dramatic stresses and pauses, and his gestures were worthy of a Barrymore.

I like this about him. He is a man of no small ego—he says so himself—but he is one of the few scientists I've met who is happy to give credit to others.

He was born in 1922 in a small Minnesota town, Crosby, one of four sons of a high school principal and a schoolteacher. He decided to be a doctor when he was five years old—for the same reason as had so many other medical men. His father had just died of cancer. It was hard going for a while. He delivered newspapers, shoveled snow, and raked leaves to help make ends meet. As a student at the University of Minnesota, he was paralyzed by a rare disease, but by the exercise of fantastic willpower, he forced himself to walk again, and he graduated with straight A's. Now he has merely a little limp left. He got both an M.D. and a Ph.D. He selected pediatrics as his specialty so he could do research in immunology. He felt that it would allow him to investigate defects in immune systems that are only seen in children (because the patients generally die before they get to be adults).

"Besides, I like children," he said. "They're tough."

For the next twenty-five years, at Rockefeller Institute and the University of Minnesota medical school, he helped make a science of immunology—an immediately valuable science that could lead to cures in cancer and other diseases.

Dr. Irving McQuarrie, who taught him pediatrics at medical school, would have applauded the way Good went about it. "Dr. McQuarrie had two great attributes," Good told me. "He was a people-watcher, and he was an interpreter of experiments in nature. He taught me to go into the clinic and make observations of those rare, unusual conditions where nature is making experiments of its own, where there is derangement of the normal function, where something is left out genetically. He taught me to see what questions these conditions raise, because very often the experiments of nature are better than any experiments we can do in the laboratory. He taught me to take the questions to the laboratory, to analyze them, and to bring back answers to test in the clinic.

"I've done that all my life. I've learned that if you pay attention to the things that don't fit, you are much more likely to make discoveries than if you try to find out things that fit. It's the things that don't fit that really count."

Science is "a fun game" to Bob Good. "You know the parlor game Twenty Questions," he said. "Well, science is a game of Twenty Questions with the unknown. If you know where to start, you can get the answer to anything by asking twenty questions, each of which bisects the remaining field. If you waste your questions by guessing or by going off in directions without orderly bisections, you don't get anywhere. But if you discipline yourself and ask questions, each of which bisects the field, you can always get the answer."

Dr. Good was the first to learn how the immune system really is organized and how it operates. He made the key discovery that the immune system consists of two separate parts each acting independently of the other, instead of just one, as scientists had erroneously believed for decades.

He told me that he came on his revolutionary thesis in this fashion: While working with Dr. Henry Kunkel at the Rockefeller Institute, he noticed that patients suffering from different cancers seemed to contract different kinds of infections. People with Hodgkin's disease were very vulnerable to viral and fungus infections, and to tuberculosis; people who had multiple myelomas, (tumors of the bone marrow) were very susceptible to bacterial infections like streptococcus and pneumococcus.

"In a kind of a vague way, I could see through this haze that there might be two major immunity systems. Myeloma patients as an experiment of nature were raising the question of what defenses they had against the streptococcus and the pneumococcus. The patients with Hodgkin's disease were raising the question of what defenses they had against viruses, funguses, and tubercle bacilli."

In 1952, Colonel Ogden C. Bruton, a U.S. Army pediatrician, discovered that a lack of gamma globulin could make people incapable of producing antibodies in their blood. But they could reject skin grafts.

As Dr. Good detailed it, "These people had one kind of immunity and not another."

It was patent that immunity was a double-barreled weapon. But how did it operate? And what parts of the body did it involve?

Good suspected the little thymus gland of collusion. He made it a point to examine forty-seven patients who came into the hospital with tumors of the thymus, and the results reinforced his suspicion. Every one had an immunological deficiency.

A freak accidental discovery involving some chickens, of all creatures, filled out the gaps in his thinking. Timothy S. Chang, a young graduate student at Ohio State University, borrowed a dozen chicks from another graduate student, Bruce Glick, to demonstrate to a class how chickens develop immunity when they are vaccinated against salmonella bacteria. Ten of the twelve chicks didn't develop any immunity, though.

"Are you playing jokes on me?" the embarrassed Chang demanded of Glick. "What's the matter with these chicks?"

Glick reviewed his laboratory records. He discovered that the bursa of Fabricius (an inconspicuous gland near the tail of the chicken—named for Girolamo Fabrizio, a seventeenth-century Italian anatomist—whose function no one understood) had been removed from the ten nonimmune chicks but not the other two.

The two graduate students realized that in some way the bursa must be essential to the development of immunity, and they hurried to write a paper on the case.

No medical journal would run it. As Dr. Good remarked, "Who the hell wanted to know about the bursa of Fabricius?"

They could only get their paper published in *Poultry Science*, where no immunologist would ever see it. However, a University of Wisconsin zoologist spotted it, and he called it to Good's attention. Good was impressed, and he assigned a team, headed by Dr. Max Cooper, to investigate it. Cooper took the bursa out of some newly hatched chicks and the thymus out of others. He subjected both groups of chicks to enough radiation to destroy any vestiges of immunity that they might have been born with.

Now everything came into line. The chicks without a bursa had no humoral immunity: they could not make antibodies to fight off infections. But they had perfectly intact cellular immunity: they could reject all foreign matter, such as transplanted kidneys and skin grafts. The chicks without a thymus had fine humoral immunity, but they didn't have any cellular immunity.

"We'd really proved it," Dr. Good said. "All the haze of malignancies cleared away, and I put forward my two-component concept of the immunological system."

He explained this concept thus: The mission of the immune system is to identify, assault, and destroy any foreign matter that dares invade the body. Its principal warriors are white blood cells called lymphocytes. There are two main kinds of them. One type consists of T-cells, which are responsible for cellular immunity. They maintain the body's biological individuality by rejecting foreign matter, and they kill certain bacteria. The other type consists of B-cells that provide humoral immunity. They produce the antibodies—special proteins—that help the body recognize and destroy millions of different disease-causing organisms. Big scavenger cells known as macrophages back up both types. They devour foreign cells.

All lymphocytes are produced in the bone marrow, but they are controlled by two totally different organs. T-cells are controlled by the thymus, and B-cells by a human counterpart of the bursa of Fabricius. Good doesn't know what this is yet. He believed for a time that it might be the tonsils, but he doesn't think so anymore.

Since he presented his two-component theory in the mid-1960s, it has become the foundation of all modern immunobiology.

Dr. Good proved the validity of the theory on an operating table in 1967. A five-month-old infant, David Camp, was carried in with a hereditary disease that had already killed twelve babies in his family. David had no lymphocytes at all. If Good's theory was correct, the deficiency lay in the infant's bone marrow, and a bone marrow transplant should give him a normal immune system.

Good's team took about a billion marrow cells from a leg bone in the baby's sister—fortunately, she had similar cells—and injected them into David. A rejection crisis boiled up, but it was surmounted. The baby's blood became immunologically perfect, at least for a while. He even had antibodies in it against chicken pox and mumps, diseases that he had never contracted but his sister had.

"What are the implications?" I asked.

"They're really tremendous," Dr. Good declared. "As a consequence of understanding this theory, we've begun to do cellular engineering. If people are born without T- or B-cells, we can give them cells from an appropriately matched donor that correct the deficit. It's like creating life, because these patients can't live without an immune system.

"Take cancer. Cancer is not so dumb. It represents an adaptive system that has been genetically interacting with bodily defense systems for four hundred million years, and it has learned how to get around our immune system. Well, now we should be able to modify the immunological parameters in cancer patients. By immunological engineering, we should be able to increase the capacity of the immune system to recognize cancer cells as foreigners and get rid of them."

Dr. Good rises at 4:00 A.M. and works a nineteen- or twenty-hour day, seven days a week. His first marriage foundered over his work addiction in 1965. (There are four children by this marriage.) He was remarried in 1967 to Joanne Finstad, a phylogeneticist who was with him at the University of Minnesota. They both dote on a farm they have in Minnesota and try to get back to it whenever they can.

"You know what I really like to do for fun?" Dr. Good said. "I really like to garden. I like to grow vegetables, I like to grow plants, and if I ever get the time, I really like to fish for trout and bass."

Good's motives are complex. "I like to discover things; I like to see things for the first time. I like competition. I like to interact with the smartest guys around. In science, there really is a very wonderful competition. Sometimes it gets a bit destructive, but not usually. I suppose, like everybody else, I also want people to recognize that I'm doing something important. And, you know, I really like to help suffering people as a doctor. I want to prevent them from suffering."

Some persons in the world of medicine consider Robert Alan Good too ambitious, "a scientific Sammy Glick who lets his ego get in the way of his intellect." They say that he acts as if he is running for the Nobel Prize, and it may be so.* But what big-time medical scientist (outside of Denis Burkitt) doesn't?

---

*Dr. Good's chances of winning a Nobel Prize were threatened when it was disclosed in the spring of 1974 that a clinical researcher at Sloan-Kettering had falsified the results of some experiments he was doing and that for a long time Dr. Good didn't realize it. The researcher said that Good was pressuring him to produce significant scientific findings.

In any case, Dr. Good's dream of defeating cancer by immunology stands a large chance of coming true. Some forms of cancer have already been cured by immunological means.

Again Dr. Edmund Klein has led the pack. As before, he took advantage of an accidental observation. One day in 1962, while he and Dr. Fred Helm, an associate at Roswell Park Memorial Institute in Buffalo, were testing some drugs against skin cancer, a patient displayed an angry allergic reaction. His skin turned a crazy red and became unbearably itchy.

"The first dictum when you see an allergic reaction," Dr. Klein said to me, "is, My God, let's get rid of the agent that caused it. And you should. These allergic reactions can be fatal. Well, we didn't. We took the allergy-producing material and dropped its concentration to a lower level. Then we tried it again. The tumor disappeared. It blistered, it swelled, it broke up, it became a mess, and it disappeared, whereas the normal skin around it showed just a little inflammation. It proved to us that the immune mechanism of the body could operate against malignant tumors and that we could control it."

This was not chemotherapy at work. It was the first demonstration of the immune system's capacity to vanquish cancer.

"For the first time," Dr. Klein testified to a committee of the U.S. Senate, "we were able to take the cause of a disease, namely allergy, and turn it into a therapeutic weapon. We were able to take it out of the hands of the devil and put it into the hands of God."

Klein developed a technique for injecting the live-bacteria vaccine BCG directly into a tumor. (Later, he was able to inject it elsewhere in the body with the same effects.) The BCG stirred up the immune system to marshal T-cells for an attack on the cancer. By 1976, Klein had treated more than five hundred skin cancer patients at Roswell Park with immunotherapy. A five-year study of his first twenty-four patients revealed that 95 percent of their five thousand tumors had gone into complete remission.

He has tried his immunotherapy against nastier cancers—tumors that originated internally and metastasized to the skin, like reticulum cell sarcoma, malignant melanoma, mycosis fungoides, and breast cancer, and he has had promising results here, too. He used immunotherapy on five women who had experienced recurrences of breast cancers after surgery. Their cancers were considered untreatable. Two years later, every one of the women was still alive. In two of them, the treated cancers had wholly disappeared.

"I think Ed Klein's work is just tremendous," Dr. Good exulted.

Dr. Georges Mathé, the distinguished French oncologist, is another who has had good results with BCG immunotherapy. Professor Mathé, who was born in 1924, is a slim, bald man with a round face. He directs research at the Institut de Cancérologie et Immunégénetique at the Hôpital Paul Brousse on the outskirts of Paris. Both Mathé and Klein have also tried to combine immunotherapy and chemotherapy. They kill off the bulk of the cancer cells with chemotherapy and use immunotherapy to get rid of those last few cells that are always so difficult to extinguish.

Dr. Klein joined with his chum, Dr. Djerassi, to bring out a whole new slant on immunotherapy in 1973. They stimulated macrophages, the scavenger cells, to destroy cancers *en masse*. Djerassi, who did the original research, activated monocytes—cells that turn into macrophages when they settle down in the tissues—and injected them near the sites of tumors. They wiped out many of them.

Immunotherapy is still in its early stages, of course, and no one is yet quite sure how it functions. Bob Good says, "It's a little bit like kicking a television set to repair it. Sometimes it doesn't work at all. But in some instances, it works really dramatically."

Gold Develops a Blood Test for Cancer

One fine by-product of the new science of immunology is a simple blood test that may be able to detect the presence of a cancer in the body well before it shows up on an X-ray film.

An exuberant young Canadian physiologist, Dr. Phil Gold, developed it. As Dr. Sidney Farber remarked, "One doesn't have to be very old in this field of cancer research to make brilliant discoveries."

Dr. Gold, a burly, black-haired man filled with happy laughter, was born in Montreal in 1936. His parents were Jewish refugees from Poland who emigrated to Canada in the 1920s.

"Being of my ethnic background," he joshed, "it was a foregone conclusion that I'd be a doctor."

I talked with him in his laboratory in the towering Montreal General Hospital. He told me that he got an M.D. and a Ph.D. at McGill University. He explained, "I grew up in a Jewish section of town where your parents expected you to go to school forever unless there was some good reason to stop."

Why research?

"I wanted to know one thing better than anybody else. I wanted to know everything I could about it."

And he added, "It's a matter of trying to leave a scratch on the rock."

Once, during his internship, he attended two lectures on cancer in a week. One described the difficulties of diagnosing cancer. The other was a discussion of tumors of the colon. They set him thinking. Working with his chief, Dr. Samuel O. Freedman, he developed a plan for a radioimmunoassay of a patient's blood to determine the presence in it of infinitesimally small quantities of a carcino-embryonic antigen (CEA) secreted by certain cancers.

He combined a sample of a patient's blood with some goat's blood known to contain antibodies to cancer, and a sample of colon cancer antigen that had been radioactively tagged. He centrifuged them and scanned them with a sensitive Geiger counter.

The results showed the concentration of CEAs in a patient's blood in amounts down to a nanogram, a billionth of a gram per cubic centimeter. A concentration of CEAs above a certain level was a danger signal. It could indicate cancer of the colon. A greater concentration of CEAs could mean that the cancer had metastasized.

In 1969, Dr. Gold tested blood samples from two hundred patients. It detected thirty-five of thirty-six patients with cancer of the colon.

"How did you feel when you saw the results?" I asked.

"Strange. My first reaction was, Keep your mouth shut, Gold, and go very slowly."

Other researchers confirmed the test's promise. John Langan of Temple University did similar radioimmunoassays of blood samples from thirty-four patients who had been diagnosed as having ulcerative colitis. Eight had high levels of CEA. Every one of the eight turned out to have cancer of the gastrointestinal tract.

Scientists at Roswell Park and other great cancer research centers around the world hastened to study and expand on the Gold concept. They have made it even more valuable. It is now in use in many cancer centers as a broad-scale screening device to detect many types of cancer far earlier than ever before. At Roswell Park, colon cancers have been spotted three and a half months before they showed up on any X-ray. It lets the Roswell Park therapists get a head start in fighting the disease.

Hoffmann-LaRoche, the drug company, made the test practical for large numbers of people. As Dr. Gold designed it, the test needed a week to do. Dr. Hans Hansen, a Hoffmann-LaRoche biochemist, streamlined it so that it takes less than a day to perform.

Dr. Gold expects a lot of his test. "The pot is just beginning to boil," he said.

Cigarettes and Lung Cancer
—*The Fatal Facts*

One thing you must say for the American Cancer Society. It thinks big. The problems it tackles are great ones, the strategies it adopts are grand scale, and the enemies it invites are brawny. The accomplishments the A.C.S. has to its credit since its resurrection in 1945 (it was not very active during the preceding thirty-two years) are big, too. It has done more than any other organization, public or private, to educate the American people to the dangers of cancer and the urgent need to seek cures for it. Its campaign to get women to take the Pap smear test has reduced the death rate from cancer of the cervix by half in a generation. Led by the indomitable Mary Lasker, the A.C.S. has persuaded Congress to appropriate billions of dollars to the National Cancer Institute for the war on cancer, and it has spent more than $300 million of its own hard-gathered funds on cancer research. Time and again, when the National Cancer Institute has been reluctant to try a new research approach, the A.C.S. has been willing to give an investigator a helping hand.

The biggest and bravest thing the American Cancer Society has ever done was to take on the issue of smoking, and the cancers in the lung some people thought it might be causing.

The first scientific evidence of the harmful effects of smoking came in 1859 from M. Bouisson, a little-known French physician in Montpellier, southern France. He reported on forty-five hospital patients with cancer of the lip, eleven patients with cancer of the mouth, seven with cancer of the tongue, and five with cancer of the tonsils. Sixty-six of them smoked pipes, and one chewed tobacco. In 1936, the New Orleans thoracic surgeon Dr. Alton Ochsner and his promising young assistant, Dr. Michael De Bakey, reported that almost all of their lung cancer patients were cigarette smokers. Two years later, the Johns Hopkins medical statistician Dr. Raymond Pearl observed that cigarette smokers had a much briefer life expectancy than nonsmokers.

No one was very impressed with this evidence until a former student of Dr. Pearl, a statistician named Edward Cuyler Hammond, who was working for the A.C.S., started thinking in even bigger terms than was the society's wont. He persuaded the A.C.S. to defy the fury of the colossal tobacco industry, the sublime disinterest of the medical profession, and the incredible addiction to nicotine ot tens of millions of people. And all this though Cuyler Hammond himself was a four-pack-a-day smoker.

Dr. Hammond has the imposing title of Vice-President, Epidemiology & Statistics. We talked in his spacious office at the A.C.S. headquarters in

New York City. I found him huskily built, with a lean, intense face and grey hair, very conservatively dressed.

"I've been interested in the sciences from my earliest recollections," he said. "As a little tot, I liked to pull apart electrical things. I used to take apart my father's car, which annoyed him no end. I like anything scientific, from bird-watching on. . . ."

He once built and operated an illegal radio-broadcasting station.

A Yale graduate who was born in 1912, Hammond got a Sc.D. at the Johns Hopkins School of Public Health, served as an Air Force statistician in World War II, and joined the staff of the A.C.S. in 1946 as director of the statistics research department. He was immediately struck by the fact that the death rates for infectious diseases were falling off sharply, the death rates for many forms of cancer were standing just about still, but the death rate for lung cancer was going up very rapidly.

"We thought it was due to air pollution. The prime suspect was coal soot. We knew it caused cancer. But its consumption was going down. We suspected automobile exhausts, too, especially since the death rate from lung cancer was higher in cities than in rural areas, but it didn't seem enough of a cause, either."

He knew that many lung cancer patients admitted to smoking heavily, but he was skeptical of it as the cause. He doubted whether these patients were giving truthful answers about their smoking.

"I could imagine this poor person lying in bed with lung cancer, in pain, frightened, maybe under opiates, and somebody comes in and starts to grill him on how much he smoked. I could imagine him admitting to anything. It's very easy to put a suggestion in somebody's mind under those conditions."

Still, as he told me, Hammond decided that there was sufficient reason to do a thorough investigation of smoking. Many members of A.C.S. board of directions had trepidations when he proposed it, but the board gave its approval.

The study started on January 1, 1952. Daniel Horn, a colleague at the A.C.A. worked on it with Hammond. Twenty-two thousand A.C.S. volunteers enrolled 187,776 men between the ages of fifty and sixty-nine without lung cancer in nine states, and kept track of them for the next forty-four months.

The big task was to keep the volunteers interested in the project: they dropped out in bunches during the first two years. Dr. Hammond's wife, Marian, spent an entire summer writing personal letters in her own handwriting to every one of the twenty-two thousand volunteers. That ended the fallout among them.

Mrs. Hammond herself was later to die of cancer.

All told, 11,870 deaths were reported during the forty-four-month span, of which 2,249 were verified as due to cancer. Dr. Hammond never smoked as many cigarettes in his life as he did while he was writing the report on the project. By 2:00 A.M., one morning, his ashtray was heaped several inches high with cigarette butts. He read what he had written and he stopped smoking cigarettes forever.

The study found that the total death rate from all causes among cigarette smokers was twice that of nonsmokers, and nearly double that of pipe and cigar smokers. It showed that the death rate increased in direct ratio to the number of cigarettes smoked. Heavy cigarette smokers had approximately nine times the death rate from lung cancer as did men who had never smoked. Even moderate cigarette smokers had to pay in sad coin for their habit. They had a death rate from lung cancer four times as great as men who had never smoked.

The report attracted wide attention. *The New York Times* published it in full, even the charts and tables. Dr. Hammond was asked to read it at the annual convention of the American Medical Association. It also brought down on Hammond's head the collective curses of the tobacco industry. The industry's defenders accused him of scientific incompetence, innumerable statistical sins, and a vicious bias against cigarettes.

Reinforcements arrived quickly from London when Drs. Richard Doll and A. Bradford Hill published the results of a study they had made of the smoking habits of forty thousand British physicians, thirty-five years old and up.

"Mild smokers are seven times as likely to die of lung cancer as nonsmokers; moderate smokers are twelve times as likely to die of lung cancer as nonsmokers; immoderate smokers are twenty-four times as likely to die of lung cancer as nonsmokers," the Britons found.

Yet the disbelievers remained. The sale of cigarettes, which had declined precipitously when the Hammond-Horn report first came out, mounted again, and the incidence of lung cancer continued to climb still more. Hammond resolved to go after statistical proof of the relationship between cigarette smoking and lung cancer that would be so convincing that no reasonable person could question it. In 1959, he launched the biggest medical investigation ever undertaken.

This was the study in which 68,116 A.C.S. volunteers enlisted 1,057,398 men and women between the ages of thirty-five and eighty-four in twenty-five states, secured their medical histories, and checked on them once a year for six years. The precise cause of death of every one who died (75,000 of them) was searched out and verified. It was, among other things, the first study ever to look into the effects of cigarette smoking on the health of women.

The study revealed the shocking consequences of smoking both to the heart and the rest of the cardiovascular system and as a cause of cancer. As will be shown in a late chapter, it found that cigarette smoking was a paramount cause of cardiovascular disease in men and women.

At the same time, this study of 459,145 men and 598,253 women proved beyond contradiction that smoking cigarettes caused cancer of the lungs. The statistics were gruesome. The death rate from lung cancer among men between forty-five and sixty-four who smoked cigarettes regularly was seven and a half times greater than that of nonsmokers. The death rate from lung cancer of women of all ages who smoked cigarettes regularly was more than twice that of women who didn't smoke.

The A.C.S. study also showed that cigarette smoking was a major cause of cancer of the mouth, pharynx, larynx, esophagus, and pancreas, and of a disease that can be even more horrible than cancer—emphysema.

There could be no more legitimate questioning now of the statistical proof of cigarettes' cancer guilt.

Some scientists had remaining doubts, though. They said to Dr. Hammond, "You haven't given us laboratory proof yet that cigarettes can produce lung cancer."

A pathologist named Dr. Oscar Auerbach settled those last doubts.

Dr. Auerbach is a senior medical investigator at the Veterans Administration Hospital in East Orange, New Jersey. He is a grey-haired, broad-shouldered man with heavy glasses who was born in 1905 and got his M.D. at New York Medical College. I found him a very enthusiastic, friendly individual. His staff worships him.

"I'm curious about everything," he said. "If I go upstairs to the lab and there's a package on the table, I have to open it. It's the feeling of wanting to see what it is, of wanting to explore."

Although he was well known for research in tuberculosis, he switched to cancer in 1953 because he wanted a new challenge. He had been a friend of Dr. Hammond for decades and collaborated with him on several research programs. Under Hammond's watchful eye, he started one of the oddest projects that cancer men have ever essayed. He taught dogs how to smoke cigarettes.

In 1967, Auerbach purchased 480,000 cigarettes and ninety-seven pedigreed beagle dogs. Tracheotomies were performed on all the dogs, and eighty-six of the ninety-seven were trained to smoke cigarettes. They were placed in special smoking cages where they breathed in smoke from lighted cigarettes through tubing connected to the breathing devices in their chests.

A small pump blew the smoke in intermittent puffs. Between each five puffs, the tube was clamped off, allowing the dog to breathe in fresh air. In a few weeks, the dogs became habituated to smoking cigarettes and enjoyed it. Their tails wagged merrily, and they jumped into the "smoking cages" without urging. The pumps were turned off and they inhaled the smoke voluntarily.

After 867 days, the fifty-eight surviving dogs were put to death. Autopsies showed that terrible things had happened to the lungs of many of them. In one group of twelve dogs that had smoked nonfiltered cigarettes, for example, eight had developed invasive malignant tumors in their lungs. The carcinogenic aftermath of cigarette smoke on the lungs was beyond dispute.

As the information on the hazards of cigarette smoking became known, thousands of people asked, "Is it too late to quit cigarettes after I've smoked them for many years?"

Auerbach proved that it was never too late to give up smoking. He paired seventy-two men who had smoked heavily for ten years or more and given up the habit for at least five years with seventy-two smokers of the same age, location, and occupation. He discovered that the incidence of lung cancer in the men who had given up smoking was one-fortieth that of the men who went on smoking.

Dr. Auerbach is at the hospital by 4:15 A.M., stays until 4:30 P.M., then often works with his microscope at home until midnight. That's seven days a week.

"I haven't had a vacation in fifteen years and I don't want one," he said. "I consider medicine a hobby."

"Are you interested in money?"

"No. For me to think that in the field of cigarette smoking, I have been responsible for saving lives is a very considerable feeling. Money can't bring you that."

He and his wife, Dora, have been married since 1932. They have two sons.

"Doesn't your wife resent your working a nineteen-and-a-half-hour day?"

He grinned. "There are times when she may be a little impatient."

Dr. Hammond works an average schedule at his office but usually takes home an attaché case full of A.C.S. papers. In his free evenings, he loves to look through a microscope. At anything, he said. He still likes to take apart electrical gadgets and to build radio sets. He has three children by his first marriage. Recently, he married again, to Katherine S. Redmond.

He smokes a pipe, but swears that he doesn't inhale.

The vast Hammond study of smoking habits—and deaths—among a million people, together with Auerbach's smoking-dog experiments, changed the world's view of cigarette smoking and lung cancer. Cigarette advertising was legally banned from television in the United States, and it became mandatory for printed advertising to carry warnings of the serious consequences of cigarette smoking. Abroad, other nations took similar action. Unprecedented triumphs, these, of the national conscience over industrial and political interests.

At the end of my interview with Dr. Robert Good at Sloan-Kettering, he was talking of his first years on a pediatric service in Minneapolis. The wards were filled with children frightfully sick with pneumonia, polio, kidney failure, rheumatic fever, and congenital heart disease.

"We lost a lot of kids," he said sadly. "But, thank God, every one of those health problems was solved by the great medical revolution that took place in the forties and fifties."

He leaned forward in his chair. "Mark my words. We're now in the beginning of a new medical revolution that will eventually permit us to control cancer and a lot of other diseases that are still plaguing us."

It may even come to pass in the next twenty-five years, he said.

6

THE WAY TO A
HUMAN'S HEART

THERE IS A MYSTIQUE TO the heart. Of all of man's organs, it is the most
dramatic. Since the start of time, poets, philosophers, and scientists have
viewed it with near-religious reverence. They have described it as the
capital of life, the soul, the emotions, the intellect. Aristotle insisted that
the heart was the domicile of thought and sensation.

In actuality, the heart is a simple four-chambered pump, shaped like a
pear, that hangs in the center of the chest. It is about six inches long and
weighs about twelve ounces, but it is the most powerful, durable pump that
has ever been built. Hour after hour, it keeps blood moving through sixty
thousand miles of blood vessels that range in size from the great aorta, as
big around as a garden hose, to capillaries so small that red blood cells can
only get through them one by one. In a normal lifetime, a man's heart
pumps 34,000,000 gallons of blood that weights 150,000 tons. It beats
more than 2,600,000,000 times.

The heart is such a vital organ, Aristotle said, it could never contract any
disease. The statistics tell a sadder story. The diseases that attack the heart
and cardiovascular system are the most deadly enemies we have. In 1973
there were 1,062,160 deaths from cardiovascular diseases in the United
States. That amounted to 54 percent of all deaths in the United States.
Some 685,000 Americans die annually of coronary attacks alone. Many of
them suffer excruciating agony; they feel as though a maddened elephant
were trampling on their chests.

Still, remarkable gains have been made in the battle against cardiovascular diseases.

The first time a surgeon purposefully operated on a human heart was in October 1872. A thirty-one-year-old man whose initials were J.E. got into a knock-down brawl in a London pub. Afterward, he couldn't find a needle he kept in the left side of his coat. He stopped in at St. Bartholomew's Hospital and told the doctors about it. They didn't see any wound and he went back to work.

Nine days later, he was in bad pain. Frightened, he returned to the hospital, and a surgeon named George Callender decided to operate. He made a neat incision between the ribs at a spot over the heart where he thought the needle had gone in. He saw no trace of the needle, so he cut into the heart again at another spot. This time, he pulled out a needle almost two inches long. J.E. recovered.

That was as far as heart surgery got for the next half century. The leading surgeons threatened professional ostracism to any surgeon who dared so much as to touch a heart. Save for an occasional operation to stitch up a stab wound, the heart was off limits to surgeons until the 1930s.

The Catheter Explores the Heart

A German, a Frenchman, and an American made surgery on the heart feasible. The German was Dr. Werner Theodor Otto Forssmann, who was born in Berlin in 1904. He had the wild notion that it might be possible to investigate the inside of a diseased heart by sticking a catheter—a thin rubber tube—into it. One night in 1929, he clandestinely punctured a vein in his arm and talked a fellow resident into working a catheter up into it. With a little more than a foot of the tube inserted into the vein, his friend refused to continue. It was too dangerous. A week later, Forssmann tried again. He did it all himself except for a nurse who held a mirror that let him watch the tube's progress on a fluoroscope. Bit by bit, Forssmann wormed twenty-five and a half inches of the tube up his elbow vein into the right atrium of his heart.

Forssmann's aim was to inject a radioactive substance through the catheter into the heart for diagnostic purposes. But that was as far as he had thought the plan through. The criticism by his German colleagues was so harsh (they called him a clown) that he quit research and became a run-of-the-mill surgeon. He joined the Nazi party and did eugenic sterilizations on anti-Nazis.

The American, Dickinson W. Richards, and the Frenchman, André F.

Cournand, took Forssmann's idea and made it into one of medicine's finest tools.

Richards was born in Orange, New Jersey, in 1895, and got an M.D. from Columbia University in 1923. In 1931, he started a close friendship with André Cournand that endured for forty-one years.

Dick Richards was as American as apple pie and ice cream. After more than four and a half decades in the United States, Cournand is still Gallic, with a conspicuous French accent and French mannerisms. He was born in Paris in 1895, the son of a physician. At nine, he made up his mind to be a surgeon. A teacher complained to him of trouble with her gallbladder.

"Do not worry yourself, madame," André promised her. "When I will be a big man, I will remove your gallbladder for you."

He was a medical corpsman at the front in World War I, bandaging wounds, carrying stretchers, burying the dead. In 1930, he obtained his M.D. at the Sorbonne and sailed to New York City for a year's training on the chest service at Bellevue Hospital. He liked the United States so much that he stayed and became a citizen.

I saw Dr. Cournand in a crowded little office at the Columbia University medical school in New York. He was small, frail, and bent, with a fringe of white hair around his bald head and thick, gold-rimmed glasses. He was wearing a lab coat that was too big for him.

He lectured as if we were in a classroom. "In the course of a clinical observation, if something doesn't respond exactly to the hypothesis you had when you started, you must always follow the new idea."

Richards and he were investigating how the respiratory gases in the lungs interact with the blood. They read Forssmann's report. Wouldn't it be wonderful, they thought, if they could use Forssmann's catheterization technique to get a sample of blood right out of the heart to measure the blood pressure there? In 1936, the pair started experimenting on the hearts of dogs and chimpanzees. To begin, they had to perfect the tube. "It had to be sufficiently stiff to transmit pressures accurately, but not so stiff that its introduction into the heart would be dangerous," Cournand said. They made it out of a woven material reinforced with plastic, about four feet long and as wide across as a small ice cream soda straw. Then they had to refine the Forssmann technique, advancing the catheter inside chimpanzees' hearts, rotating it, pulling it back, and going forward again.

In 1941, Cournand did the first cardiac catheterization on a human at Bellevue. The patient was an old man, very sick with hypertension.

"How nervous were you?" I asked Dr. Cournand.

"Very nervous," he admitted.

The procedure was a success. Cournand and Richards became so adept at doing it that they could keep a catheter in a patient's heart for seven hours at a time. They could pass the catheter through abnormal defects in the wall between the two sides of the heart without causing any clotting. The patients felt nothing.

"A little nick in the arm, that's all," Cournand said.

With this technique, Cournand and Richards could investigate a patient's heart as it had never before been investigated. They could measure the volume, pressure, and rate of flow of the blood in the heart, its oxygen content, and the flow of blood through the lungs. They could locate faulty connections between the aorta and the pulmonary artery that no one knew existed. They could detect congenital flaws in the hearts of tiny children. Conditions that inevitably spelled death could be diagnosed and remedied.

The three, Forssmann, Cournand, and Richards, were jointly awarded the 1956 Nobel Prize in medicine and physiology for their work. To Cournand and Richards, "It was like a fairy tale," Cournand said. To Forssmann, it was equally gratifying. As a former Nazi, Forssmann could only find work in postwar Germany as a lumberjack. After that, he had to support his wife and six children as a small-town doctor. When he heard about his Nobel Prize, he relaxed. "I feel like a village pastor who is suddenly informed that he has been named a cardinal," he said. Lately, he has published a book saying he meant no harm by joining the Nazis.

A heart attack took Dr. Richards in 1973. Dr. Cournand is going strong in New York City. His first wife died in 1959 and he married a former laboratory assistant in 1963. He is still a mountain climber and an ardent collector of modern art.

Cournand has now embarked on a new venture. He is doing research on the future.

"You can extrapolate from the future to the present," he says. "You imagine a future, you create a future, and then you shape today to match it."

Blue Babies
—*Taussig and Blalock to the Rescue*

While André Cournand and Dick Richards were experimenting on their chimpanzees, something else big was happening in the cardiac field. Dr. Robert E. Gross, a thirty-three-year-old specialist at Children's Hospital in Boston, defied the *diktat* that surgeons must never operate upon the heart. In 1938, he went in to the sick heart of a seven-and-a-half-year-old girl with his scalpel and repaired her ductus arteriosus, the blood vessel that connects the pulmonary artery to the aorta. Its job is to divert blood from the inactive lungs of the child during the embryonic period. After birth, it is supposed to close automatically. If it remains open, it can cause serious infections of the heart. That is what befell the little girl. Dr. Gross closed off her ductus arteriosus and gave her a normal circulation.

"Blue babies" stood a chance now.

You could see them in a few hospitals—sad little babies and children whose lips and fingertips were colored a strange blue because their blood didn't get enough oxygen. Many were so pathetically weak that they couldn't totter across the room. They would go a few faltering steps and squat on the floor, exhausted. These were blue babies who had been born with malformed hearts. The passageways between their hearts and the big pulmonary arteries that carried blood to the lungs for oxygenation were too small or were obstructed. They could look forward to nothing but early death or chronic invalidism.

A tender, compassionate woman physician, who wasn't even a surgeon, devised an operation that has given tens of thousands of these blue babies normal lives. Her name is Helen Taussig.

I met Dr. Taussig on a wild, rainy December afternoon in her homey office at Johns Hopkins Hospital in Baltimore. The records stated that she was in her middle seventies, but she looked to be in her early sixties at the most—very tall, with bright blue eyes and a beautiful profile under her trimly bobbed grey hair. She was charmingly, youthfully dressed in a low-cut blue silk blouse and a blue woolen skirt beneath the usual white lab coat. She poured coffee for me with the elegant grace of an embassy hostess.

She was born in Cambridge, Massachusetts, in 1898, the daughter of a world-famous Harvard economist whom she worshiped. She chose medicine and public health as a career and, naturally, applied for admission to Harvard medical school. The dean had no use for women doctors, so she went to Johns Hopkins medical school. In 1930, she was made chief of the new children's cardiac clinic at Hopkins. She ran it for thirty-three years.

Dr. Taussig was the first to recognize that different malformations can cause different shapes of a child's heart. Her superiors at Hopkins didn't believe her, but she had the X-rays to prove it.

She studied scores of blue babies—"cyanotic" is the medical term for them—throughout their tragic lives. Most of these infants were not dying of cardiac arrest, she found. They were losing their lives to anoxemia—a lack of oxygen.

The pioneering operation on the ductus arteriosus by Dr. Gross came to Dr. Taussig's mind. "Dr. Gross operated and showed that you could close off a blood vessel in the heart," she said. "I said to myself, If you can close off a blood vessel, why can't you put one in?"

In the spring of 1940, she went to Boston to see Gross. "I tried to interest Dr. Gross in building a blood vessel," she said, "but he'd just heard how wonderful it was to close one. Everyone was congratulating him, and nothing seemed more foolish than to turn around and put one in."

Her thought was to build a new passageway from the aorta to a pulmonary artery that would shunt blood into the lung. She believed that the subclavian artery, the trunk of the arterial system that leads to the arm, could be used for this purpose.

The man who was to do this for her joined the Johns Hopkins staff in 1942. He was Dr. Alfred Blalock, a chain-smoking forty-three-year-old Georgian with a national reputation for his surgery on blood vessels. He was medium-tall, slender, with a scholarly face and an explosive temper. Rub his fiery temper against Helen Taussig's New England forthrightness and clashes were certain. Yet the two got along well, in the main.

After Dr. Blalock did his first ductus arteriosus operation at Hopkins, Dr. Taussig made her pitch. "I stand in awe and admiration of your surgical skill," she said to him. "But the really great day will come when you build me a ductus for a child who is dying because too little blood is going to the lungs, not tying one off for a child who is getting too much blood."

"When that day comes," he sighed, "this will seem like child's play."

Her challenge piqued Blalock's professional interest. He tried the idea on dogs—two hundred of them. Actually, most of the dog surgery was done by a black medical technician, Vivian Thomas. Although he operated exclusively on animals, Mr. Thomas was reputed to be the best vascular surgeon in America.

Blalock first tried the operation on a human blue baby on November 29, 1944. The patient was a miserably ill baby girl. At fifteen months of age, she weighed only ten pounds. Dr. Taussig was very worried because the baby was in such bad shape, but Blalock reassured her.

"That's the type of a patient you should try a new operation on," he declared.

With Dr. Taussig looking on, Dr. Blalock made an incision in the baby's puny chest, exposing her tiny heart. It was so small that it was difficult to find the left subclavian artery—"It was just a little matchstick of a vessel," Dr. Taussig said—but Dr. Blalock picked it out, clamped it to halt the flow of blood, slit through it, and tied off the lower end. Next, he cut a miniscule hole in the left pulmonary artery. He drew the lower end of the subclavian artery down, fitted it into the tiny hole he had made in the pulmonary artery, and patiently stitched it in place, therewith bypassing the obstruction to the pulmonary artery. It was a risky business. A lung had to be collapsed throughout the entire procedure, and the pulmonary artery had to be clamped shut for a half hour while Blalock was doing the stitching. The operation took almost three hours. Finally, Blalock removed the clamps. Blood started flowing from the aorta through the bypass, and into the pulmonary artery and the lung. It was a comforting sight.

The outcome was disappointing. The baby survived the operation but had a stormy postoperative course. Although her color improved, she didn't maintain her progress. The subclavian artery was too small to handle the extra blood pressure. A second operation was necessary, and the child died.

On February 1, 1945, Blalock operated on an eleven-year-old girl who was so feeble that she could scarcely walk. This time, he used a larger artery for the bypass, and the little girl made a good recovery. She lived sixteen years, long enough to graduate from college, get happily married, and travel through Europe.

The third operation was performed on February 8, 1945, on a six-year-old boy who was even weaker than the little girl. And bluer. He no longer could walk. This was the operation that really proved the worth of the procedure.

"When Dr. Blalock took off the clamps, he got a terrific hemorrhage," Dr. Taussig recalled. "I thought this time I might have to go down and tell the parents that their child had died. Dr. Blalock warned me that I might. But he located the hemorrhage, controlled it, and sewed it up. When he took the clamps off again, we got a beautiful thrill. The anesthesiologist called out. 'There's a lovely color now!' We walked around to the end of the operating table and there the youngster was, perfectly normal, with high pink lips.''

The little boy awakened from the anesthesia while Blalock was bandaging the gaping wound in his chest. "Is the operation over?" he inquired.

"Yes," Dr. Blalock told him.

"May I get up now?" he asked.

Dr. Taussig smiled at the memory. "We knew then that we'd really won.''

The little boy got a total correction of his anoxemia. He lived healthily for twenty years, and he might be living yet if he hadn't insisted on acting in an amateur production shortly after he had recovered from the flu. His wife begged him not to go on, but he wouldn't listen to her. It was a very exciting play, and he dropped dead on stage.

In six years, the blue baby operation was performed a thousand times at John Hopkins, and 780 patients survived. Ninety-three percent of them lived ten years; 88 percent lived fifteen years; and 80 percent lived twenty years.

Dr. Taussig got to be the most honored woman doctor alive. President Lyndon B. Johnson presented her with the Medal of Freedom, the highest civilian award of the U.S. government, and the French government made her a Chevalier of the Legion of Honor. She received more than twenty honorary degrees. It didn't turn her head. Both she and Blalock persisted at their endless hospital schedules. Occasionally, she would take a few minutes off for gardening—that was all. His only recreation was chopping down trees or a few holes of golf.

Dr. Blalock's wife, Mary, was once asked how he spent his summers. She answered, "Why, he spends them the same way he spends his winters—working."

He worked too hard. He died when he was sixty-five.

Dr. Taussig retired as head of the children's cardiac clinic at Hopkins in 1963, but she continues to put in a full day at the hospital. She just tries to leave at 4:30 P.M. in order to beat the rush-hour traffic. She won't go home if any one of her little patients is in the operating room. It was night when I departed her office, but she was still waiting for a child to come down from the "O.R."

She has not been married. "I've never had any children except the thousands I've taken care of," she smiled.

Why did she work so hard?

She looked off into the distance. "Two things make us scientists work. One is that we live in the future. There is always more ahead. There is always something around the corner. The other thing that probably motivates us is that we want to be wanted. More than anything else in the world, one wants to be wanted, and you've got to contribute something, somewhere, if you are to be wanted. As soon as you drop back, nobody wants you."

It is easy to set off an argument in scientific circles over who made the greater contribution to the successful development of the blue baby operation—Blalock, the daring genius with a scalpel, or Taussig, the original medical thinker. Blalock had the courage to try an untried operation on dying children and the surgical skill to rebuild their faltering hearts. But there would have been no blue baby operation without Helen Taussig's creative thinking. One suspects it was her idea that meant the most. In the sciences as in the arts, creativity assesses high.

An Artificial Valve for the Aorta

Now that a heart could be rebuilt, surgeons everywhere felt free to work inside sickly hearts and blood vessels.

Up in Boston, Robert Gross was a leader again, along with a Swedish surgeon, Clarence Crafoord. Early in 1945, each reported independently that he had cut out an obstructed section of the aorta and sewn the two ends together. When the two ends couldn't be stretched into place, Gross took a piece of an artery out of a corpse and grafted it into the excised aorta. It was the first graft ever used on a blood vessel. A Canadian pioneer, Dr. Gordon Murray, soon inserted grafts in coronary arteries. In June 1948, Dr. Charles Bailey, a talented if flamboyant Philadelphia surgeon, opened a scarred mitral valve. His patient was Claire Ward, a chronic invalid who had been given six months to live. Nine years afterward, Mrs. Ward was gaily scampering upstairs to her second-floor apartment in East Orange, New Jersey. Off in Soviet Russia, Vladamir Demikhov was performing surgical legerdemain. He connected the left internal mammary artery to the left descending artery in dogs. The dogs had normal lives thereafter.

Dr. Charles A. Hufnagel, a thirty-six-year-old Kentuckian, soon developed the first artificial heart valve. It consisted of a small lucite tube containing a float the size of a mothball that rose and fell with the beat of the heart. When the pressure relaxed, the ball sank down and prevented the blood from flowing back from the aorta into the heart.

In September 1952, Hufnagel successfully inserted this artificial heart valve into the descending aorta of a miserably ill thirty-year-old former student nurse at Georgetown University Hospital in Washington, D.C. Her own valve was hopelessly diseased. It couldn't guard the entrance to the aorta from her heart anymore.

Would the new valve stay put, people worried?

"Patients will be able to stand on their heads," Hufnagel promised. Justifiably, time showed.

That same year, a different kind of research was going on off the coast of Alaska. Dr. Paul Dudley White, a famous Boston cardiologist (President Dwight D. Eisenhower was his patient) made the first electrocardiogram of a whale. The sixty-six-year-old White and two associates pulled alongside a two-ton white Beluga whale in a small boat and shot a harpoon into its blubber, with wires trailing back to an EKG machine. They found that the whale's huge heart beat fifteen times a minute. A mouse's heart beats one thousand times a minute, a human heart about seventy.

Gibbon Builds the First Heart-Lung Machine

A French surgeon, André Juvenelle, proved the feasibility of hypothermia—lowering the body temperature to slow the flow of blood through the heart—in 1952. Dr. Juvenelle and two confrères in Sweden kept a dog in icy water until his body temperature was down to fifty-four degrees, then reduced the flow of the dog's blood to one twentieth of its normal volume. It made possible the first open-heart surgery. Surgeons could operate on the heart and see what they were doing, unimpeded by gushing blood.

Hypothermia only allowed a few minutes in an open heart, not enough for complicated surgery. Something was needed that would let a patient live without his heart for several hours while a surgeon was repairing it—some kind of machine that could take over the work of the heart and the lungs. A frustrated poet who became a chest surgeon, Dr. John H. Gibbon, Jr., invented it.

He was sixty-eight years old on the spring morning in 1971 when I met him. Tall, husky, and bald, he had finally retired from surgery and was writing the poetry he had always wanted to write, painting portraits, and enjoying life on a fine estate in Media, Pennsylvania, on the Philadelphia Main Line. He and his wife, Mary, the former medical technician who helped him develop the heart-lung machine, seemed inseparable. They played tennis together every day, always at noon. Two loving dogs, a majestic old collie and a joyous golden retriever puppy, frolicked around us as we talked in the dining room of their 275-year-old grey stone house. Sprays of forsythia framed the windows.

For four generations, Gibbons were surgeons. John would have preferred to be a poet, but his father pointed out that poetry was a poor way to make a living. So John went to Princeton and to Thomas Jefferson Medical College in Philadelphia.

He was a research fellow under the great Dr. Edward D. Churchill at Massachusetts General Hospital in Boston. (He married Mary while she was a technician for Churchill.) One February afternoon in 1931, a middle-aged woman who had had her gallbladder taken out fifteen days before, felt cruel pains in her chest, accompanied by nausea and vomiting. Her blood pressure dwindled and her pulse raced. It was a massive pulmonary emoblism, and almost sure death. A pulmonary embolus had never been successfully removed in the United States by surgical means.

Every fifteen minutes through an endless night, Gibbon took the woman's blood pressure and pulse. In the morning, Dr. Churchill operated. He clamped off the pulmonary artery, cut out the clot, and closed the opening, all in six and a half minutes, but it was too long. There was no way to keep the woman alive while the flow of blood was halted. She died on the table.

"I kept thinking that we could have saved that poor woman's life," Dr. Gibbon recalled, "if we could just have taken some blue blood out of her veins, put oxygen in, and let the carbon dioxide escape."

He and his wife set to developing a heart-lung machine that would do all three jobs. The hardest part was designing something to do the lung's work: making the blood take up oxygen and give up carbon dioxide. The Gibbons fabricated an apparatus that would have made Rube Goldberg jealous. They made valves by slicing three quarters of the way through rubber corks, leaving little flaps, and boring a hole through the center of the corks to make a channel for the blood. They put finger cots between the valves to pump the blood, squeezing and compressing the cots alternately by compressed air and vacuum. They oxygenated the blood by passing a thin film of it down the inner surface of a vertical rotating cylinder. It was a weird-looking object with its metal, glass, water baths, and electric motors. The plan was to bypass the patient's blood through the machine while surgeons worked on his idle heart and lungs.

Cats were the first animals on which they used it. "I'd go prowling over Beacon Hill at night with tunafish as bait and a gunnysack, to catch any of the stray cats that were swarming over Boston," Dr. Gibbon said.

One night in 1935, they were able to shut off a cat's heart and lungs and keep it alive, for the first time, with their machine.

"My wife and I threw our arms around each other and danced around the laboratory, laughing and shouting," Dr. Gibbon remembered.

None of the cats they used suffered any harm from having their hearts and lungs temporarily turned off. One cat delivered a litter of nine lively kittens a few weeks later.

The Gibbons returned to Philadelphia in 1935, convinced that they had the problem in hand. They had eighteen years to go, though, before they could try their machine on a human. Things got tougher when they progressed to dogs. As late as 1950, 80 percent of their dogs were dying.

Other heart surgeons became impatient. "Come on, Jack," Dr. Blalock said. "When are you going to stop working on dogs and start working on man?"

Gibbon couldn't be rushed. "As soon as I can do it on enough animals without mortality, I'll go ahead. Not before," he insisted.

He first tried the heart-lung machine on a human in 1952. He operated with it on a baby girl who had severe congestive heart failure. The poor little thing was so pathetically small that at fifteen months she weighed only eleven pounds. She died shortly after the operation.

The following year, Gibbon tried again. On May 6, 1953, Cecilia Bavolek, a pretty eighteen-year-old girl with an atrial septal defect—a hole in her heart—was hooked up to Gibbon's heart-lung machine at the Thomas Jefferson University Hospital in Philadelphia. Cecilia had experienced three heart failures in the preceding six months; she would surely have died without this operation. Her heart was completely shut off for twenty-seven minutes as Gibbon and three more surgeons worked on her. (It required six other persons to operate the heart-lung machine.) The hole in her heart was fully repaired, and Cecilia pulled through the operation excellently. Twenty years after, she was flourishing.

That was the extent of Gibbon's triumph. In July 1953, he tried the heart-lung machine in operations on two male cardiac patients. Both died. In despair, Gibbon went back to the laboratory and more work on the machine. Before he could perfect it, someone else, Dr. C. Walton Lillehei, developed a simpler, more dependable heart-lung machine. Nevertheless, no one can take away from John Gibbon the fact that he invented the first successful heart-lung machine.

I've rarely met a more contented man than John Gibbon. "I've always wanted to help people," he said, "and I've always been curious about everything. It's a great combination."

He died of a heart attack while he was playing tennis in February 1973. It was sad news, for he loved living so much.

Lillehei's Contributions
—*From Safe Open-Heart Surgery to Pacemaker*

The taboos were done with. The best surgeons were not afraid of the heart anymore. They had some remarkable new techniques and diagnostic tools to assist them in the struggle against heart disease and its related agonies. They knew the body's great secret: the heart could stand still while they worked on it. The time was ready for someone to come forward and climax this magnificent progress. Dr. Clarence Walton Lillehei was the man. He gave open-heart surgery its first full dimensions as a saver of threatened lives.

Lillehei developed the first fully practical heart-lung machine, designed the first complete artificial valve to be inserted inside a human heart, and invented the first internal pacemaker to keep a limping heart in tempo. Few surgeons have had as many original ideas as he.

I met Dr. Lillehei on an autumn afternoon in his office at the New York Hospital-Cornell Medical Center in New York City. He was a very tall, husky man with dark hair, dwindling in front and very long in the back. Under his white lab coat, he wore a garish yellow striped shirt and necktie. He laughed a lot as he spoke, almost like punctuation.

The Lillehei *curriculum vitae*—ten single-spaced pages of it—listed the titles of 542 medical papers he had written and thirty-two awards he had received, including decorations from the governments of Belgium and Ecuador and an appointment as an honorary admiral of the Texas navy. He was born in Minneapolis in 1918 and graduated from the University of Minnesota medical school just in time for World War II. He made four D-Day landings—in North Africa, in Sicily, at murderous Salerno, and at Anzio. He returned to a surgical residency and research at the University of Minnesota Hospital in Minneapolis under the best surgical teacher of them all, Dr. Owen H. Wangensteen.

Lillehei's biggest problem during his residency was cancer. His own.

"One day, in February 1949," he told me, "I noticed this little lump in front of my ear. I didn't pay much attention to it. I made my own diagnosis that it was probably a common benign tumor of the parotid gland. On Lincoln's Birthday, I said to another surgeon, 'Dave, it's a holiday. Why don't you take this out for me under a local?' He did, and I didn't think about it again. I didn't even look in the book to see what it was." The pathology book, he meant.

The pathologists found that it was a malignant lymphosarcoma—cancer of the lymph nodes. You usually can figure on living one to two years with a diagnosis like that. And Lillehei was only thirty-one years old.

"What did the news do to you psychologically?" I asked him.

"Well, it was a little difficult for a couple of days."

The conventional treatment was X-rays, but Dr. Wangensteen urged Lillehei to gamble on surgery. It was an extraordinary operation. Three teams of surgeons operated on him for twelve hours. One team cut out all the lymph glands from the left side of his jaw. Another team did a radical neck excision. Dr. Wangensteen and a third platoon of surgeons split his breastbone down the center and removed all the lymph glands from the middle of his chest between the lungs, both above and below the heart and the big blood vessels.

By great good fortune, they were able to clean out every trace of the cancer. "I don't know whether they got out all the cancer or just scared it away," Lillehei laughed, "but I've never had any trouble since. I don't even go for a chest X-ray anymore."

The operation taught him something very useful. "I learned how patients feel when they are looking at death," he declared.

A lovely seventeen-year-old girl, Dorothy Eustace, got Dr. Lillehei interested in open-heart surgery. A distant relative of his mother, Dorothy was in the hospital with severe heart failure. At his mother's request, Lillehei visited her and tried to cheer her up. After her death, he watched the autopsy. She had a ventricular septum defect—a small hole in her heart.

My God, here we are, Dr. Lillehei said to himself. We've got good anesthesia, blood transfusions, electrolytes. Operations for cancer can last twelve hours. We can take out all sorts of things. But we can't sew up a stinking little hole in there.

He went to the dog laboratory and started looking for ways to perform open-heart surgery without killing the patient. Gibbon's heart-lung machine gave him hope, but it was obviously too complex to do the job safely.

In March 1954, Lillehei came out with something different, very different. It was clumsy, it was makeshift, but it permitted complicated open-heart surgery. Lillehei took Gregory Glidden, a thirteen-month-old baby boy, to the operating room for surgery to repair a hole between the ventricles of his heart. There he hooked up Greg's heart and lungs to his father's heart and lungs by means of plastic tubes passing through a mechanical pump. The son's used blood was pumped to the father, and clean, oxygenated blood went from the father to the son. In effect, the father's lungs were doing the work of his son's lungs while the pump was performing the functions of the baby's heart.

Greg's heart continued to beat during the operation, but it was in plain view and dry for seventeen and a half minutes while Lillehei closed the hole in it. Although Greg survived the operation by just a few days, the operation was deemed a success. It demonstrated conclusively that open-heart surgery was feasible. By means of this cross-circulation technique, operations inside the heart could last as long as fifty minutes.

The next step followed fast. In June 1955, Dr. Lillehei and Dr. Richard A. DeWall, a colleague at Minnesota, came out with the bubble-oxygenator. It was a beautifully simple affair, consisting of a cheap, disposable artificial oxygenator made of plastic sheeting and an electronically controlled pump. Two catheters took blood from the patient's venae cavae (the large veins that carry blood into the right atrium of the heart) to a mixing unit, where the blood was permeated with little bubbles of oxygen. A debubbler then took out the bubbles, and the oxygenated blood ran into a spiral-shaped reservoir from which it flowed gently back into the patient's femoral artery.

"Of course, everyone else in the world said that the bubble-oxygenator was a death trap," Dr. Lillehei recalled. "They said you'd never get the bubbles out and there wouldn't be any brain left."

"Everyone else" was wrong. Lillehei's buggle-oxygenator worked perfectly, and safely allowed surgeons hours of time, not minutes, with the heart shut down. Open-heart surgery became an international fact.

In 1957, Lillehei inserted the aortic valve he had designed directly into the heart of a fifty-seven-year-old New Zealand woman. (Dr. Hufnagel had placed his valve in the aorta artery outside the patient's heart.) Lillehei's valve was made of an ultrapowerful plastic. The plastic had to be strong inasmuch as a normal aortic valve opens and closes 115,000 times a day. No valve is more important.

"A person would live less than a minute if this valve stopped functioning," Dr. Lillehei declared.

The new valve lasted the New Zealand woman five years before she needed a replacement.

The year 1957 was also the year of an even greater Lillehei contribution: the pacemaker, the admirable little electronic device that can be inserted inside the cardiac patient's chest to jolt his heart electrically to a normal rhythm.

Dr. Paul M. Zoll, a Harvard professor, had the first idea for a pacemaker. His pacemaker sat outside the body, though. It delivered mighty jabs of electric current to the heart through flat electrodes set on top of the chest.

That was too painful. Said Dr. Lillehei, "It took from seventy to a hundred and fifty volts with electrodes on the skin to drive the heart, and the pain was intolerable. You just couldn't do it. You just couldn't keep those electrodes on, not even if you tied them down physically. They burnt the skin."

Lillehei said to himself, Why don't we put the electricity right into the heart? Why don't we put a wire right in the heart?

Lillehei and his staff rigged up a big electricity-dispensing machine in the operating room. A month later, they were ready when a patient had a heart block during an open-heart operation. They hooked the wires to the patient's heart, and the machine started the heart beating with just two volts of electricity. The difficulty was that they could not move the patient without shifting the whole massive apparatus.

A *bona fide* Horatio Alger story unfolded. "There was a student around who said to me, 'You need a little transistorized box with some batteries in it,' and he promised to build it for me," Dr. Lillehei said. "He always had it half done, but we never saw the box. About three months went by, and a fellow came into the operating room to fix the very modest electronic equipment we had. He had a part-time repair shop in his garage for television sets. His name was Earl Bakk.

"I told him what I needed. Ten days later, he came back with a little box that was just what I wanted. That guy, Bakk, is now president of an electronics company. I saw their last stock statement. He is worth about $30 million."

Lillehei first inserted his little pacemaker inside the chest of a seven-year-old girl. He pierced a hole in her chest wall with a hollow needle and passed an electrode through it directly into her skitterish heart. The pacemaker stimulated the heart to near-normalcy with 1.5 to 1.8 volts of electricity. It didn't pain the child at all.

Today, more than three hundred thousand patients with dangerously irregular heart rhythms are alive and comfortably walking around with pacemakers inside their chests. All you see is a small bulge near the shoulder. Some pacemakers are powered by nuclear energy.

Dr. Lillehei moved to New York City and an appointment as chief of surgery at New York-Cornell Hospital. The transfer did not work out well, and he stepped down to a professorship of surgery.

In 1946, he was married to a nurse, Katherine R. Lindberg. They have three sons and a daughter. He likes golf, skiing, water sports, and dancing, but he said that he wasn't expert at any of them.

What are the motives of a Lillehei?

"A curiosity, a desire to explore the unknown, to do things successfully that haven't been done before," he declared. "Possibly to make money. It's not a motive to be totally ignored or decried. And to achieve fame, I guess."*

Sones Makes Movies Inside the Arteries

One more thing was needed for the open-heart surgeons to do their dexterous best: a diagnostic tool that could tell them exactly where in the

---

*In February 1973, Dr. Lillehei was convicted of income tax evasion. A federal jury found him guilty of omitting more than $250,000 from his tax returns for 1964 through 1968, and of owing more than $125,000 in taxes. One witness at his trial, a gum-chewing prostitute from Las Vegas, testified that a $100 check Lillehei had sought to deduct for "typing expenses" had been paid her for her services to him at a medical convention.

Lillehei faced a twenty-five-year prison sentence. Because of his great medical talents, U.S. Judge Philip Neville placed him on probation for five years provided he agreed to perform "charitable medical services, teaching or an equivalent allied activity," for six months. He agreed. The judge also fined him $50,000.

Lillehei served his sentence at the Brooklyn Veterans Hospital in New York City. His license to practice medicine in Minnesota was restored in 1975 and he returned to St. Paul to practice.

heart to operate. X-rays and fluoroscopes didn't give enough detail for the infinitely delicate surgery that was now possible. A Cleveland cardiologist, Dr. F. Mason Sones, Jr., came up with the solution: coronary arteriography—moving pictures inside the arteries.

I talked with Mason Sones after midnight in a dimly lit, shabby bar in a run-down section of Brooklyn, New York. He had lectured that evening at an overflow meeting of Brooklyn cardiologists, and this was the only place we could find to talk in. I found him medium-tall, stocky, with a pug nose on a very square face. He was a very friendly person, willing to share his innermost feelings.

Sones was born in Baltimore in 1919, a mechanic's son. He chose cardiology as his field while he was at the University of Maryland medical school even though his chief professor urged him against it. The professor thought cardiology was "a nothing specialty."

"There'll never be any great discoveries in cardiology," the professor dourly predicted.

Dr. Sones is now a ranking cardiologist at the highly esteemed Cleveland Clinic. His interest initially was pediatric cardiology. Children enchant him. He lovingly refers to them as "the little people," and says, often, how much he wants to help them.

He started working on coronary arteriography in 1955.

"It upset the hell out of me when I was working on infants with heart disease because I practically had to work in the dark," he said. "The damned fluoroscope didn't show me enough of what I needed to see to make a decent diagnosis."

In the early fifties, a new way to amplify light produced by X-rays was achieved in Holland that gave a thousand times more light. Sones immediately saw that this made movies inside the coronary arteries possible. If only a way existed to combine Cournand and Richards's catheterization with high-speed X-ray motion pictures!

He set to work with cameras, lenses, and lights, about which he knew nothing. The big companies were not very disposed to help him. He went to a huge electronics manufacturer, a household name in America, and asked for help in producing a special closed-circuit television camera. It could save many lives, he pledged.

"How many doctors might buy this?" a company official said.

"Maybe a hundred," Sones answered.

Not interested, they said.

He asked a leading company in the photographic field for assistance in creating a special kind of 35-mm film. "How many doctors might buy it?" a company man inquired.

"I dunno," Sones said. "Maybe two hundred."

Not interested, the company man said. Sones had to fashion the necessary equipment and film himself.

Together with Dr. Earl Shirey, Sones developed a technique for taking a catheter farther than Cournand and Richards dreamed possible. He guided it through the right brachial artery and the heart directly into the openings of the coronary arteries. Then he injected small quantities of dye into these arteries. While the heart was pumping the dye-streaked blood along the arteries, he took movies of it through a fluoroscope image intensifier with the 35-mm motion picture camera and film he had perfected.

Sones tested his coronary arteriography on human patients first in October 1958. His movies clearly showed the precise location of any significant obstruction and lesion in a coronary artery. They revealed how much damage had been done to the artery. The detail they contained was amazing. Sones could follow blood vessels as small as 80 microns in diameter. (A micron is a millionth of a meter.)

Today, coronary arteriography is considered "a must" by most outstanding heart surgeons before they undertake any major operation on the coronary arteries or on the aortic valve, or before operations to improve the blood circulation in cases of brutal angina pectoris.

Some heart specialists claim that coronary arteriography is too perilous. That infuriates Sones. He says it is dangerous only in inept, amateurish hands.

Dr. Sones used to work eighteen hours a day. His compulsive concentration on his research, admittedly, played havoc with his first marriage. It led to a bitter divorce after twenty-three years of marriage and four children. Following five years of unhappy bachelorhood, Sones found a new wife with whom he said he was divinely happy. Now he gets to the hospital no earlier than 8:30 A.M. and makes it a point to drop everything and go home at 7:30 P.M.

Not that he is any less absorbed in his work. "Doing research is like kicking down a door," Mason Sones said in the grubby Brooklyn bar that night. "Every time you kick down one door, you find seven more doors waiting to be kicked down."

The Big Risk Factors Behind Heart Attacks

Back in 1949, the National Heart Institute launched an historic epidemiological study of heart disease in Framingham, Massachusetts, a factory town of 28,000 people which, sociologically and ethnically, represented a cross section of the American population. More than 5,200 men and women between the ages of thirty-six and fifty-nine with no trace of heart disease were selected for the study. For fourteen years, all of them (save 900 or so who died) were given regular physical examinations while their cardiovascular systems were watched with hawk-eyes.

The Framingham study was the first to identify the key "risk factors" that led to heart attacks. It proved that individuals with high levels of cholesterol in their blood, high blood pressure, abnormal electrocardiograms, a "low vital capacity" (that's the amount of air that can be expelled from the lungs), who smoke cigarettes, or who have a history of heart disease in their families, are much more likely to have heart attacks than other people.

The most significant of these "risk factors" were found to be high blood pressure, cholesterol, and smoking.

The study proved that coronary heart disease occurred three to five times as often among people with high blood pressure as among those with normal blood pressure. Furthermore, it proved that the likelihood of a cardiovascular accident—a stroke, in other words—was four times as great among people with hypertension as among those without it.

When you consider that over twenty-three million people in the United States have high blood pressure, you can see how critical this situation is.

Cholesterol is a white fatty alcohol, without taste or odor, that is mainly found in eggs, meat, shellfish, and butterfat. The more you eat of these foods, the higher the cholesterol level in your body, especially if you also eat a lot of saturated fats—the kind that commonly are solid at room temperature. For some strange reason, saturated fats make the level of cholesterol in your blood rise.

The higher your blood cholesterol level, the more probable it is that atherosclerotic plaques will form on the walls of your arteries and choke off your blood flow.

Medical scientists have been concerned about cholesterol since 1913, when a twenty-eight-year-old Russian pathologist Nikolai Anchkov, served some rabbits a cholesterol-high fat diet. His bunnies soon were suffering from serious hardening of their arteries. No one could be sure, though, that rabbits and humans would respond alike to cholesterol.

The findings at Framingham showed that they did.

Incidentally, the Framingham findings on the harm done to the heart by cigarette smoking were incontrovertibly confirmed by the great American Cancer Society study of 1,057,398 people in 1959-1965. It established that the death rate from aortic aneurysms among men between forty-five and sixty-four years of age who smoked regularly was nearly three times as great as that for men who never smoked regularly. For men between sixty-five and seventy-nine who smoked regularly, the death rate from aortic aneurysms was almost five times as great.

Almost three times as many men between forty-five and sixty-four who smoked regularly were dying of coronary heart disease as men who didn't smoke. Among women forty-five to sixty-four who smoked regularly, the death toll of coronary heart disease was twice as high as that of women who had never smoked regularly.

Nor was that all that cigarettes were guilty of. It was discovered that cigarette smoking was a major cause of emphysema, a horrible respiratory disease that chokes people to death. Among the men forty-five to sixty-four years of age with a cigarette-smoking history in this study, the death rate from emphysema was more than six and a half times that of nonsmokers. Among men sixty-five to seventy-nine, the emphysema death rate was eleven times as big.

Dangerous things, cigarettes.

Drugs that Control Hypertension

The horror is that so many die of heart attacks, strokes, and other cardiovascular disturbances. The wonder is that so many millions of people with diseased hearts and circulatory systems can now live full, normal lives. Several drugs have helped mightily here.

Let us start with Dr. Edward R. Freis. When a Lasker Award for Clinical Research was presented to Freis in 1971, the citation read, ''Dr. Freis has demonstrated the lifesaving effectiveness of the use of drugs in the treatment of moderate hypertension, and the dramatic reduction of deaths from stroke and congestive heart failure which can be realized when blood pressure is kept within normal limits. . . .'' It was a demonstration that was urgently needed. Until Freis did his stint, most doctors ignored moderate high blood pressure in their patients. They didn't realize that it could kill them.

Dr. Freis, a short, cheerful man with longish, greying hair, was born in 1912 in Chicago. He had a wealthy father who wanted him to go into his real estate business, and he might have if he hadn't watched some of his fraternity brothers at the University of Arizona dissect a cat. It interested him in medicine and he got an M.D. at Columbia. During a residency in Boston, he started research on drugs that might help hypertensive patients.

"I'm a very patient guy," he remarked. "You realize that I've stuck to the same thing from 1946 to the present. That's a long time."

Today, Dr. Freis is senior medical investigator at the Veterans Administration Hospital in Washington, D.C., a position created by the V.A. just for him. We talked in his wood-paneled office at the rear of the hospital. He was wearing stained slacks, a blue checked shirt, and a green woolen tie. A very relaxed man.

In 1946, he said, physicians, by and large, had no use for drugs for hypertension. They didn't think that any drug would ever affect high blood pressure. Freis's chief, Dr. James A. Shannon, had some faith in chemotherapy, though, and he had Freis investigate a drug called penaquin. Freis was to try it only on patients desperately ill with hypertension, too far gone for surgery.

"I gave it to one physician from California who had malignant hypertension. He was horribly depressed over the fact that there was no hope for him. I gave him the penaquin and his blood pressure came right down. The signs of malignant hypertension in his eye blood vessels cleared up. So did his congestive heart failure. It was almost unbelievable. Unfortunately, his kidney damage was so far advanced that we couldn't keep him going. But he did survive long enough to go back to California, and he was much more comfortable than he would have been.

"Seeing the changes in that man's eyes was a tremendously exciting thing to me. I said, 'Golly, this is it. We're on the right track.' But I couldn't get anyone else excited about it. When I talked about it at medical meetings, the other physicians thought I was a charlatan. Or they thought I was a sincere but overly enthusiastic young man. The drug was too toxic to be used, they insisted. It took five years before people began to believe that you could treat malignant hypertension with drugs."

As Freis continued his research, he became convinced that the best way to treat the consequences of hypertension was to prevent blood pressure from getting too high.

In 1964, he inaugurated a research project that changed most cardiologists' concept of high blood pressure. He organized a study of 523 middle-aged men with varying degrees of hypertension in seventeen Veterans Administration hospitals. They were all carefully checked to make sure that they were conscientious types who could be depended upon to take their pills regularly.

The study lasted five years, and it proved that moderate hypertension was a potentially fatal disease. Left untreated, it led to cerebral hemorrhages, congestive heart failure, kidney collapse, and more.

But drug treatment, the evidence showed, could completely alter the outcome in cases of both mild and severe hypertension. Among patients with severe hypertension, the risk of death fell from one in five to practically zero if the right antihypertensive drugs were used. Proper medication reduced the risk of serious complications—strokes, congestive heart failures, kidney failures, and the like—for people with moderately high blood pressure by as much as 300 percent. It could prevent these complications in two out of every three people with moderate hypertension.

"The impact of this study was fantastic," Dr. Freis said. "The academicians simply couldn't argue the thing anymore. They used to say that you were not treating the patient when you lowered his blood pressure. You were just treating the blood pressure monometer. They couldn't use that argument anymore."

Freis is one researcher who lives a resasonable life. He works from 8:30 A.M. to 4:30 P.M., five days a week. That leaves time for converting an old schoolhouse in West Virginia into a country home—and for golf. He's very serious about golf. He is a tournament player.

He is married to small, blue-eyed Willa Hussey, whom he met as a student at the University of Arizona. They have three grown children.

He thinks his research is, essentially, an expression of his artistic nature. "Basically, I'm a creative person. If I were a peon in Mexico, I'd probably be doing handicrafts, making silver ornaments."

I said, "A cardiologist in private practice can earn a helluva lot of money in Washington. You could be rich, living in a mansion on Massachusetts Avenue. Yet you prefer research to that?"

"Right."

"Why?"

"My wife isn't demanding. If I'd had a different kind of wife who wanted a higher style of living, I probably wouldn't have done it. We've talked about it. She's told me that she's prouder of me for doing research than if I'd gone into private practice and made mountains of money."

Today, most American medical schools are teaching their students that they cannot safely ignore moderate hypertension in their patients anymore.

Reserpine and chlorothiazide—these are two drugs that have become household words in the medical world in the treatment of hypertension. Many years of research went into their development.

For thousands of years, Indian herb doctors have used *Rauwolfia serpentina*, a climbing vine with lovely pink blossoms and snakelike roots that flourishes on the tropical Himalaya Mountains, for snakebite, cholera, epilepsy, insanity, and a myriad of other conditions. In 1931, Indian physicians began to use *Rauwolfia serpentina* to treat hypertension. They had excellent results and published them in the best Indian medical journals.

No one in the West paid the least attention. In 1949, Dr. Rustom Jal Vakil of King Edward Memorial Hospital in Bombay wrote an article for a British heart journal that reviewed ten years of his careful research with *Rauwolfia serpentina* and cited the supporting views of fifty other Indian physicians. At last, Western medical men woke up.

In 1952, three scientists at the Ciba pharmaceutical company in Basel, Switzerland—Drs. J. M. Muller, Emil Schlitter, and Hugo J. Bein—isolated reserpine, the specific element in the herb that reduces blood pressure. Across the Atlantic Dr. Robert W. Wilkins, a forty-six-year-old cardiologist at the Boston University medical school tested it. He found that reserpine greatly helped his hypertensive patients.

Western medicine had finally caught up with traditional Indian herb medicine. Since then, reserpine has helped millions of people in the Western world to control their high blood pressure.

Chlorothiazide is a double-barreled weapon against cardiovascular disease. It relieves the body of the oceans of excess fluid that come from kidney and liver diseases or congestive heart failure, and it helps to restore normal blood pressure in hypertension.

The scientists at Sharp & Dohme Research Laboratories in West Point, Pennsylvania, who developed it, were not looking to do any of those things in the beginning. And they certainly weren't hunting for a drug that would help control gout, which they found along the way. They were seeking a drug that would retain penicillin in the body longer. Patients were excreting it in their urine so fast that its effects were being squandered. That was in the mid-1940s, when penicillin was in such short supply that hospitals were retrieving it from patients' urine and using it over again.

The Sharp & Dohme quartet that discovered chlorothiazide consisted of a couple of chemists, Drs. James M. Sprague and Frederick C. Novello, Dr. Karl H. Beyer, Jr., a physician and pharmacologist, and Dr. John E. Baer, another pharmacologist. That was no coincidence.

"I'd like to stress the game of intellectual Ping-Pong that goes on between the chemists and the pharmacologists," Dr. Sprague said to me. "The chemist has an idea, the pharmacologist evaluates it, turns back the results and some ideas of his. The chemist takes these and incorporates them into his thinking, and passes them back to the pharmacologist to evaluate all over again until they can come up with something valuable."

Just for the record, let it be noted that Dr. Sprague was born in 1908, Dr. Novello in 1916, Dr. Beyer in 1914, and Dr. Baer in 1917.

After years of basic research on the kidney, Beyer recognized the same excretion pattern in penicillin and para-aminhippuric acid. He got an idea that one might compete with the other. Perhaps if you administered them together to a patient, the para-aminhippuric acid would block the egress of the penicillin, like two molecules trying to get out of the same hole at the same time.

The theory turned out to be true. Para-aminhippuric acid did block the excretion of penicillin. However, it took vast amounts of the acid to do so. The Sharp & Dohme men, therefore, set out to find an agent that would do a more effective job. Their quest led them to a new type of benzoic acid called probenecid that served the purpose admirably.

It was ironic. By the time they had found probenecid, the need for it was gone. Penicillin was in ample supply. Probenecid was just another new drug looking for a disease to cure.

Quite by accident, it achieved a role for itself. Probenecid has a very provocative property. It facilitates the excretion of uric acid by the kidneys. At the outset, no one could see any practical worth to this, but a few years later, it was discovered that the elimination of uric acid was important to the control of gout. Immediately, probenecid became a drug of choice for this purpose.

"There's a hell of a lot of luck involved in this business," Dr. Sprague said.

Meanwhile, Beyer and his associates were off on a new quest—for a diuretic, a drug that would help get rid of the excess fluid in a patient's body by increasing his output of urine. It was needed urgently. Aside from mercury compounds, which had serious side effects, medical science had no diuretic that could do this with effectiveness.

Beyer and the others made big demands of their diuretic. It had to eliminate chloride as well as sodium from the body since it is sodium chloride—salt—that keeps fluid in the body tissues. It had to be administered by mouth. It had to finish its work in the daytime so the patient could sleep at night. Instead of screening thousands of chemicals as researchers generally do, they decided to tailor-make a compound to their specifications.

Dr. Novello was the man who did the creative chemical work inside the laboratory, maneuvering the molecules of the various chemicals under Sprague's direction. It was a heartbreaking task for him. Years of work and millions of dollars went into it without results. The powers-that-be at Merck, Sharp & Dohme (Sharp & Dohme merged with Merck & Co. in 1953) nearly canceled out the whole project because it looked so hopeless. Then in 1955, Novello created a new compound called chlorothiazide that seemed to work. Dr. Baer tried it on a hundred dogs and every dog excreted streams of fluid with sodium and chloride. As an added dividend, the new compound seemed to increase the effects of other drugs against hypertension.

The first human patient received chlorothiazide in November 1956. He was a sixty-year-old man hospitalized for congestive heart failure and hypertension, so short of breath that he could scarcely breathe. His feet and ankles were swollen grotesquely, and his blood pressure was dangerously high, 196/144. Digitalis and rauwolfia didn't help him.

On November 15, he was given chlorothiazide along with the other two drugs. In one week, he had urinated away ten pounds of fluid. In the following five weeks, he lost ten more pounds. The shortness of breath and the swelling disappeared. His blood pressure dropped to 148/110. Five years afterward, he was still doing well.

The introduction of chlorothiazide into medical practice in 1958, under the brand name of Diuril, transformed the treatment of congestive heart failure and hypertension.

All four scientists were still with Merck, Sharp & Dohme Research Laboratories when I visited its rolling Pennsylvania campus, and at least three of them seemed quite content with life. Dr. Beyer, brawny and bald, was the highly paid executive vice-president for research. He proved unique among scientists in the variety of his extracurricular activities. He flew his own twin-engine Cessna, rode horseback, golfed, played the piano, and built handsome furniture for his wife and two daughters.

Dr. Sprague, white-haired and short, was director of medicinal chemistry, with an expensive, paneled office, too. A quiet academic type, he happily divided his spare time between his wife, his grandchildren, and his gardening.

Dr. Baer, medium tall and slender, with white hair, was senior director of drug metabolism. He loved his life with his wife, his four children, and his sailboat.

Dr. Novello, who was granted the actual patent on chlorothiazide, was something else. A short, thin man with greying hair, he was unsmiling, tense, and suspicious while we talked. He relaxed only when he spoke of his wife, a former scientist, their children, and the garden that he loved.

In 1975, all four shared a Lasker Award.

Krasno Finds a Way to Prevent Coronary Attacks

Dr. Louis R. Krasno tried for an even bigger jackpot in the crusade against heart attacks, and he "collected" on it. He proved that there was a drug that could prevent atherosclerosis—a major cause of heart attacks. Its name was clofibrate, and Dr. Krasno showed that it prevented 60-70 percent of coronary attacks.

To his mind, "Prevention is the only logical answer to a disease that does not give you a second opportunity—because twenty-five to thirty percent of people die of heart attacks in the first hour before they even get to the hospital."

Dr. Krasno is director of clinical research for United Airlines. I found him a stocky, good-looking man with iron-grey hair. Were it not for his shiny, dark eyes, you would never guess that he has Gypsy blood in him. You feel very comfortable with him. He acts like your family physician.

He is a very neat man, carefully dressed, with a very orderly office in the medical building at the United Airlines base at San Francisco International Airport. The walls are covered with framed diplomas, tributes, and photographs of him in U.S. Navy uniform taken while he was serving on an aircraft carrier.

His father was a fur trapper in Rumania who emigrated to the United States, made money as a fur tanner, and lost it all in the 1929 crash. Louis, born in 1914, was very close to him. He resolved to be a heart doctor as a boy when he saw his father almost die of a massive coronary attack.

"I'll never forget that night. The doctor called the whole family in to talk to my father because he was afraid he might be gone by morning."

Krasno got a Ph.D in physiology and an M.D. at Northwestern University. He was in private practice for a while, and in 1957 went to United Airlines to do research. He needed a healthy captive audience for what he had in mind.

Drugs were known that helped, somewhat, to counteract the strangling effects of atherosclerosis after it had developed. But there was no way known to keep atherosclerosis from developing, except the ordinary things like diet and exercise that most people find impossible. The pharmacists had nothing on their shelves that could keep cholesterol from running rampant with dangerous atherosclerotic consequences.

After years of preliminary investigation, Krasno decided in 1963 to match clofibrate against cholesterol. It was a synthetic drug created by Dr. J.M. Thorp, a Britisher, and its effectiveness in lowering high serum cholesterol and triglyceride counts had been demonstrated by several physicians. However, they had used it only on people who had experienced heart attacks or whose cholesterol levels were already alarmingly high. No one had tested it for preventive purposes.

Krasno used his captive audience at United Airlines for the test. He enlisted over 3,200 of the airline's male ground employees in San Francisco between the ages of thirty and sixty and gave them all very thorough physical examinations—blood tests, X-rays, EKGs, everything. For the next eight years, each participant got an examination annually. Rarely has so extensive a study been so well orchestrated. Sixty-seven men with heart disease and a thousand and one without it, whose average age came to 47.5 years, were divided into two groups and pair-matched for risk factors such as age, blood pressure, cholesterol level, EKG results, weight, cigarette smoking, and alcohol consumption, even urban versus suburban living. Approximately half received the brownish clofibrate capsules four times a day; half remained untreated.

Two more groups were formed of the 2,100 younger men without any evidence of heart disease. Their average age was 37.5 years. The men in one of these groups received clofibrate; the others got none.

The study started in 1964. In January 1972, Dr. Krasno reported his first results in the *Journal of the American Medical Association*. They were impressive.

Among the older men who had taken clofibrate, the heart attack rate was less than one-third that of the men who had not taken it—1.89 versus 6.6 per 1,000 each year. The difference was even more striking among the younger men. The heart attack rate for the men who didn't take clofibrate was 5 per 1,000 each year. For those who did, it was only .64 per 1,000 each year. That was one-eighth as much.

The men who took clofibrate were spared 70 percent of the heart attacks they probably would have suffered without it.

Heart men were enthusiastic over Dr. Krasno's news. Thousands of requests for reprints rained on him from Russia to Rhode Island. The American Heart Association called the study "a real step forward!" The eminent cardiologist Dr. Irvine Page heartily endorsed Krasno's findings. He had been on clofibrate himself for five years, he said. His wife was taking it, too.

Curiously, clofibrate has not yet proven to be helpful for persons who have had a heart attack before. It does not deter them from having a second attack. It may be of great value in forestalling strokes, though. The early data suggests to Krasno that clofibrate is as effective in averting strokes as it is with many heart attacks. It has eliminated 70 percent of strokes, so far.

A marathon worker, Dr. Krasno reaches his airport office at 5:30 A.M. and stays till 4:00 P.M., with no lunch—he doesn't take time out for it. At four o'clock, he goes home and labors hours more. He and his singer-wife, Elaine, have been married for more than three decades. They have one son.

Krasno is a gifted violinist who has recorded for Decca with an excellent San Francisco trio. His special interest is Gypsy music. Whenever he goes to Europe, he tries to unearth authentic Gypsy melodies.

"I want to preserve the Gypsy musical idiom," he told me. "It would be a shame to lose it. It is very romantic and nostalgic. It has great excitement."

There is an ancient Gypsy superstition that says—these are Krasno's words—"When a performer and audience are united as one, then Duende, the Romany Devil, visits the musicians and makes them play above their heads."

Krasno said that it's true. It's happened to him. But Duende rates no credit for Krasno's medical research.

The greatest heart doctors are still to make their appearance in this book: surgeons who can clean the muck out of your choked blood vessels, or create new blood vessels for you; surgeons who can take a beating heart out of a dead person and set it to work inside your body. Many of these surgeons look bigger than life, bigger than death even, while they compete for public acclaim with scalpels inside your body.

7

A HEART FOR A HEART

IT WAS HOUSTON, TEXAS, ON a chilly afternoon in April. I was watching Michael Ellis DeBakey, the famed pioneer in heart surgery, operate at glistening Methodist Hospital.

A white-haired old man lay stretched out, anesthetized, on an operating table in a large green-colored operating room, his body slit open from his groin to the breastbone. Most of his abdominal organs were slung out over the outside of his body haphazardly, like reddish bean bags.

I was standing next to Dr. DeBakey, a gaunt-faced little man in his sixties, amid a cluster of assisting surgeons and nurses in green scrub suits. I moved to the other side of the table and looked down into the old man's belly. He had an aneurysm—a horrible big bulge in his aorta where the weakened wall of the artery had ballooned outward. Blood was oozing from it. He would have been dead in another week.

Dr. DeBakey cut through the aorta. A geyser of blood shot up in the air and hit me in the face. The blood smeared my eyeglasses red.

Swiftly, DeBakey clamped off the flow. He laid a long stretch of fine-spun Dacron pipe inside the old man's belly and started to suture it to the healthy portions of the aorta with little black stitches. He was making a detour for the old man's blood around the aneurysm, utilizing a bypass he had invented.

I glanced at a clock on the wall. It was 5:00 P.M. This was Mike DeBakey's sixth major operation since 7:30 that morning. He hadn't even taken a moment for lunch.

"Are you tired?" I asked across the operating table.

"I haven't done enough yet to be tired," he growled.

He operated until ten o'clock that night.

It was midnight when DeBakey got home. At 4:30 A.M., he was back in the hospital, writing a medical paper. I met him at 7:30 A.M. in his small cluttered office. He looked older and more haggard than ever. Proudly, he enumerated his accomplishments to me. Then he spoke of his bitter feud with Dr. Denton A. Cooley, once his student but now his rival for recognition as the best heart surgeon in the world. He despised Cooley. He scornfully said that Cooley was a mediocre surgeon.

Houston, on an icy winter evening. I was making rounds with Denton Cooley in the magnificent Texas Heart Institute that was built especially for him. This was the Cooley who had implanted the first artificial heart into a living man, who had done the first successful heart transplant in America. He is probably the deftest, fastest heart surgeon on earth.

I found Cooley tall, fair-haired, and handsome, as friendly as DeBakey was irritable. "Dr. Wonderful," his scrub nurses called him. It had been a slow day for him. He had only done fourteen major operations because he had to see his dentist. The following day, he had nineteen operations scheduled. Some estimates place his income at $100,000 a week.

Ten white-coated residents and other doctors trailed after him as he strode briskly from room to room. To the bedside of a young girl gasping for breath. To a fat, middle-aged man whose belly was distorted uglily by an embolism. To an old woman with merely a stump of a leg left her by her shattered circulation. To some who appeared healthy although their hearts were close to death. They all looked imploringly at Dr. Cooley as he walked into their rooms.

He promised each of them, "Don't worry. We'll take good care of you."

He saw thirty patients in forty minutes.

Later, we talked for hours. He proudly enumerated his attainments. He spoke openly of his celebrated feud with DeBakey.

I asked him. "Would you let Dr. DeBakey operate on your heart?"

He thought for a moment. "Yes—if he didn't know it was me."

A ghetto neighborhood in Brooklyn, New York, on a sultry summer afternoon. I was sitting with Dr. Philip N. Sawyer, a burly, bald man, in a drab office at the New York State University Downstate Medical Center. Sawyer was another of the world's distinguished cardiovascular surgeons and had no doubt of it. He developed the revolutionary gas endarterectomy procedure utilizing jet streams of carbon dioxide to loosen fatty deposits that clog coronary arteries.

"How do you feel when a patient dies?" I asked him.

"God, horrible," he replied in his broad Maine accent. "It's an insult to the doctor's ego, if nothing else. He's lost a battle in this continuing fight to prove that mankind has some function on the earth. That's what it's really all about. All the rest of it is just so much garbage. What a physician is doing is trying to prove in this world of paradoxes that man has some function in the universe. That man isn't just a funny bunch of blubbery protoplasm. That man is a mean, irascible, tough, malignant, carnivorous, hunting, murdering son-of-a-bitch. . . ."

"With ideals?"

"With ideals. The last remaining vestige of man's humanity to man is the commitment of one man to the salvage of another man's health."

DeBakey, Pioneer in Cardiovascular Surgery

Thin, waxen-faced Dr. DeBakey may be the best heart surgeon of all. Certainly, he likes to think so.

Unquestionably, he has a high degree of genius in his head and his hands, along with vision and guts. His energy and drive are almost beyond credulity. He can put in a nineteen-hour day, examining, operating, making rounds, writing, politicking, and be back in his hospital at 4:30 A.M. the next morning, ready for nineteen more hours. His idea of a vacation is more work. He says he went fishing once and was bored to pieces. He can be gentle with his frightened patients and cruelly choleric to his fellow doctors and nurses. His conceit and his appetite for publicity are colossal, yet he is an honest liberal, genuinely anxious to provide better, cheaper medical care to poor people.

Dr. DeBakey performed the first successful carotid endarterectomy. This is the crucial operation in which the atherosclerotic debris that blocks blood from flowing through the carotid artery to the brain is cleaned out. He created a substitute for sick blood vessels. He devised the roller-pump used in the first heart-lung machine. He built a substitute for the main pumping station to the heart. Beyond that, DeBakey has invented more than fifty surgical instruments, and performed over fifteen thousand critical operations on people's cardiovascular systems, including one on the Duke of Windsor. He took an aneurysm the size of a grapefruit out of the duke's distended belly.

I saw DeBakey all of a Saturday and again the next morning. The first day, I followed him pantingly from operating room to operating room at Methodist Hospital. The next day, we talked in his littered office.

"As far back as I can remember, I wanted to be a doctor," he said. "When I was a little boy, I used to work in my father's drugstores and I met all the doctors in town. They were my heroes."

He was born in 1908 in Lake Charles, Louisiana, the son of a Lebanese businessman who hit it rich in the United States. Michael DeBakey had always liked to do things with his hands. He worked as a carpenter in his teens, did professional drawing, played in the college orchestra. His mother even taught him to sew.

DeBakey became interested in the circulatory system while he was a medical student at Tulane. There must be some way to minimize the need for the heart, he believed. After he received his M.D. in 1932, he became an expert on blood transfusions, and he invented a roller-pump as an aid in blood transfusing. Decades later, he met John Gibbon at a medical meeting. He told him about the roller-pump and Gibbon incorporated it in his heart-lung machine.

DeBakey taught at Tulane, carved out a sizable name with his scalpel, and was invited to head the department of surgery at the Baylor College of Medicine in Houston in 1948. An enthusiastic salesman, he got the local Texas millionaires as excited about heart surgery as they were about football. Houston had to be the heart capital of the world, he told them, and they poured millions into Methodist Hospital for glittering new buildings and heart-saving equipment.

A venturous Portuguese surgeon, Dr. J.C. dos Santos, performed the first endarterectomy in 1947, cutting a sodden clot out of a blood vessel. DeBakey carried the technique to its most delicate extreme in 1953 with his carotid endarterectomy.

The DeBakey operation was intended to prevent a stroke due to a blood clot in any of the four carotid arteries that feed blood to the brain. It was an extremely difficult procedure. For one reason, it was almost impossible to obtain a clear X-ray view of the carotids. For another, after he had scraped out the repulsive porridgelike goo in the artery (calcium and cholesterol, mainly), DeBakey couldn't close up the wound in the usual fashion. That would have narrowed the artery and raised the risk of a later blockage. He had to enlarge the artery by inserting a patch of Dacron in the slit.

A school-bus driver who had been having a series of little strokes underwent the first carotid endarterectomy. Following the operation, his strokes stopped.

DeBakey went searching for a new material that could be used to patch human blood vessels, or to make new ones. It was a long-term mission with him and many other researchers. The politically evil Frenchman Alexis Carrell* used aluminum and glass tubes lined with paraffin. Other researchers tried tubes contrived of silver, gold, rigid plastics, and flexible plastic sponge. Segments of human blood vessels were the most generally employed. They were obtained from cadavers.

None worked satisfactorily.

DeBakey haunted the morgues to get blood vessels from corpses. "But I was aware that they weren't adequate. I had to have something that you could take off the shelf any time you needed it."

He approached a giant chemical company with a request that they make up a new material for him that could move blood around a human body without leaking or clotting.

"They wouldn't touch it. They were afraid they might be sued for damages if something went wrong."

Through a wealthy patient whose life he had saved, DeBakey got a textile manufacturers' association in Philadelphia to knit the material he wanted—a white, seamless, flexible tubing made of crimped Dacron. The ex-patient donated $15,000 to build the new machinery that was needed.

DeBakey tried the tubing first to get around a blocked aorta in a patient's abdomen. Before the operation, the patient couldn't walk a city block without crippling pain. Ten days after DeBakey had made him a Dacron bypass around his blocked aorta, the patient could walk a mile.

Four years of intense work at the Baylor labs by Dr. DeBakey and Dr. Domingo Liotta, a modest, good-looking surgeon from Argentina, went into the creation of the artificial left ventricle. (Remember that name, Liotta. The mere mention of it can set off violent arguments in Houston medical circles.)

The artificial left ventricle was half of a new heart, enough, DeBakey hoped, to tide over a patient while his natural heart was recovering from surgery.

In essence, the artificial left ventricle was a pump inside a plastic shell the size of a small grapefruit. With its dangling Dacron and silicone tubes, it looked like an octopus. DeBakey gave it a fearsome challenge to start. Michael DeRudder, a sixty-five-year-old coal miner, was dying after twenty-five years of incessant heart trouble. His single chance was a new aortic valve, but implanting one in him was difficult with his sagging heart.

*One of the most innovative surgeons of his time, Carrell spent twenty-eight years at the Rockefeller Institute for Medical Research in New York City, won a Nobel Prize in 1912 for his work in vascular surgery and transplantation, but later became a focus of controversy and opprobrium as a Nazi collaborator under the Vichy regime in France.

The artificial left ventricle was asked to keep him alive until a new valve could get into stride in his heart.

There was a circus atmosphere at Methodist Hospital on the April morning in 1966 when Dr. DeBakey operated on DeRudder. A mob of newspaper and TV reporters and cameramen milled through the hospital corridors.

At 9:00 A.M., DeBakey knifed open DeRudder's chest, hooked up a heart-lung machine, and rapidly implanted the new aortic valve. He cut into DeRudder's left atrium. Daintily, he inserted his artificial ventribular pump and began stitching its tubes to DeRudder's empty blood vessels. At 11:17 A.M., DeRudder's blood started to flow through the artificial pump. Three minutes later, DeRudder was taken off the heart-lung machine. The pump behaved ideally. Each time DeRudder's natural right ventricle pulsed, a Silastic diaphragm in the pump pushed down and moved blood into his waiting aorta. DeRudder's left ventricle was getting the rest it had begged for.

DeRudder never regained consciousness. His ravaged heart and kidneys were too sick to survive the new ordeal. But the DeBakey half heart kept the unconscious man alive for five days.

"It was all that kept him going," Dr. DeBakey declared with no little pride.

A completely artificial heart was possible now.

A Day in the Operating Rooms with DeBakey

I stood close to Mike DeBakey for the better part of eight hours while he operated on eight men, each dismayingly ill of cardiovascular disease. It was an amazing display of surgical skill, physical endurance, and ferocious artistic temperament.

Dr. DeBakey keeps four different operating rooms going day and night at Methodist. The O.R.s are set in a row with wide windows between them that let you look from one into another and see the green-clad surgeons wielding their knives. This day, I was also green-clad in scrub suit, cap, mask, and apron. My apron was quickly covered with bloody blotches.

The first patient was sixty-eight, white-haired, and gnarled. He had a blockage in his right femoral artery, the artery that passes blood to the leg. Unless DeBakey could build a bypass around the obstruction, he was going to lose the leg. His body was swathed in white except for the groin and the upper leg. Gaping, bloody incisions were there. One of DeBakey's assistants—there were three—made the incisions before DeBakey ran in. At the end of the operating table, a meticulous anesthesiologist eyed a small screen overhead on which three dancing dots of white light told how the patient's heart was holding out. This was the electrocardiograph. Now and then, the anesthesiologist reinforced the anesthesia. He had started the old man on nitrous oxide and curare, a South American Indian poison that utterly paralyzes the muscles. You can't risk the slightest move when you are carving up an artery. Two nurses looked on. In the background, a radio softly played show music. Every hour, the news came on. No one seemed to pay it any attention except me.

Now DeBakey was raptly working, hunched over the table, eyes riveted to the incisions. He guided a great needle, pulling a two-foot-long stretch of Dacron tubing into the opening at the groin, down through the hollow in the thigh, to the incision in the leg. He clamped off the artery and cut away the blocked segment. He sewed the Dacron tubing to the artery with small, neat stitches. His mother had taught him well.

The trouble was the blood. The wound kept filling up with blood so DeBakey couldn't see what he was sewing. The younger assistants tried to draw off the blood through their rubber suction tubes as though they were housewives using a vacuum cleaner to tidy up a mess. But the blood kept gaining.

DeBakey shouted angrily at a young doctor, accused him of incompetence, carelessness, stupidity. He grabbed the suction tube right out of his hand and demonstrated how he wanted him to use it.

"Why can't you do it my way? Why do you change your hand around? It should be like a chicken picking at corn. See. Do it my way."

The blood got ahead of the young doctor again and DeBakey shrieked furiously at him, shaming him in front of everybody. The young doctor paled. He had heard—everyone had—that DeBakey had thrown residents out of his operating room and never let them back again. It could end a career.

DeBakey went out of the room and let the assistants complete the bypass. As he put in the final stitches, one of them hopefully said, "DeBakey will like this."

Dr. DeBakey didn't. On his return, his experienced eye recognized that something was wrong. Blood was clotting in the new bypass. DeBakey immediately cut apart the stitches and sucked out the clot. He sewed the artery and the bypass together again himself. This time, it was satisfactory. There was no threat of a leak. DeBakey left the assistants to close the wound and raced off to the next operation.

Later, I watched his *chef d'oeuvre*, the carotid endarterectomy. The patient was in his fifties, black-haired, but with deep pain lines etched in his face. He had had a severe stroke, and DeBakey wanted to stave off the killing one that threatened. He made the incision himself in the right side of the patient's neck. He clamped the clogged carotid, rerouting its trickle of blood to the brain through a thin tube. He opened the artery and began to bore into the brown muck. He held up some muck for me to see. Silently, I vowed to retrench on cholesterol. Knifeful by knifeful, he dug out the muck until the artery was a freeway. He took a small Dacron patch and daintily sewed it into the wall of the artery like a seamstress letting out a dress with an extra gore of cloth.

Tension in the O.R. Dr. DeBakey had halted the operation on an aneurysm. All nine of us in the O.R., DeBakey, his assistants, the resourceful anesthesiologist, Dr. William B. Gerecke, the two nurses, me, were holding our breath. Our eyes were fixed on the flashing numbers on the EKG screen. The patient's blood pressure was dropping lower and lower. Gerecke gave him an injection. And another. At last, the blood pressure started up again. I heard a collective sigh of relief, and DeBakey resumed the operation.

Sunday morning, I asked Dr. DeBakey about those eight patients.
"All of them are doing fine," he said. "They'll all be okay. I'll have them sitting up in two days."
I checked in the middle of the week. Every one of the eight was sitting up.
That Sunday morning, Dr. DeBakey and I talked of many things. Of the DeBakey survival rate. From 95 to 98 percent, he said. Of DeBakey's splenetic temper in the O.R. "I'm a perfectionist, I suppose. I have to teach these fellows to concentrate on what they're doing. In surgery, every little thing is critical." Of DeBakey's relations with his patients. He showed me stacks of letters from adoring patients. "You were kinder to me than a father," one wrote. Of the many poor people he had operated on for nothing. How he gave the Baylor College of Medicine half of the $2 million he made a year. It was one cause for his feud with Denton Cooley. Cooley insisted on keeping all his fees for himself, DeBakey scornfully said.
"I've been invited to every major country in the world," he boasted. "I've won the Lasker Award. That's second only to the Nobel Prize, you know."
"How does someone forge ahead as a surgeon?" I asked.
"By developing new techniques, new methods that were not known before. By pioneering. When you're successful in that, you become recognized in the profession."
Big doses of publicity help, he conceded.

Stress doesn't worry Dr. DeBakey. "Man is made to work hard. I don't think it ever hurt anyone." He does his scientific writing and his correspondence from 4:30 A.M. until 6:30 A.M., then starts his rounds, is in the O.R. by 7:30, rarely gets home much before midnight. Work is his recreation. "I like what I do more than anything else. I find it fascinating, challenging, enjoyable."

He was married to a pretty Louisiana nurse, Diana Cooper, for thirty-five years until her sudden death of a heart attack in 1972. None of their four sons is interested in medicine. In 1975, DeBakey married again, this time to Katrin Fehlhaber, a thirty-three-year-old German actress.

One can be sure that Mike DeBakey, the surgeon, wants to heal sick people—as many as his flying fingers can reach. One just can speculate as to what interests Mike DeBakey, the medical researcher, the most. Is it a passion for discovery, or a yearning for acclaim?

In parting, Dr. DeBakey remarked, "You must be a huminatarian to be a great surgeon. Above all, you must have faith in God and be a good Christian. You must love people."

He did not mention Dr. Cooley then.

Cooley, Master Surgeon, Breaks with DeBakey

Drs. DeBakey and Cooley have two things in common: 1) Both are grand masters with a scalpel, and 2) Both are determined to "get thar fustest with the mostest headlines." Beyond this, the differences between the two are large. Good-looking Denton Cooley, six feet four inches tall, slim, and blue-eyed, is as soft-spoken and easy to get along with as Mike DeBakey is difficult.

Outside of DeBakey, Cooley has few peers in an operating room. His long slender fingers can do virtually anything in and around the human heart. He devised many of the newest techniques for treating anomalies of the heart. He demonstrated that the most intricate open-heart surgery is feasible on newborn infants; he has operated on more than one thousand of them successfully. He eliminated the need for full blood transfusions in open-heart surgery. He proved that glucose serves as well as full blood for priming heart-lung machines, thereby reducing the risk of hepatitis and adverse blood reactions. It's been a boon to Jehovah's Witnesses, whose religion prohibits blood transfusions. They flock to Cooley when their hearts go bad. Cooley has also turned out his own synthetic bypass to rival the renowned DeBakey bypass. Naturally.

More than anyone else, save Dr. Christiaan Barnard, who did the first, Dr. Cooley dramatized heart transplants. He did twenty-two in one year.

He cut the time of the operation from about four and a half hours to one hour and forty-five minutes, "skin to skin."

Dr. Barnard watched Cooley operate on a heart. "It was the most beautiful surgery that I ever saw in my life," he wrote. "Every movement had a purpose and achieved its aim. Where most surgeons would have taken three hours, he could do the same operation in one hour."

I met Dr. Cooley at seven-thirty in the evening at the Texas Heart Institute. His office could have been a stage set: a spacious room done all in white, with an unhospital-like hardwood floor, colonial furniture, and lovely oriental paintings. A portable television set and a hi-fi were set in the white bookshelves. It was a homey room with nothing medical showing, not even an X-ray rack. Rumor had it that it cost $15,000 to decorate the office.

"I spend so much time here that I want it to be like home," Dr. Cooley said.

He came directly from the operating room in a rumpled green scrub suit. He had had one bag of potato chips to eat all day, so we ran down to the hospital cafeteria for a quick dinner. His consisted of a cheeseburger, a piece of cake, and a cup of coffee—total cost, $1.24. He didn't have enough money with him, and he had to borrow twenty-five cents from me to pay his check.

After dinner, Cooley made rounds. He loaned me a long white lab coat, and I joined the procession of residents, interns, and other medicos who followed him. The patients would turn entreating eyes on him as he entered their rooms. "We're going to operate on you tomorrow morning," he would say in a matter-of-fact voice, and strangely, the patients all seemed relieved, happy to put their lives in his hands. Here and there, he would take hold of a patient's foot or touch a groin with the tips of his fingers to note the strength of the circulation.

A frightened old woman whose husband was sitting alongside the bed holding her hand begged Dr. Cooley not to cut too much off the stump of her rotted leg. He promised. A fully dressed man with an ashen, pain-streaked face was sitting on a chair at the window of his room, breathing in gasps. He didn't say a word.

"There's not much we can do for him," Dr. Cooley said regretfully when we were out in the corridor again.

"How much time has he?"

"Four or five days."

"Does he know it?"

"Yes. But if they'd let me do a heart transplant for him, I could give him six months, maybe a year, maybe two years more of good life."

A beautiful little girl with golden curls, no more than four years of age, came running up to Cooley in the corridor. He leaned down and she kissed him. The child had had open-heart surgery the day before.

We went into the recovery room, the one place in the hospital where death seemed present. A couple of dozen newly operated patients lay in bed, still asleep or with their eyes staring dully into space, covered with blood-stained bandages, wound in a maze of wires connected to a mass of electronic apparatus that was checking their condition moment by moment. Above each bed dancing lights on an EKG monitor revealed the truth about the patient's postoperative heart currents. A very fat old woman, with one huge, shapeless breast exposed, was dying hard, but all the others were going to make it.

It was 9:00 P.M. when we finished rounds. Dr. Cooley quipped to his staff, who had been working since 6:00 that morning, "You can have the rest of the day off."

We sat down in his comfortable white office to talk about him. He said that he was born in Houston in 1920, the son of a wealthy, socially prominent dentist. "My father would have preferred to be a surgeon, but he settled for dentistry. I decided that I wouldn't compromise my future. I would do whatever challenged me the most."

He played varsity basketball all four years at college, was active in fraternity affairs, and still made straight As. He did as well at Johns Hopkins medical school.

"I've always been an achiever," he boasted.

He obtained his first real schooling in heart surgery at Hopkins under Dr. Blalock, whom he assisted at the first blue baby operation. He got his polishing under the best heart surgeon in England. When he returned to Houston in 1951, he had perhaps the most training in congenital heart surgery of any young man in the country. DeBakey grabbed him for his staff at Baylor.

The two of them set records in cardiovascular pioneering and surgical volume. Said Cooley, "Dr. DeBakey is a tireless worker and, as you can see, I have some energy myself. Together, we accumulated the largest experience and developed a lot of new techniques and did many things for the first time in operations on the aorta."

Now comes the murky area. Who did what first? A case in point: Who originated the brilliant surgical techniques that are employed to remove fatal aneurysms from weakened thoracic aortas? As Dr. DeBakey recounts the story, he was the first. He told me that he cut a big spindle-shaped aneurysm out of a descending thoracic aorta in 1953 and replaced the diseased segment with a piece of an aorta taken from a corpse. He had been keeping a dead man's aorta in a freezer for the purpose. According to DeBakey, this operation opened the entire field of aorta surgery.

Dr. Cooley tells it differently.

"One of the first operations I did in Houston was on a fellow named Joe Mitchell. Joe was a black man over at the county hospital. He had a big, bulging aneurysm sticking out of his chest. On ward rounds, Dr. DeBakey said, 'Let's ask Dr. Cooley what he would do. He's a new man on the staff.' I said, 'I'd take it out.' 'Well,' he said, 'why don't you go ahead and try it?' The next day, I took it out.

"From that time on, Dr. DeBakey and I began to resect aneurysms wherever they could be resected. We were the first to develop the technique for removing thoracic aneurysms in all locations."

You can make up your own mind as to who deserves the credit.

By 1960, Denton Cooley was a full professor at Baylor, famous, and, to quote his colleagues, "tired of sucking hind tit with DeBakey." Without so much as a by-your-leave, he upped and transferred his burgeoning surgical practice from Methodist Hospital to the St. Luke's Episcopal-Texas Children's hospitals, something for which DeBakey never forgave him. After DeBakey got his millionaires to build him a $20 million cardiovascular research and training center at Methodist Hospital, Cooley got his millionaires to construct the lush Texas Heart Institute for him. DeBakey hasn't forgiven him for that, either.

The stages were set for an Olympic competition in heart surgery, plus a feud between two heart surgeons that would make the hostilities between Sigmund Freud and Carl Jung look like an exercise in amiability.

Dr. Cooley doesn't work as many hours as Dr. DeBakey each day—who does?—but he is so fast with a knife that he tallies many more operations. He can accurately brag, "I've done more open-heart surgery than anybody else in the world." On an average day, he may do eight to ten open-heart operations, and ten to twelve vascular jobs. By 7:10 A.M., he is at the hospital, checking his patients in the recovery room. Fifteen minutes of that and then twenty minutes on his correspondence. At 7:45, he is in the operating room, where his assistants will have at least two, possibly four, patients asleep, awaiting his scalpel. He operates steadily till mid-evening, often later.

"Do you blow up at the people in the O.R.?"

"No, I stay pretty calm. The biggest criticism of me is that I get a little sarcastic if things aren't done well. But it doesn't happen often."

Does he still get a thrill out of operating?

"An enormous satisfaction from an operation that is well done technically if the patient gets well. Particularly if other surgeons and cardiologists said that the patient was too sick for me to operate on."

He gets some recreation on weekends—tennis and horseback riding. He used to play double bass in the Heartbeats, a crack combo composed of heart doctors, and he faithfully practiced with them one night a week. Now he just shows up for concerts and plays along on his bull fiddle. He has been married since 1949 to Louise Thomas, a blonde, blue-eyed nurse he met at Hopkins. They have five daughters. One of the girls is a pre-med student, another a medical illustrator.

How long can Dr. Cooley stand the strain of twenty operations a day?

"I suppose I should deescalate, but it's hard for a surgeon to do that before he's sick. If he's worth his salt, he'd rather be in the operating room than doing anything else."

How long since he had had an EKG himself?

"Ten years," he said. He couldn't have been less concerned about the health of his own heart.

One can pose the same question about Denton Cooley's innermost motivations as was raised about Mike DeBakey. Which interests him most—a passion for discovery or the love of acclaim? The answer is moot. However, one can be sure that Cooley likes people and wants to cure more of them than anybody else.

There remains to be told the most exciting pages of Dr. Cooley's life—his part in the great heart transplant sweepstakes, and the jugular feud with Dr. DeBakey to which it led.

"I have a theory," Dr. Cooley said, "that the love between two heart surgeons is measured by the distance that separates them."

Definitely, Drs. DeBakey and Cooley worked too closely too long.

Shumway Originates Heart Transplant Techniques

Chinese legend has it that a surgeon named Pien Ch'iao who lived in the third century B.C. had an assistant that most present-day surgeons would envy. The assistant was an elf who could see through the human body and identify the symptoms of any disease. With the elf's aid, Dr. Pien performed the first human transplant. He dropped a Mickey Finn into the wine of two soldiers. While they slept, he cut them both open and exchanged their hearts and several other organs.

Seventy-two hours later, the two soldiers woke up, as good as new. Alas, neither Dr. Pien nor the elf ever wrote up the case for a medical journal.

The modern transplant era is better documented. Its foundations were laid at the University of Chicago in the first years of this century by Alexis Carrell and his American collaborator, Dr. Charles Guthrie. Together, they transplanted kidneys, thyroid glands, adrenals, ovaries, arms, legs, lungs, and hearts from one animal to another. Particularly dogs and cats.

One cat that received a new pair of kidneys survived with them for two years. Among other things, Carrell and Guthrie shifted the head of a small dog onto the neck of a larger dog.

The Russian Vladamir Demikhov did more than 250 animal transplants between 1940 and 1958. He switched kidneys, livers, the entire gastrointestinal tract. He also gave dogs new heads. One of his dogs lived twenty-nine days with a different head, playing spiritedly with other dogs until he was sacrificed. A beautiful furry dog named Borzoi lived thirty-two days with an extra heart that Demikhov gave him. Demikhov cut out part of Borzoi's lung to make room for the second heart.

At the University of Mississippi Medical Center, Dr. James D. Hardy transplanted the ovaries and the uteri of ten female dogs to ten others with good success. Three of the bitches became pregnant and gave birth to fine, healthy puppies. And in Palo Alto, California, Dr. Norman Shumway, of Stanford University, began the heart transplants on dogs that made human heart transplants possible. He developed the techniques used by all heart transplanters.

In 1958, Shumway was thirty-five years old, a slim, dark-haired man who spoke in whispers. Born in Kalamazoo, Michigan, he got his M.D. at Vanderbilt University and did his residency at the University of Minnesota Hospital under Walt Lillehei.

Dr. Lillehei thinks the world of him. "A great surgeon and a great guy, with a tremendous sense of humor," he said. "A cynical sense of humor. If he thinks you're full of bullshit, he'll tell you. And he'll tell you why."

Shumway started his dog experiments at Stanford in 1958, working with Dr. Richard R. Lower. He perfected a way to take out the entire heart, leaving only the common posterior atrial wall. He decided just where to cut off the aorta and pulmonary arteries—about a centimeter distal to the commissures. He figured out which nerves had to be preserved so the transplanted heart could function. He determined the right immunosuppressant drugs to be used. He worked out a method for cooling the donor's heart safely before it goes into its new home—dipping it for five minutes in a saline solution whose temperature is 39° Fahrenheit.

After Shumway published his findings in the early 1960s, the door was open for human heart transplants.

It was a race. Shumway and Lower were the favorites. Hardy was a prime contender. Lillehei was raring to go in Minneapolis. Adrian Kantrowitz, another surgical star (who is reputed to be as sharp-tempered as Mike DeBakey), was poised to try in Brooklyn, New York. DeBakey and Cooley were entrants. Far off in South Africa, another of Lillehei's students was waiting for the right moment. His name was Barnard.

Barnard Does the First Human-Heart Transplant

Slim, dark, and very handsome, Christiaan Barnard won the big race. He successfully transplanted a human heart on December 3, 1967.

Barnard was born in 1923 in the little village of Beauford West in South Africa. His father was a Dutch Reformed minister who never earned more than $59 a month. Barnard and his three brothers grew up in poverty.

His mother used to repeat one thing to Chris: "I expect you to be first. Not second or third, but first."

He obtained his medical degree at Cape Town University and went to the United States to study surgery with Dr. Lillehei. Lillehei was impressed with his photographic memory.

"It used to worry me when we made rounds that Barnard never wrote down my instructions. You know, we saw twenty-five to thirty postop patients and there might be a hundred orders for them, but Barnard never took a note. One day, I burst out, 'Chris, write that down, goddamn it.' He asked me, 'Has anything ever failed to get done?' I had to say no."

When Barnard returned to South Africa, he brought with him an $8,000 grant from the U.S. government to help him with his research. He and his surgeon brother, Marius, started doing heart transplants on dogs, using the Shumway technique. They did forty-eight of them. By late 1967, Barnard felt he was ready. All he needed were the right patient and the right donor at the right time.

Louis Washansky, a fifty-four-year-old greengrocer, was picked to be the first recipient of another person's heart. Washansky was dying of gross heart failure. He had already suffered two brutal heart attacks, and his heart was two thirds dead. On top of that, he had liver failure, kidney failure, and diabetes. His legs were swollen fat with excess fluid. He had to sleep sitting up in a chair so he wouldn't drown in his own fluid. Louis should have been dead long ago but refused to die. He was a fighter.

He knew he had little time left to live. Still, someone had to explain to him the fearful risks of a heart transplant. To a dying man, a couple of months can seem like a lot of life compared to a couple of hours.

"Louis," Dr. Barry Kaplan, his physician at suburban Groote Schuur Hospital, said to Washansky, "something may be able to be done for you, but it entails a terrible risk. It is such a gamble you may not come out of it alive."

"What is it?"

"There is a possibility they may be able to transplant somebody's heart into you."

"If that's the only chance, I'll take it."

"Louis, don't you want to think about it? Don't you want to discuss this with your wife?"

"No, no. There's nothing to think about. I can't go on living like this. The way I am now is not living."

Late on Saturday afternoon, December 2, 1967, a speeding automobile smashed into twenty-five-year-old Denise Ann Darvall and her mother as they walked across a Cape Town street to buy a cake for dinner. Mrs. Darvall was killed instantly. Denise was barely alive when they carried her into the Groote Schuur Hospital. Her head and her brain were almost totally destroyed. Her weeping father, Edward G. Darvall, was asked for Denise's heart.

"Well, doctor, if you can't save my daughter, try and save this man," he said through his tears.

The blood types matched. Washansky's was ARh-positive, Denise's was ORh-negative. Dr. Barnard was summoned from his home. Driving into the hospital, he prayed, "Dear Lord, help me in this operation."

At 2:15 A.M., Sunday morning, December 3, it commenced. Dr. Barnard was assisted by his brother, Marius, Dr. Terry O'Donovan, Dr. Francois Hitchcock, and a distinguished surgeon, Rodney Hewitson. While Hewitson opened Washansky's chest in operating theater A, Marius, O'Donovan, and Hitchcock waited in operating theater B for Denise Darvall to die.

"I'll not lift an instrument until the EKG line is flat," Terry Donovan declared, and the others agreed.

Washanksy lay in theater A with his chest open, his bloated, scarred heart in full view, while the others waited helplessly for Denise to expire. Ten, fifteen, eighteen minutes went by. At last, she died. O'Donovan immediately opened her chest and attached her undersized heart to the heart-lung machine. Now Barnard took over. He severed the eight blood vessels to the heart and separated the heart from the ligaments holding it in place. Quickly, Denise's tiny heart was taken off the pump, borne in a bowl into theatre A, and hooked onto another pump. There it rested, chilled and perfused in oxygenated blood, waiting its turn.

Dr. Barnard strode into theater A, scrubbed, and picked up a new scalpel. He cut out almost all of Washansky's ruined heart, leaving behind only the grey, red-streaked atrial lid. Into the strange cavity, he dropped Denise's firm, pink heart. Slowly, he stitched the heart into Washansky's body, the left auricle first, next the right. He varied some from the Shumway technique by leaving the septum of the donor heart intact. Instead of cutting off the entire atrial lid, he merely cut off the two sections of the heart where the veins feed into the two separate chambers. That left

Denise's heart with two holes at the top. Barnard sewed them to the atrial lid of Washansky's heart, which he had kept in place. It allowed him to compensate for the difference in size between the two hearts. He was able to enlarge the openings in Denise's heart to match Washansky's bigger heart without injuring her septum.

The stitching took more than three hours. At the end, Barnard and Hewitson inspected the lines of sutures. There was no leak.

"Pump off," Dr. Barnard ordered.

The borrowed heart started beating on its own—slowly, then a little faster. Barnard turned the pump on, off, on, and off again, testing the new heart. The blood pressure climbed, to 90, to 95. Barnard pulled out the last catheter, tied the final pursestring suture, and checked for air in the heart. All was well. The beat stayed steady, the EKG lights danced up and down with perfect rhythm.

"We made it," the exhausted Barnard said to Hewitson. "I need a cup of tea."

It was 7:00 A.M.

An hour later, Washansky awakened and tried to speak. Within thirty-six hours, he was complaining that he was hungry. He ate a soft-boiled egg.

The fight for Washansky's life had just started. Barnard had to find ways to keep the body from rejecting its new heart, and to stave off other killers. He tried immunosuppressant drugs and cobalt irradiation of the heart, but they failed. Brave Louis Washansky died eighteen days later of a lung infection.

Dr. Barnard was grief-stricken. "I crash-landed," he said.

He could take some comfort from the autopsy. It showed that the stitches in Washansky's new heart had held fast and that there were no indications of serious rejection although the measures taken to prevent rejection obviously had lowered Washansky's resistance to infection.

Barnard had better fortune with his second transplant. He gave Dr. Philip Blaiberg, a fifty-eight-year-old white dentist, 593 days of good life with the heart of a twenty-four-year-old black man who had died of a brain hemmorrhage. Blaiberg had been a bedridden cardiac cripple, scarcely able to breathe. The new heart let him live almost normally, able to drive a car, even to swim in the ocean.

The first successful human heart transplant was the biggest medical news of the decade—of the century, probably. The thought that a person could live with someone else's heart captured the imagination of the world. Television and radio networks bulletined the news. Eight-column headlines emblazoned newspapers. The news magazines ran ecstatic cover stories. Throngs of reporters and photographers descended on the startled

Groote Schuur Hospital, ferreting out every wisp of fact or fancy about Washansky and Barnard. The obscure South African surgeon became a world-famous celebrity, a familiar figure on TV screens and in gossip columns. He went dancing with glamorous movie stars. He had a private audience with the Pope. He published a best-selling autobiography called *One Life*. The title could well have been "Two Lives," for Barnard's life would never be the same again.

According to his former wife, Louwtjie, public adulation made a different man of Barnard. She divorced him after thirty-one years of marriage and two children and wrote her own book, *Heartbreak*, in which she told "how fame lost me my husband and broke the hearts of myself and my children." Among other things, she accused Barnard of repeated, flagrant adultery.

"I do not believe there is another man in the world who has the ability to charm a woman that Chris has," Mrs. Barnard ruefully wrote. Soon after their divorce, he married Barbara Zoellner, a beautiful brunette half his age.

Many medical men in Cape Town do not like Christiaan Barnard. "He is arrogant, rides roughshod over his colleagues, and makes distasteful use of publicity," a Cape Town physician declared to a *Newsweek* reporter. Yet nobody could gainsay the fact that Dr. Barnard was a daring and conscientious researcher who achieved one of surgery's most noteworthy "firsts."

The Heart Transplant Derby that Faltered

After Barnard's triumph, almost every big-name heart surgeon had to show that he could do a transplant. It was a matter of prestige. Dr. Kantrowitz was quickest to get on the bandwagon. Within three days, Kantrowitz took a seventeen-day-old baby into the O.R. at the Maimonides Hospital in Brooklyn, N.Y., and gave him the heart of a two-day-old baby. The child lived six and a half hours. On January 6, 1968, the pioneering Norman Shumway, no doubt a bit disappointed that Barnard had gotten ahead of him, transplanted the heart of a forty-three-year-old man into Michael Kasperak, a fifty-four-year-old man near death from chronic viral myocarditis. Kasperak lived only sixteen days. (It cost $28,845, including $7,200 for 288 pints of blood, to keep him alive for those sixteen days.) The Indian P.K. Sen did a heart transplant in Bombay on February 16, 1968, but his patient survived a mere three hours. A French surgeon named Cabrol went at it in Paris on April 27. His patient died in two days.

Not until Dr. Cooley tried his hand on May 3 in Houston did anyone have the success that Barnard had had. Cooley gave a dying forty-seven-year-old man the heart of a fifteen-year-old girl. The recipient was a certified public accountant, Everett Thomas, who had had two heart attacks and two strokes, and was petrified at the prospect of another. The donor was a new bride who had shot out her brains with a .22 rifle because she believed her nineteen-year-old husband didn't love her anymore. With her heart—and another that Cooley transplanted later—Thomas obtained 204 more days of life. Dr. Donald N. Ross did Britain's first heart transplant on the same day in London. His forty-five-year-old patient survived forty-five days.

It got to be a three-ring circus. Everywhere, surgeons rushed to do heart transplants to the beat of the publicity drums and the glare of the TV lights. From the U.S.S.R., Poland, Czechoslovakia, Germany, Switzerland, Spain, Israel, Turkey, Venezuela, Brazil, Argentina, Chile, Canada, Australia, and Japan came more reports of heart transplants. Before the craze was over, Barnard did nine, Shumway dozens, Cooley a score or more, Lillehei eight, DeBakey twelve. DeBakey was late getting into the competition; he didn't do his first until August 31, 1968.

Shumway's old-time partner, Dr. Richard Lower, set the top record for patient longevity. He gave Louis Russell, a forty-three-year-old industrial arts teacher, the heart of a seventeen-year-old gunshot wound victim in August 1968, at the Medical College of Virginia in Richmond. Russell lived a cheerful life in Indianapolis for more than six years. He taught, rode his bicycle every day, and delivered reassuring lectures on family life until his new heart finally gave out in November 1974.

By April 1, 1976, 305 persons throughout the world had received heart transplants, and fifty-seven of them were alive. However, the early, exciting dreams of new hearts for all who needed them were forgotten, and the technique was largely in disrepute. In 1968, 101 people were transplanted; in 1971, just seventeen. Dr. Helen Taussig was one of many who criticized the technique severely. "Any new drug placed on the market, no matter how great the beneficial effects, would be promptly withdrawn if after four months fifty percent of the people who had taken it were dead," she wrote. Dr. DeBakey was appalled by the continued lack of understanding of the rejection process. "I've done twelve transplants," he told me. "Two of them are still alive, but I have absolutely no idea why they're alive and the others died." The logistics problem seemed insoluble. No one knew how to get the thousands of dying cardiac patients the healthy hearts they needed when they needed them. The public itself was frightened of transplants. Few were willing to donate their hearts anymore.

Dr. Barnard blamed the fiasco on the sensationalism that had accompanied the first transplants. "By exploiting the public taste for the macabre, the press did a great deal of harm. . . ." he angrily charged. He claimed that "the publicity sparked off a spate of bandwagon transplants by teams ill equipped to perform them but constrained to try by motives that are far from medical." He insisted that heart transplants were "a serious therapeutic technique."

Dr. Cooley also retained faith in the technique. "Half of our patients would have lived less than two days had we not transplanted," he said to me. "If they lived for six months or twelve months after that, you've offered them something worthwhile. To a dying man, six months more of life could be worthwhile. He may want to see his daughter graduate from college, his son get married, or hold his first grandson in his arms. You and me being healthy, we don't think that the next six months mean so much. But, by George, if you're only looking forward to two or three days of life, you'd be more interested in six months."

Cooley was not performing transplants anymore, though. Cooley quit doing them because he couldn't get any more hearts, he said.

Dr. Barnard was to startle the medical world again. On November 25, 1974, he performed the first double-heart transplant. He implanted the heart of a ten-year-old child in a fifty-eight-year-old man without removing the patient's own diseased heart. The two hearts were supposed to work in tandem in the one chest. Early in 1975, Barnard gave a second patient a second heart. The two patients lived for a few months. Four other patients who received extra hearts at Barnard's hospital survived somewhat longer.

Dr. Barnard made no protest against the publicity he got.

By the end of 1975, Norman Shumway was the only prominent surgeon doing heart transplants regularly. He and his Stanford team had done ninety-five transplants quietly, carefully, without fanfare. They were getting more encouraging results; 60 percent of their patients were living a year or more.

"The trick is to recognize early rejection, and know when to give drugs to prevent it," Dr. Shumway stated.

Still, it was doubtful whether the exchange of one human heart for another would ever be generally accepted as valid therapy for heart disease. The risks were too high for the small results you got. Not that the great transplant derby of the late 1960s and early 1970s was wasted effort. It firmly established that surgeons could safely give a dying man a substitute for his blighted heart.

Heart transplants became part of the national consciousness. Even former-President Lyndon B. Johnson had his favorite transplant joke. He told it at an educational symposium at the University of Texas in January

1973. It concerned an old Texas cowboy who had a heart transplant performed in Houston. The surgeons gave him his choice of the heart of a virile young movie star, a husky young ski instructor, or a sixty-nine-year-old Republican banker. He selected the heart of the old Republican banker.

"Why'd you pick the heart of that old Republican banker when you could have had a heart from one of those young fellows?" the doctors asked.

The cowboy said, "I wanted to make sure I got one that had never been used."

Ironically, Mr. Johnson died of a coronary attack a few days after the symposium.

Cooley Implants an Artificial Heart
—and Starts a Furor

If a hale human heart can't be substituted for a dying one, what can? The need is immense. The Blue Cross estimates that between 100,000 and 300,000 lives a year could be saved if substitute hearts were available.

Some medical greats, Dr. Taussig, for one, have suggested that animals might be bred specifically for this purpose, but the proposal has not won much support. The rejection problem is as difficult with an animal's heart as a human heart.

Some kind of an artificial heart is needed.

Many outstanding scientists have tried to develop one. In 1937, Russia's Vladamir Demikhov took the hearts out of dogs and replaced them with mechanical pumps. Some of his dogs lived five and a half days. Kazuhiko Arsumi built an artificial heart at the Tokyo University School of Medicine out of two little roller-type pumps operated by a Lilliputian motor. In January 1960, he kept a dog alive with it for thirteen hours. Dr. Willem Kolff's artificial heart kept a calf named Latina (Cherokee for "long-lived") alive for 174 hours at the University of Utah Medical Center.

Making an artificial heart for a human is something else. Three big problems are involved: a power source small enough to fit inside a human body; a way to stop human blood from clotting; and some way to overcome the body's rejection mechanism.

Dr. DeBakey pointed out the path. His half-heart helped keep a human alive for five days in 1965, you'll remember. Adrian Kantrowitz went a little further.

A heavy-set six-footer who was born in New York City in 1918, Dr. Kantrowitz is a medical inventor par excellence; he designed his own heart-lung machine and a fine pacemaker. Early in 1966, he perfected an artificial left ventricle that kept an elderly woman with congestive heart failure alive for twelve days. This, though she was suffering from diabetes, a diseased kidney, and a sick liver. Kantrowitz's half-heart was cigar-shaped and constructed of plastic without any moving parts. Like the DeBakey half-heart, it was powered by compressed air, but it was linked by wires to a control unit outside the body. Kantrowitz stitched it into the descending aorta, where it behaved as an extra heart for the woman.

Kantrowitz also developed a remarkable sausage-shaped "balloon pump" that he implanted in the patient's thigh to help the heart to function immediately after a coronary attack. It was connected to the heart by a plastic tube that he ran up through the femoral artery and the aorta. In June 1967, a forty-five-year-old woman was treated with the "balloon pump" at Maimonides Hospital for seven hours. She got better.

Techniques that could save hundreds of thousands of lives may come from these devices, Dr. Kantrowitz said.

But not at Maimonides. Kantrowitz resentfully transferred his research to Sinai Hospital in Detroit in 1970. To secure greater freedom for his experiments, he said.

Were you forbidden to do such work at Maimonides?, he was asked.

"I wouldn't say 'forbidden,' but I certainly was not encouraged," he growled.

Now it was a race again. Who among the big-name heart surgeons—DeBakey, Cooley, Kantrowitz, Barnard, Lower, or the others—would be first to introduce a whole artificial heart?

Cooley won the race. Or did he?

All one can write with sureness is this: The race provoked a roaring public feud between DeBakey and Cooley that rocked Houston and a lot of other cities where heart surgeons congregate.

On April 4, 1969, Dr. Cooley took Haskell Karp, a forty-seven-year-old printing estimator from Illinois, dying of heart disease, into the operating room at the Texas Heart Institute. Karp had suffered a half-dozen bad heart attacks over the past ten years. He couldn't shave himself or clean his teeth—the pain was too awful. Cooley proposed a human heart transplant to him, but Karp wouldn't have one. He was too frightened of transplants. Besides, Cooley couldn't get a matching heart for him.

"Please, doctor," Karp begged, "can't you do something to repair my heart instead?"

"I don't believe it's going to work to repair your heart," Dr. Cooley told him. "I can almost guarantee it won't."

"Well, I still want to try it."

"Listen, Mr. Karp, I can't just take you into the operating room unless I have some assurance I can get you out," Dr. Cooley said. "You've got to give me permission to use an artificial heart so we can get you out of the operating room alive. It would be on my conscience, operating on one as sick as you are, if I didn't have something to fall back on."

At last, Karp agreed.

Cooley operated on Karp for three hours with the assistance of Dr. Domingo Liotta. (Remember that name?) No matter what Cooley tried, he couldn't get Karp's heart to support his circulation. He decided he had no other option. He took out all of Karp's heart and inserted a whole artificial heart in its place. The artificial heart was about the same size as a normal heart. It contained four chambers and valves, was made of Silastic with a Dacron lining, and was pneumatic. It had been developed by Dr. Liotta.

Two hours after the operation, Karp was fully conscious. He was talking, and moving his arms and legs freely. For the first time in human experience, a man was being kept alive by a totally self-contained artificial heart.

Dr. Cooley's face lit up when he spoke of it to me. "The excitement and the thrill when this man woke up and talked to us with his artificial heart in place was one of the most stimulating things that's ever happened to me in all my professional career."

For sixty-five hours, the artificial heart sustained Karp. Cooley then removed it and replaced it with the heart of a forty-year-old Massachusetts woman whose body had been raced to Houston in a chartered jet plane after Cooley went on television and appealed for a heart donor. Karp lived twenty more hours.

It was an extraordinary performance that was hailed by worldwide headlines and cheers. It became even more extraordinary when Dr. DeBakey charged that the artificial heart used by Dr. Cooley had been stolen from his laboratory! He claimed that the heart had been developed by Dr. Liotta with his funds under his direction in his Baylor laboratory. He further accused Cooley of violating medical ethics and U.S. government regulations by using an unproven device on a human being without first getting the approval of the Baylor Committee on Research Involving Human Beings.

It was a *bona fide* scandal, especially when it became known that Liotta had been secretly working for Cooley at the Texas Heart Institute while he was on DeBakey's staff at Baylor.

DeBakey flayed Cooley in speeches and in statements to the press. Years later, he criticized him vitriolically to me for this.

"Cooley put a heart in a human that was stolen from my laboratory, a heart that I developed," he said. "I trained Cooley. I even wrote his papers for him because he can't write. Then he did this."

The reverberations reached right to Washington. The National Heart Institute expressed its official concern and ordered Baylor to conduct a thorough investigation.

The Establishment came down hard on both Cooley and Liotta. Spurred by DeBakey, the Baylor Committee on Research Involving Human Beings found Cooley guilty of seducing Liotta away from DeBakey's staff, of using an artificial heart created in DeBakey's laboratory, and of trying an unproven device on a human being. (The artificial heart had only been tested in seven calves. The longest that one had survived was a mere forty-four hours.) And Cooley was found guilty by the Houston medical society of unseemly publicity.

Cooley had to resign from the Baylor faculty. Liotta was dismissed, and then immediately employed full-time by Cooley at his Texas Heart Institute.

Dr. DeBakey wasn't satisfied yet. He sent out a raft of furious letters to doctors and hospitals in the United States and abroad attacking Cooley for his actions. He would never speak to Cooley again.

Dr. Cooley still feels he was justified. He said that Dr. Liotta had worked on his artificial heart for years, but could not persuade DeBakey to give it a trial.

"Dr. DeBakey had never even seen the heart; he'd never even been in the Liotta laboratory," Dr. Cooley declared.

"Dr. Liotta came to me and said he thought the thing deserved a clinical trial. I thought it over and proposed to him that we work on the artificial heart ourselves, using our own funds. I said we wouldn't hamper ourselves by seeking permission because I felt we were better qualified to do clinical work than anyone else."

It would have been futile to apply for approval to the Baylor Committee on Research Involving Human Beings, Cooley said; the DeBakey-dominated committee would inevitably have refused him.

What about the use of an unproven device?

It was an emergency, with a human life at stake, Cooley maintained.

He went on, "Maybe DeBakey was insanely upset about it, but he didn't have to cause all the repercussions. All that has been done is to obscure an important scientific fact—that a man's circulation can be maintained by an artificial heart.

"That was years ago, and we'll have to wait many years more before anyone will have the nerve to try it again."

Sawyer Uses Streams of Gas to Open Plugged Arteries

Some unfinished surgical business remained. Important business such as a neat bypass inside the heart itself that has remitted the pain of angina pectoris for thousands of sufferers. The foundation for this bypass was laid by Dr. Arthur Vineberg at the Royal Victoria Hospital in Montreal. He had an idea for utilizing the internal mammary artery as a detour around an obstructed coronary artery. He tried it in 1950, inserting the severed, bleeding end of the mammary artery directly into a patient's heart muscle. It worked magic. "From a condition of complete disability," Dr. Vineberg reported three years after, the patient now "can walk ten miles through the bush." There was a drawback, though. It meant diverting the mammary artery from its regular duties.

An Argentine, Dr. René Favoloro, who was training at the Cleveland Clinic, thought of a more sophisticated way to get blood past an obstructed coronary artery to a starving heart. In May 1967, he cut out the blocked section of a patient's coronary artery. He took a long strip of the patient's saphenous vein—the big blood vessel that reaches the length of each leg—and sewed it in place of the blocked segment of the artery. The heart could get enough blood now, and the crushing chest pains of angina desisted.

Favoloro did this more than a hundred times before he returned to Argentina. Dr. Sones, the coronary movie man, begged him to settle permanently in America, but Favoloro felt he was needed more at home. He opened his own cardiovascular clinic in Buenos Aires.

Fourteen months later, Dr. W. Dudley Johnson, a professor of surgery at Marquette University in Milwaukee, was still more audacious. Utilizing Favoloro's technique, he took out a stretch of saphenous vein and connected one end to the aorta, the other to the small arteries at the back of the heart. These arteries are so tiny, scarcely one sixteenth of an inch in diameter, that no one before had ever dared work on them. The operation let Dr. Johnson bypass the dreadful fatty goo in the coronary artery and feed oxygen-rich blood to the heart through those healthy little arteries in the rear.

By the mid 1970's, more than thirty-five thousand saphenous vein bypasses had been performed in the United States. Some cardiologists considered the operation too dangerous. But done well, with carefully selected patients, it seemed comparatively safe. The Cleveland Clinic did two thousand saphenous vein bypasses in 1972 with a mortality of less than 4 percent.

Now it was the turn of the vivid Dr. Philip Sawyer and his gas endarterectomy. Along with Dr. DeBakey, Sawyer is of Lebanese extraction. His aunt, who recently died at the age of ninety-seven, was the first woman physician in the Middle East. (She had to obtain a special dispensation from the Sultan of Turkey in order to practice.) Sawyer was born in Bangor, Maine, in 1925, the son of a wealthy lumberman and a strong-minded mother. He wanted engineering, but his mother preferred medicine, so he went to the University of Pennsylvania medical school.

I met Dr. Sawyer in a small factory-like office at Downstate Medical Center in Brooklyn. His bulk seemed to fill the room to overflowing.

How did he come to select surgery?

"I knew the only way I was going to get a look at what happened inside of a living human was to be a surgeon."

"Are you as temperamental in the O.R. as Dr. DeBakey?"

Dr. Sawyer laughed uproariously. "Not quite. But I'm as irascible as he is. I'm intolerant of stupidity. I'm intolerant of slowness."

He started his experiments with high-pressure devices in the 1950s. He tried to separate the layers of the arterial walls by forcing air between them with a syringe plunger. It didn't work.

In 1961, the hospital was hit by a rash of deaths following endarterec-tomies. They were doing them the standard way, using a circular knife to gouge out the atheroma—the fatty deposits—from clogged arteries. This worked satisfactorily for freeing the core of the main artery, but it did nothing for the fine branches of the artery. They stayed clogged with muck.

Dr. Sol Sobel, one of Sawyer's assistant's was disgusted. "Why in hell are we using mechanical picks and shovels to do endarterectomies?" he asked Sawyer. "Why not use a hydraulic ram?"

They tried it. It didn't work.

Word came that a Salt Lake City researcher had separated whole organs from scar tissue by use of carbon dioxide. Perhaps the carbon dioxide would do for a plugged artery what the hydraulic ram wouldn't do. Hesitantly, Drs. Sobel and Martin Kaplitt, another Sawyer assistant, proposed it. Sawyer grabbed at the suggestion. He designed and built the equipment almost entirely himself. He tested it on cadavers in the postmortem room. He tested it on thirty dogs, and on clogged arteries in human legs, abdomens and necks. On June 5, 1967, he tried it inside a living human heart.

The patient was a forty-four-year-old housewife so tortured by heart disease that she couldn't walk. She had had two serious heart attacks in a month. One more and she would certainly die. Her right coronary artery was solidly blocked by the mushy deposits for inches.

Sawyer operated for three and a half hours at Kings County Hospital. He split the sternum and hooked her up to a heart-lung machine. Exposing the clogged artery, he inserted a hypodermic needle into it that was connected to a cylinder of carbon dioxide. He blew a few powerful jets of gas into the artery. They successfully loosened the fatty deposits from the walls of the artery.

Sawyer made a small incision in the wall of the artery, a mere quarter inch long. With a pair of tiny forceps, he was able to remove more than three inches of waxy materials. He even got out the blood clot that had set off the second heart attack.

Three days later, the woman was up from bed, walking without pain.

The Sawyer operation not only cleaned out the main artery but the branches as well, and it did it in half the time of a conventional endarterectomy.

Dr. Sawyer is married to a tall, willowy schoolteacher, Grace. They have three daughters and a son. He doesn't see any of the five very much. Between the operating room and the laboratories, he works a 120-hour week.

"How do you keep a marriage going with a schedule like yours?" I asked.

"My wife is not particularly in love with my work, I will say that. But she knows that I'm not philandering. She knows that I'm not carrying on or doing something inappropriate."

He has strong convictions on why people do scientific research.

"Man is a primitive buccaneer underneath his superficial veneer of civilization," he says. "The frontiers that are available for his restless, curious, predatory mind to explore are limited. He cannot discover the Great West anymore. He can't have a running battle with some Sioux Indians while discovering the Painted Desert. All he can do is roam around the mental vacuums that exist in the world today, and those mental vacuums are largely scientific."

8

OUT OF THE MIND'S DARKNESS

SHE WAS A MENTALLY ILL woman in her mid-forties, unkempt and slovenly dressed, who cradled a big teddy bear in her arms wherever she went. She raged and screamed endlessly because she didn't want to swallow the tranquilizers that the psychiatrists at Boston State Hospital prescribed. She spit out the pills when no one was looking.

In seventeen years, she had only been outside the hospital grounds once. She ran away one evening and rang her ex-husband's doorbell. He wouldn't let her in. After the hospital attendants came for her, she was confined again to the back wards, hopeless and forgotten.

Then in 1973, a new long-acting drug, fluphenazine enanthate, was tried on her. She couldn't dupe the psychiatrists about it because they injected it into her arm with a hypodermic syringe. The calming effects lasted two weeks or more. Soon she was living a comparatively normal life out of the hospital and holding down a paid job. She merely reported to the outpatient service every two weeks for an injection. She dressed neatly and had thrown away her teddy bear. She typified a new era in the treatment and relief of mental illness.

Some prime advances have been made in recent years in the treatment of mental disorders. Antipsychotic drugs have resurrected millions of people from living death in mental hospitals. Other great gains have come through electric shock and new methods of psychotherapy.

Dr. Bertram D. Brown, director of the National Institute of Mental Health in Bethesda, Maryland, told me:

"We now have cures—in the true sense of the word—for some of the worst forms of mental illness. Depression, for example. Twenty years ago, if you had a severe depression, it was a saddening, death-dealing fact. The likelihood was that you'd have to spend many months or years in a state institution. That is, if you didn't commit suicide first. Now, with the new drugs and other techniques at our disposal, a severely depressed person has an eighty to ninety percent chance of being back home, functioning in full health, inside of a month or two."

The mental hospital records capsulate the story. In 1955, 559,000 patients were hospitalized in state and county mental insitutions in the United States, and the number was growing rapidly. Statisticians predicted that the total would top 800,000 by 1975. Instead, less than 216,000 patients were in our public mental hospitals at the start of 1975.

Mental illness is still an appalling problem, though—the biggest, most threatening health problem we have. More than 5,200,000 people have to seek professional mental health care in the United States each year. "At least one out of every ten Americans alive today will have to get professional psychiatric treatment during the course of his or her life," Dr. Brown said. (As a side note, he pointed out that several of the U.S. astronauts who landed on the moon have since suffered serious emotional problems.)

Many people do not realize how painful a disease mental illness can be. They think of mental patients as funny nuts who imagine they're Napoleon and rather enjoy the charade. They couldn't be more cruelly mistaken. The thing that struck me hardest as I traveled around the United States visiting mental hospitals was the agony of mental patients. They hurt. They constantly feel torturously, achingly sick in body as well as mind.

Dr. Henry Brill, then the director of Pilgrim State Hospital in West Brentwood, New York, one of the largest mental hospitals in the world, said to me: "The experience of mental illness is among the most difficult that human flesh is heir to. I've seen all kinds of suffering, and the suffering that goes with mental illness impresses me more than the suffering that goes with any other illness I know. It can go on for a longer time. It attacks the individual as an individual, and it destroys him if it is not controlled. It tends to alienate those near to him."

"Does a mental patient hurt the way a cancer patient hurts?" I asked.

"I've treated people with both diseases," Dr. Brill declared, "and I honestly believe that the mental patient hurts more deeply."

The most serious form of mental disease is schizophrenia. It can cause the total crumbling of an individual's personality, with hallucinations, disordered thinking, and sometimes fearful violence. It is very prevalent; one out of every two beds in our mental hospitals is occupied by a schizophrenia patient. Depression is the other major class of mental illness, and it is extremely widespread, too. Hundreds of thousands of people have manic depression, with its unreinable highs and miserable lows, or unipolar depression, which solely has the Stygian lows. Depression is a fatal illness. It is a principal cause of suicides in the United States, recently running at above 26,000 reported cases annually, plus more than twice that number that were unreported.

Mental illness is most common among elderly men and women. People over sixty-five occupy 30 percent of the beds in public mental hospitals. However, mental illness respects no age limits. It is estimated that 500,000 children in America are afflicted with psychoses and borderline psychotic conditions. This total does not include some 830,000 mentally retarded children. As a rule, these children are listed in a separate category from the mentally ill. They are usually kept in special institutions and treated by different sorts of specialists. The nine million to ten million alcoholics and problem drinkers under treatment, the 60,000 narcotic addicts, and the 200,000 to 400,000 persons caught on non-narcotic drugs can also be considered part of the mentally ill, although they generally receive therapy different from ordinary mental patients.

The hordes of people with less severe mental illnesses—the anxiety neuroses, compulsive neuroses, and other neurotic conditions that do not require hospitalization but can ruin a person's career, marriage, and family—must be included. There is no knowing exactly how many people are anguished by these neurotic disturbances. Some notion of the dimensions of the problem can be gathered from the fact that 223,200,000 prescriptions were written for psychotropic drugs (drugs for mental conditions) in one year, 1973. The N.I.M.H. says that a great mass of them was prescribed for people with neurotic difficulties.

That adds up to torrents of pills for many millions of troubled people.

Old-Time Mental Hospitals

Some diseases have been more difficult for the public mind to grasp and sympathize with than others. Leprosy is one. Syphilis and gonorrhea are two others. The sorriest has been mental illness. Through most of recorded time, people who behaved strangely were thought to be possessed by the devil. Or, at the least, to be magicians. Many were burned at the stake as witches. They were chained in dungeons, flogged, and tortured.

An Italian, Vincenzio Chiarugi, took the first step toward reform. He laid down a radical rule at Bonifacio Hospital in Florence in 1788, stating, "It is a supreme moral duty and medical obligation to respect the insane person as an individual." Dr. Philippe Pinel, a physician at the Bicêtre prison in Paris, took mental patients out of their chains in 1793. "In lunatic hospitals, as in despotic governments," Dr. Pinel wrote, "it is no doubt possible to maintain by unlimited confinement and barbarous treatment, the appearance of order and loyalty. The stillness of the grave and the silence of death, however, are not to be expected in a residence consecrated for the reception of madmen." The Englishman John Conolly taught that for mental patients restraint was even worse than neglect. In the United States, a determined nurse, Dorothea Lynde Dix, put up a magnificent battle in the middle years of the nineteenth century to halt the mistreatment of the "pauper insane." She got thirty state hospitals built for the mentally ill.

No one had a treatment for helping the insane, though. When King George III of England went into a deep psychotic depression in 1788, his doctors debated vehemently as to whether they should bleed His Majesty, purge his intestines, give him something to make him vomit, blister his skull, or walk him around the royal gardens to the accompaniment of calming music.

A century and a half later, not much more was known. Dr. Frank J. Ayd has provided a vivid picture of the conditions in most mental hospitals before the introduction of psychotropic drugs in the 1950s.

Within the bare walls of isolated, overcrowded, prisonlike asylums were housed many screaming, combative individuals whose animalistic behavior required restraint and seclusion. Catatonic patients stood day after day, rigid as statues, their legs swollen and bursting with dependent edema. Their comrades idled week after week, lying on hard benches or the floor, aware only of their delusions and hallucinations. Others were incessantly restive, pacing back and forth like caged animals in a zoo. Periodically, the air was pierced by the shouts of a raving maniac. Suddenly, without notice, like an erupting volcano, an anergic schizophrenic bursts into frenetic behavior, lashing out at others or striking himself with his fists, or running wildly and aimlessly about.

Nurses and attendants, ever in danger, spent their time protecting patients from harming themselves or others. . . . For lack of more effective remedies, they secluded dangerously frenetic individuals behind thick doors in barred rooms stripped of all furniture and lacking toilet facilities. They restrained many others in cuffs and jackets or chained them to floors and walls. Daily they sent patients for hydrotherapy, where they were immersed for long hours in tubs, or were packed in wet sheets until their disturbed behavior subsided. These measures, barbaric and inhumane as they appear in retrospect, euphemistically called therapy, at best offered protection to patient and personnel and a temporary respite from the most distressing symptoms of psychoses.

Schizophrenia and Depression

Let us take a closer look at the two most terrifying disorders, schizophrenia and depression.

Schizophrenia is a relatively new term for an old disease. It used to be known as dementia praecox. This is an ogreish disease in which the patient can lose all contact with reality. The individual symptoms may vary. One patient may go into catatonic trances while another keeps on the move ceaselessly, from ward wall to ward wall. One may gorge herself, another may refuse to eat and have to be force-fed. No single cause for the disorder is known. No evil gene, no one chemical, no one stressful occurrence (such as the death of a loved one) seems able by itself to cause this shattering disorder, but a combination of these factors can lead to it. Ordinarily, schizophrenia manifests itself in early adolescence or young adulthood.

Depression comes at any age. In manic depressive disorders, the patient swings between the wildest psychic elation and the darkest, numbing melancholia. The unipolar depressive knows only the black melancholia. He feels mountainous despair, fear, tension, guilt, and hopelessness. He is apt to have physical symptoms like nausea, stomach cramps, headaches, chest pains, and a feeling of overwhelming exhaustion. He may lie in bed, inert, for long periods, curled up in a fetal position.

Some authorities believe that the causes of depression are biochemical. They say that depression stems from abnormal chemical processes in the brain and body. Other authorities feel that depressions are produced by psychological defects resulting from ''unfortunate events in human relationships.'' A third group thinks that the causes are a combination of biochemical and psychological factors. No one really knows the answer with scientific certainty.

Like so many diseases, mental illness is punctuated mostly with question marks.

Sigmund Freud, who was born in Austria in 1856 and died in England in 1939, a refugee from Nazi terror, turned the first shining light into the murky regions of mental illness. Dr. Freud suggested that many abnormal mental states were due to psychic trauma that the patients had suffered in early youth and repressed or forgotten. He placed immense stress on infantile sexuality and Oedipus complexes. Dreams were an unconscious revelation of repressed desires, he maintained, primarily sexual desires.

Freud developed a probing method of psychoanalytic treatment for mental conditions. Under this treatment, a patient allowed emotionally disturbing material to escape from his subconscious through the free association of ideas. The patient underwent a catharsis in this way that effected a cure, Freud believed.

Controversy has raged around Freud and his theories of psychoanalysis ever since he promulgated them. His two chief disciples, Carl Gustav Jung and Alfred Adler, set up competing schools of psychoanalysis, and many others have emulated them. But nobody can rightly discount the impact that Freud has had on psychiatry. He stands with the titans.

Psychoanalysis can only help a comparatively few patients, though. It is very costly and time-consuming.

A Portuguese surgeon, Dr. Egas Moniz, devised a different approach to the problem of mental illness in the 1930s. It was far more drastic. Inhuman, many have charged.

Moniz bored two small holes in the patient's forehead and destroyed the frontal lobe areas of the patient's brain. The operation, called lobotomy, was supposed to make a chronic schizophrenic suffer less from his hallucinations and delusions. In fact, it was useful mostly for making unruly patients manageable. The hospital attendants were the principal beneficiaries.

This kind of psychosurgery was widely employed for some years. Finally, the side effects became too glaring to countenance. The operation could completely change a patient's personality. It often turned him into a lazy, cowlike creature. A modified version of the operation continues to be used in some British, Scandinavian, and other foreign hospitals, but it is rarely done in the United States.

Kalinowsky Suggests Electric Shock Therapy

Shock therapy was something else. It furnished the first real, large-scale help for the mentally ill.

In 1933, Dr. Manfred Sakel, a Viennese physician, administered enough insulin to some agitated mental patients to render them unconscious. When these patients came out of their comas, they were markedly improved for a time. All their symptoms temporarily vanished. In 1934, the Hungarian Lazlo von Meduna found that the drug Metrazol was even more effective than insulin. It sent the patients into convulsions that greatly alleviated their symptoms for a while.

Two Italian physicians did it still better—with electricity. Drs. Ugo Cerletti and Lucio Bini heard about the Metrazol shock treatments from Dr. Lothar B. Kalinowsky, a German psychiatrist who had fled Nazi Germany to Rome. He had seen Meduna perform the Metrazol shock treatments.

"Why doesn't Meduna give these convulsions with electricity?" Cerletti immediately asked him.

"It would surely seem to be easier," Dr. Kalinowsky agreed.

In November 1937, the two Italians placed electrodes on both sides of the forehead of a schizophrenic patient and sent electricity jolting into his brain. Their treatment proved far superior to the Metrazol therapy. Schizophrenics stopped hallucinating, mute patients began to talk, and the convulsions were no more violent.

Across the Atlantic, the American Medical Association was horrified. It published a strident warning that patients might be electrocuted. (The A.M.A.'s experts mistakenly assumed that the electric current went to the heart instead of the brain.) Nevertheless, electroshock quickly became standard therapy for schizophrenia in Europe.

Dr. Kalinowsky did more than anyone to introduce electroshock to the United States. He came to America in 1940, on the run again from the Nazis, and he conducted the first large-scale clinical evaluation of electroshock at Pilgrim State Hospital. It was a pivotal study. It showed that electroshock was actually more helpful for depression than for schizophrenia. The fact was that electroshock could help schizophrenics in the very early stages of their illness, but it had nothing to offer the chronic schizophrenic. On the other hand, electroshock could be of great value for most types of depression.

I talked with Dr. Kalinowsky about it more than thirty years later in his New York City office. He was a man in the early seventies, white-haired, with a very thin face and unusually big ears.

"It was one of the most spectacular things in the history of medicine," he declared. "We found that the endogenous type of depression—the kind that's not caused by outside emotional factors—usually cleared up after three or four electroshock treatments. A series of six treatments was generally sufficient to clear up most other types of depression. It worked with young persons, middle-aged persons, or even old persons, the sort who frequently have depressions that are sometimes misdiagnosed as senile psychosis."

A manic depressive might have a new episode several years later, he stated, but a few shock treatments could easily bring him out of it again.

At the outset, electroshock had the scent of the rack, and was feared as much. At times, a patient was completely conscious when the electric current surged into him. Attendants had to hold him down to keep him from breaking an arm, a leg, or his spine while he thrashed madly about. With the passage of time, kinder techniques were perfected. A patient is now put gently to sleep with an intravenous anesthetic and is given an injection that relaxes his muscles. He sleeps through the procedure and awakens gradually. Usually, he is up and walking within a half hour. The electricity merely causes mild muscular contractions. The most that shows is a slight twitching of the toes. Some patients suffer a temporary loss of memory, but they customarily recover it in a few weeks. Physicians don't refer to it as electroshock therapy anymore. They call it electroconvulsive therapy, or ECT.

Joshua Logan, the celebrated Broadway director and playwright, who has been a manic depressive for more than thirty years, was given ECT to bring him down from a manic high. It was, he recalls, a remarkable experience.

"I cannot describe to you what a peaceful, quiet, almost miraculous effect it had," he told me. "I had no sense of electricity or shock or hurt or jerking. I just went to sleep. When I woke up a half hour later, I felt marvelous. Absolutely marvelous. I couldn't wait to have it happen again. I think they gave me either four or five treatments. I welcomed them like a baby reaching for candy. In three weeks, I was well."

It must be said that other patients have had different reactions. They dread ECT treatments.

ECT has now been largely replaced by drug therapy. However, it is still used in very severe cases when there isn't time to wait for drugs to take effect—when suicide is an immediate threat, say, or for patients who don't respond to antidepressant drugs. U.S. Senator Thomas F. Eagleton, of Missouri, underwent ECT twice for depression before he got to the Senate in 1969. With fine results, I must note.

Dr. Kalinowsky is a rarity among medical pioneers: a man who shies away from credit. When his colleagues hail him as "a father of electroshock therapy," he adamantly denies paternity.

"Maybe a godfather, but no more," he says.

He was born in Berlin in 1899 of an old Prussian family, but ran afoul of the Nazis because his mother was Jewish. He chose psychiatry after he graduated from medical school because it was easier to land a job in a mental institution than a general hospital. Besides, mental institutions paid wages to their interns.

At seventy-six, Dr. Kalinowsky still had an active psychiatric practice in New York City. "A certain curiosity" motivated him. That and the necessity to find scientific proof to convince other physicians of the right kind of treatment for the mentally ill.

He married Hilda Pohl, a Berlin girl who typed his doctoral dissertation and who continues to be his secretary. They have two daughters. Music and travel are his twin loves. His idea of the perfect vacation is visiting one psychiatric hospital after another.

"In what mental hospitals do we have tea tomorrow?" his wife has to ask him daily when they are abroad on a vacation.

Dr. Kalinowsky holds that the cause of most mental illness is chemical.

"If only we knew what chemical changes in the brain cause the schizophrenic and the depressive psychoses, we could develop drugs to counteract them," he said.

A Triple Play for CPZ
—*Revolutionary Tranquilizer*

When the city of Paris paid excited tribute to Sir Alexander Fleming in 1945 for his splendid discovery of penicillin, the British scientist remarked, "I have been accused of having invented penicillin. But I didn't. And nobody could have invented it because penicillin was always there."

Chlorpromazine, the greatest of the tranquilizing drugs, was not always there. It was created out of nothingness, carefully designed in the laboratories of a pharmaceutical company for three specific medical purposes.

The three purposes had nothing whatsoever to do with tranquilizing medical patients, though.

On December 11, 1950, French chemist Paul Charpentier, who was employed in the Rhône-Poulenc laboratories of the drug firm Specia, synthesized a new phenothiazine derivative. It took him only three months to do it. This was chlorpromazine, or CPZ for short.

CPZ was tailor-made to have maximum effect on the involuntary nervous system. Specia saw it as a drug that would make anesthetics, painkillers, and hypnotics more powerful. No one was very impressed by it, and it would probably have wound up on a back shelf if a thirty-six-year-old French navy doctor, Dr. Henri-Marie Laborit, had not recommended a different use for it.

Peppery Dr. Laborit is a physician who has always been intensely concerned with alleviating pain. "Our profession, in the laboratory as at the patient's bedside—keeping us increasingly in contact with life, with suffering, and with death—forbids indifference," he wrote. "Can one remain insensate and not revolt if one sees how life leaves a body it animated and that nothing in the world can prohibit this? Can one remain insensate if one sees physical pain so unjustly dealt out. . . ?"

Laborit was born of French parents in Indo-China, graduated from a university in Paris, and got his medical schooling at the Naval Health Service in Bordeaux. During World War II, he heard gunfire in torpedo boats and cruisers, and helped patch up the wounded at Dakar and Anzio.

Anesthesiology was his specialty—the field most directly occupied with easing pain.

While on duty in a naval hospital in Tunisia in 1949, Laborit started to study a synthetic antihistamine named promethazine. It was a derivative of phenothiazine. He found that it was "eminently precious in the prevention of surgical shock." But it did something else. "For reasons we had not suspected," he reported, "the promethazine produced 'euphoric quietude' in patients undergoing surgery." After patients were given promethazine, they became "calm, somewhat somnolent, relaxed, and looked rested." Even after they underwent major surgery, the patients were euphoric, never excited, uncomplaining, and they appeared to suffer less.

A new medical term was coined for this reaction—ataraxia. The medical dictionaries define it as "complete calmness and peace of mind." It comes from the Greek word for that cold-blooded indifference which the Stoics exalted.

The Labroit report had immediate effects on surgery. French anesthesiologists began to substitute promethazine for barbiturates on the evening before surgery, and to use it instead of morphine following the operation. It made matters a lot easier for the surgeons as well.

"Gone is the time of not so long ago when a surgeon who wanted to work quietly loved to hear his deeply anesthetized patient's sonorous snore," Dr. Laborit commented.

But Laborit wanted more. Surgeons often need to operate with the patient fully conscious, so Laborit sought a drug that had no sedative effects but would still anesthetize the patient and stave off shock. At his prodding, Charpentier went to work on the problem. CPZ was the speedy solution.

Early in 1951, the navy transferred Laborit to its Val-de-Grâce hospital in Paris and told him to concentrate on his research. In September 1951, he reported that CPZ was far superior to promethazine as an anesthetic. Injected intravenously, CPZ produced satisfactory anesthesia without loss of consciousness, and it could bring patients out of severe traumatic shock. Large doses could be administered to patients without detrimental side effects.

He concocted a "lyptic cocktail" composed of CPZ and two other drugs, pethidine and promethazine, that made it possible to produce a state of artificial hibernation in a patient in the operating room. After the lyptic cocktail was administered, a patient could be swathed in ice bags and his temperature safely lowered to 80° Fahrenheit, or even less. It permitted surgeons to do very complicated operations on poor-risk patients without danger of surgical shock.

Laborit had more on his mind, though. He was a genuine scientist with an eye always open for other therapeutic possibilities. In his paper on CPZ, he made an observation that hatched a golden era in the treatment of the mentally ill.

"In doses of 50-100 mg intravenously," he wrote, "[CPZ] does not provoke any loss in consciousness, not any change in the patient's mentality but a slight tendency to sleep and above all 'disinterest' for all that goes on around him. . . ."

At the end, Laborit added twelve historic words: "These facts let us see certain indications for this drug in psychiatry."

It was the first suggestion that CPZ would be valuable in treating mentally ill patients.

The first test was a flop. Psychiatrists at Val-de-Grâe tried the lyptic cocktail on manic patients and got nowhere with it. They judged its effects interesting, but not strong enough. They contentedly resumed their regular electroshock therapy.

Another Paris psychiatrist was not so easily put off. Dr. Pierre G. Deniker, a thirty-four-year-old friend of Laborit who taught at the University of Paris medical school, decided to let some patients have the CPZ alone. A young intern, Dr. J.M. Harl, started the experiment with him but didn't live to finish it. He was killed in a mountain-climbing accident. Laborit's chief, Dr. Jean Delay, kept a supervisory eye on the experiment from afar.

Deniker gave the CPZ to thirty-eight patients. He used big doses by early standards, tiny by today's thinking, about 150 mg daily in four well-spaced injections.

The results were unprecedented, and rapid. After the first ten patients, the outcome was certain. Deniker reported to a medical meeting in Luxembourg in May 1952 that CPZ did away with "agitation, aggressiveness, and delusive conditions" in schizophrenics. It enabled psychiatrists to reestablish contact with far-gone schizophrenics. Psychotics who were resistant to shock and sleep therapy responded to CPZ. Mental wards that had been arenas of raucous noise and violence became peaceful, quiet refuges.

CPZ was not very helpful to depressives. Deniker reported that it just gave some symptomatic relief. Four and a half more years had to pass before real antidepressant drugs were discovered in an American mental hospital.

Dr. Laborit referred to CPZ as "a stabilizer," but that name never caught on. By 1954, most medical people were calling drugs of this type "tranquilizers," and they still do. It is a dangerously bad use of the language.

The word "tranquilizer" entered the medical vocabulary in 1810 when Dr. Benjamin Rush, the father of American psychiatry, designed an uncomfortable wooden chair, fitted it out with harsh restraining straps, and euphemistically dubbed it "a tranquilizer." As the term "tranquilizer" is employed in most medical circles today, it is a misnomer. Tranquilizing is only a partial description of what drugs like CPZ do. The word "tranquilizer" implies that these drugs are solely sedatives, to be used to calm excitement. They do considerably more than that. They have a distinctly curative, antipsychotic effect on the schizophrenic's brain. They decrease his fears and lessen his acute symptoms. Even if delusions or hallucinations remain, they are less scary and disturbing to the patient. The drugs enable the schizophrenic patient to think more clearly and function more appropriately.

According to Dr. Brill, a pioneer in the use of tranquilizers, countless physicians have been misled by the name into prescribing these drugs principally as sedatives.

"Most doctors have shockingly underestimated the usefulness of these medications," Dr. Brill declared.

Which is not to denigrate the magnificent help that CPZ and other tranquilizers have given countless numbers of psychotic patients. Or their sedative value to millions of nonpsychotic people whose tensions have gotten the best of them.

Drs. Laborit and Deniker are still active in their Paris laboratories. Laborit is a Gallic type, of average height, who cuts a dashing figure in his naval uniform. He has risen to be a colonel and director of all medical research for the French military. He and Genevieve de Saint-Mart were married in 1936. They have had five children. Deniker is a heavy-set man, slow and steady-going, more Teutonic than Gallic in manner. He has been married to Nadine Vincent since 1941. He teaches at the Sorbonne (where he obtained his M.D. in 1945), and is physician-in-chief at the Hôpitaux Psychologiques. Both Laborit and Deniker have been made Chevaliers de la Légion d'Honneur.

The tranquilizer story now shifts from Paris to Canada. A French-speaking German refugee from Nazism with a near-holy consecration to research introduced tranquilizers to the North American continent. On a Sunday morning in 1953, Dr. Heinz E. Lehmann, clinical director of the Verdun Protestant Hospital, a mental institution in Montreal that is now called Douglas Hospital, happened to glance at some reprints of French medical reports. One was on CPZ. He tried it on seventy schizophrenic patients, and within a week saw that "it was revolutionary."

Lehmann was born in Berlin in 1911. His school grades were so bad that his teacher urged his mother to take him out of school and have him learn a trade.

"Let Heinz be a plumber or a carpenter," the teacher said. "I tell you, Frau Lehmann, he's no good for anything else."

Frau Lehmann would not listen to him.

By the time Heinz was fifteen, he had read most of Freud's writings. By sixteen, he had decided to become a psychiatrist. It was much against his father's wishes. A surgeon, Dr. Lehmann, Sr., thought psychotherapy was fine as a theory but not very effective as treatment. Heinz secured his M.D. at the University of Berlin in 1935, but he was half Jewish so he couldn't practice medicine in Nazi Germany. He emigrated to Canada in 1937 and learned English. He married a French-Canadian nurse, Annette Joyal, in 1940 and learned French. Their only son is a family physician who works in a storefront clinic in a Montreal slum.

A short, white-haired man, Dr. Lehmann is now a professor of psychiatry at the McGill University medical school, director of medical education and research at Douglas Hospital, and the most respected man in Canadian psychiatry.

He has no private practice. "I can't afford to make money," he told me. "If I made money, I'd be at the beck and call of people who might not interest me or really need serious treatment."

He is deeply, emotionally committed to his patients. "I have a personal battle against sickness," he said. "I hate suffering. As soon as I see suffering, I am personally enraged."

Drs. Laborit, Deniker and Lehmann each received a Lasker Award for their work with CPZ. As the Lasker Awards committee said, "The problems of psychiatry had been brought within reach of the experimental laboratory as never before and the future was suddenly more bright and promising."

Kline Discovers the Antidepressants

Now, a scene change and a switch of cast. We are going to the rolling campus of Rockland State Hospital in Orangeburg, New York, to meet one of the most Promethean men in medicine, the only person ever to win two Lasker Awards. This is Dr. Nathan S. Kline, the psychiatrist who first discovered the infinite worth of antidepressant drugs. It was the most significant development in the treatment of the mentally ill during the past half century. Dr. Kline also gave the Western world a new class of tranquilizers.

I confess to a certain enthusiasm in Dr. Kline's favor. I've seen the near-miraculous results he has attained in caring for patients with depression. I saw him treat a highly intelligent, well-educated woman in her forties who was so depressed that she had virtually become a zombi. She was in continuous black despair, unable to talk or think coherently. She could scarcely move. She was without hope.

Kline tried several antidepressant drugs on her. If one didn't help or had upsetting side effects, he switched to another. Swiftly, he found the combination of drugs that was right for her. At the same time, he talked with her and gave her hope that she could recover. In a month, she was showing signs of real improvement. Inside of two months, her depression was completely gone, she was her attractive self again. Six years later, she was living a thoroughly normal, satisfying life.

Needless to say, the woman worships Dr. Kline. She says that he saved her life. In fact, he did. She had tried suicide twice before she got to him.

Kline is a man in his early sixties, middle-tall, with a mane of thick grey hair and, always, a wonderful coat of tan. He fairly bursts with energy. He can get along on four and a half hours' sleep a night and crowd a week's activity into the other nineteen and a half hours. He holds down three important positions in the psychiatric field. He is director of the Rockland Research Institute at Rockland State Hospital, clinical professor of psychiatry at Columbia University medical school, and director of psychiatric services at a New Jersey hospital. Important jobs, each of them. He is a consultant to WHO and a half dozen foreign governments such as Haiti and Nepal. On top of this, he has the largest private psychiatric practice in the United States. He also finds time to collect modern paintings, abstract sculpture, and primitive artifacts. A speed-reader, he can gobble up two or three books a day. He is a storehouse of esoteric facts about medicine and practically everything else. He can quote poetry for hours on end. He writes poetry, too.

"It's another kind of reality for me," he says.

He was born to a wealthy family in Philadelphia in 1916, but his family's money was no help. His father died when he was sixteen and his guardian refused to give him any money for college. He insisted that the boy go into the family's department store business instead. Kline worked his way through Swarthmore College by waiting on tables.

He started psychology at Harvard Graduate School with no thought of becoming a physician. However, Professor McFie Campbell, chairman of the Harvard psychiatry department, got him aside.

"Kline," he growled in his Scottish burr, "I've never seen a psychologist who didn't have an inferiority complex. For God's sake, go to medical school."

He enrolled in N.Y.U. medical school and was "bored to hell" by most of his classes. He was in the bottom 10 percent of the class when he graduated in 1943. An internship at St. Elizabeth's, the U.S. mental hospital in Washington, D.C., followed, and wartime service in the merchant marine. In 1952, he reported to Rockland State Hospital as research director. The hospital authorities had promised him a free hand.

Why did he go into research?

"I have a kind of obsessive curiosity about everything," he said to me. "Whatever goes on, I like to stick my rather long nose into. Particularly into what makes people behave the way they do."

He continued. "I'm like Will Rogers. I never met a person I didn't really like. Some of them I grew to hate, but they never stopped interesting me."

He has been accused of intellectual snobbery. He scoffs at the idea. "I have prejudices, but no snobbery. Most people are very interesting if you ask them the right questions."

Dr. Kline stumbled into his tranquilizers. In the spring of 1953, his laboratory needed money to purchase some apparatus for analyzing gases. He applied to E.R. Squibb & Sons, the pharmaceutical manufacturers, for a research grant. Squibb's told him that it only gave money to researchers for product development or for goodwill, and that no drug manufacturer cared much about the goodwill of mental hospitals.

Kline scouted about for a new product and brought up one that was two thousand years old. It was *Rauwolfia serpentina*, the ancient Indian remedy for cholera, epilepsy, and a host of other maladies. An Indian scientist had reported that it might be of use in schizophrenia. Kline got a $1,000 grant from Squibb's to evaluate it as a sedative for psychotic patients.

While he was organizing the study, Dr. Kline heard that scientists of the Ciba company of Switzerland had isolated the rauwolfia alkaloid, reserpine. (As we've already learned, reserpine was soon to prove of great value in reducing high blood pressure.) Kline raced over to the Ciba division in Summit, New Jersey, and persuaded them to give him a few thousand dollars more to include reserpine in his study.

Remember, no one in the United States was yet aware of CPZ and its remarkable effects on schizophrenic patients.

Kline's study started with 710 severely disturbed schizophrenic patients. Each patient was tested with the whole rauwolfia, the reserpine, and a placebo. Instead of employing subjective criteria, such as "The patient seems better today," Kline set up objective standards. How many windows in the ward were broken this week? How many patients had to be sent for ice packs? What other sedatives were needed?

Toward the close of the nine-month trials, Ciba came out with a new, concentrated, intramuscular form of reserpine. It produced the most vivid results. In a matter of hours, severely demented patients were calm.

"I remember one woman who was convinced that she was in hell and burning," Dr. Kline said. "We gave her an injection and within an hour or two she quieted down. Within a day or two the psychosis was relatively relieved."

More than four hundred schizophrenic patients were observed from start to finish, and the biggest number of them were vastly benefited by the reserpine. They calmed down. They largely lost their delusions and hallucinations. They were able to cope with their environment.

Dr. Kline reported his results in 1954 shortly after Dr. Lehmann published his findings on CPZ. According to Kline, "There was general and universal skepticism."

He relished the fray. "I must say that it was one of the most enjoyable periods of my existence. By this time, I was positive that all of the angels were on my side, and I didn't really give a damn whether people agreed or disagreed."

The Kline and Lehmann reports reinforced each other. Together, they proved the value of tranquilizers in the treatment of mental disease. Reluctantly, the psychotherapists had to accept them. No aspect of mental hospital life was left untouched. Inside of a year, the population of mental hospitals had commenced to fall. Rockland had 8,150 patients in 1954. In 1957, it had 7,600. On April 1, 1975, it had 2,251.

Dr. Kline received his first Lasker Award in 1957 for his work with reserpine. It was well earned even though reserpine has now been supplanted by CPZ in mental hospitals inasmuch as CPZ's side effects are less dangerous. In its time, reserpine helped tens of thousands of psychotic patients to refind their lives.

Unlike his research with tranquilizers, there was nothing accidental about Dr. Kline's discovery of the antidepressant drugs. He went hunting for them.

"If you can treat schizophrenics with drugs," he argued, "there must be something you can do with drugs for depressives."

He was looking for something that he named a "psychic energizer": a drug that would generate enough psychic energy in the patients to bring them out of the sadness and inertia of melancholia. Kline outlined the clinical properties he wanted in a paper for the American Psychoanalytic Association in the spring of 1956.

Such a drug, he said, "would reduce the sleep requirements and delay the onset of fatigue. It would increase appetite and sexual desire and increase behavioral drive in general. Motor and intellectual activity would be speeded up. It would heighten responsiveness to stimuli, both pleasant and noxious. . . . [It] would result in a sense of joyousness and optimism.''

The psychoanalysts thought Kline was himself out of his mind. But the fates were with him even if the psychoanalysts weren't.

In April 1956, Kline gave a lecture at Warner-Chilcott Laboratories in Morris Plains, New Jersey. Afterward, Dr. Charles P. Scott, a company scientist, described to him the strange outcome of an experiment of his. Scott had injected laboratory mice with iproniazid, the drug that had such salutary effects on tuberculosis patients. It made the mice as lively as it had the TB patients. Scott followed it up with an injection of reserpine to see how well it could tranquilize the mice. It couldn't. Instead of calming down, the mice became hyperactive and hyperalert.

Scott was interested in the functioning of reserpine. Kline saw something more to the experiment. Maybe this was the psychic energizer he had been chasing.

''I was fascinated by the photos of the experimental animals,'' he said. ''One of them had become a veritable supermouse. I was glad that he was inside the cage.''

He searched through the medical literature on iproniazid, back to the first tests on tuberculosis patients. In report after report, he found, clinicians treating tubercular patients had noted the euphoria produced by iproniazid. But . . .

''This went right by everybody's nose,'' Dr. Kline declared. ''Here all the psychiatrists in the world and everybody looked at this, and not a single person had the thought that it might be useful in treating depression.''

Dr. Evert Svenson, the assistant medical director of Hoffmann-LaRoche, the manufacturers of iproniazid, had the same good inspiration. He suggested to his chief that iproniazid might be valuable as an antidepressant. His chief laughed him out of his office. Svenson later had a hard fight to get his company to supply enough iproniazid for Kline's experiments.

In November 1956, Dr. Kline launched his depression trials. This time, he didn't go after big numbers of patients. He started seventeen patients at Rockland State on iproniazid. The hospital didn't have enough depressives on its rolls, so these were just ''burnt-out schizophrenic patients, flattened, blah.'' In January 1957, Kline broadened the experiment to include nine real depressives from his private practice in New York City.

In three weeks, he had the answer from the really depressed patients. One patient who had a physical ailment didn't respond to the iproniazid, and another only feebly, but the other seven showed extraordinary improvement. Their melancholia and its accompanying horrors melted away. They became normal human beings.

Was a sampling of seven patients enough to prove that a drug could dissipate depression? Was this scientific evidence, or was it merely an anecdote?

Dr. Kline has a provocative theory here. "Frequently, the question arises as to how many patients you need to prove something," he said. "My reply is that it really depends on what you want to prove, and how dramatic the proof is. If you had a drug that would revive someone postmortem, one case is all that you would need. If you were an absolute purist, you might ask for a second case. Anything beyond that would be nonsense. You wouldn't have to do any statistical analyses."

He first reported his findings with iproniazid at a public hearing of a U.S. Senate appropriations subcommittee in May 1957, and he encountered more skepticism in the psychiatric community than he did with his reserpine findings.

"A lot of people were waiting to get me," he says. "This time, they were sure that I'd come a cropper. People announced that they had disproved my facts before they'd even tried the drug."

It was a medication whose time had come, though. No drug in history has been so widely used so soon after the announcement of its usefulness. As estimated four hundred thousand people were treated with iproniazid in the United States in the first year.

Kline won his second Lasker Award in 1964 for the introduction of iproniazid. The citation read, "Dr. Kline more than any other single psychiatrist has been responsible for one of the greatest revolutions ever to occur in the care and treatment of the mentally ill. Literally hundreds of thousands of people are leading productive, normal lives who—but for Dr. Kline's work—would be leading lives of fruitless despair and frustration."

Apparently iproniazid inhibits a key enzyme, monamine oxidase, that prolongs the life of a chemical that probably serves as a transmitter between nerve cells in the brain. Iproniazid and antidepressants that work like it are therefore called MAO inhibitors. There is a small clan of them now.

Some orthodox psychotherapists discount the value of psychotropic drugs on the grounds that they don't cure the disease. They merely ameliorate the symptoms, it is claimed. Kline thinks these critics are psychiatric nit-pickers.

"No one knows what causes psychiatric disorders," he delcares. "We have some nice theories, sure, but we still don't know the cause of any of the major mental diseases and emotional disorders. So no one can talk about cures. It's meaningless. How are you going to tell whether you've affected a cure, or not, if you don't know what the cause of a disease is? You can't tell if you've done away with it.

"Let's say that someone discovered penicillin and didn't know that bacteria existed. You'd give the patient the antibiotic and the symptoms would disappear. Then someone would say, 'Did you cure the patient?' If you're unable to tell what's causing the sickness, how can you tell whether you've cured the patient? All you can say is that the symptoms are totally gone.

"With antidepressant drugs, the symptoms usually disappear and, for the most part, don't recur. The psychotherapists and the electroshock therapists can say no more than that."

Today, Dr. Kline is the most influential psychopharmacologist alive, and I must say that he enjoys his eminence. He revels in his frequent TV appearances, his testimony "on the Hill," his darting trips about the world for lectures and conferences.

He continues his research at Rockland State. He is seeking a blood test for schizophrenia, for example. And trying to establish whether the month of a person's birth has anything to do with his development of schizophrenia. Seemingly, it does. More schizophrenics are born in January, February, and March than in any other month. In the Northern Hemisphere, that is. He is trying to find out if it is true of July, August, and September in the Southern Hemisphere.

He is principally interested in research methodology. What is science? What is the scientific method? How do you prove something? How do you demonstrate a truth?

"I write articles on this for learned journals that no one reads but myself," he ruefully remarks.

Chess used to be an outlet for him, but no more. It eats up too much time. "Music, I like," he says. "Theater, I'm mad for. I read a lot, both fiction as well as nonfiction. I have an inordinate interest in early cultures.

"Travel, of course. The universe is my hobby. In a sense, I have a problem because I get so curious about anything I do. I get so intensely involved in it that I have to pull myself away. Otherwise, I'd keep on almost indefinitely in almost anything you set me to looking at."

After more than thirty years, his marriage to Margot Hess broke up in 1973. They have a very attractive daughter, Marna, in her twenties.

His private offices on the chic East Side are a bit like a subway car in a rush hour. On an average day, Kline and his assistants treat as many as seventy-five patients, and the jam can be colossal.

Dr. Kline doesn't like to admit it, but he seems to get far better results with the same psychotropic drugs than do other physicians. Dr. Brill has an interesting explanation for this phenomenon.

"If a drug is to have the optimal effect, the doctor must have a high degree of charisma," Brill declares. "The charismatic doctor can get two to three times the value of a drug that another doctor can who is not as good."

If there is one thing Nate Kline has, it is charisma.

Kuhn and Cade Bring More Help to the Depressed

More solace for the depressed was emerging during these years in Switzerland and Australia.

Claude Bernard, the nineteenth-century Frenchman who sired the science of physiology, liked to say, "An experiment is nothing but a provoked experience." Dr. Roland Kuhn, a Swiss psychiatrist, provoked some clinical "experiences" that led to a new type of antidepressant. Dr. John F.J. Cade, an obscure Australian psychiatrist, did the same thing "down under." He chanced on a use for the chemical element lithium that no one had ever suspected.

Kuhn, a tall white-haired man who stands very erect, was born in 1912 in Bienne and obtained his education at the University of Berne and the Sorbonne. In childhood, he yearned to find new drugs for the sick. "As a schoolboy," he recalls, "I used to collect plants and believed that these or even just bright green water colors would cure all sorts of dangerous diseases I had read or heard about."

In 1950, the Swiss drug firm J.R. Geigy went to Kuhn at the Münsterlingen Psychiatric Clinic in Münsterlingen and asked him to test a new antihistamine for use as a hypnotic, a sleep-inducing drug. The results were utterly negative. Still, it seemed to Kuhn that the antihistamine might have some special antidepressive value, and he proposed to Geigy that he follow up on this. No thanks, the company said. It wasn't interested.

By 1954, CPZ had been discovered, and the psychiatric climate had changed. Kuhn wrote to Geigy, urging again that the antihistamine be run through some more tests. Geigy agreed, but the results were as fruitless. The antihistamine proved useless against depression.

The following year, Geigy sent Kuhn another substance to test. Its only name was substance G 22355. Later, it would be known to physicians as imipramine, to the lay public as Tofranil. It belonged to the dibenazepine group of compounds, and its chemical structure was notable in that it had a three-membered branch side chain.

Geigy thought that G 22355 would be valuable in schizophrenia. It wasn't. Schizophrenic symptoms weren't at all alleviated. However, something else happened, and Kuhn spotted it. The symptoms of depression that are also seen in some schizophrenics cleared up. Kuhn was not one to let something like that slip by him. He gave G 22355 to a group of patients with endogenous depression. The first three told him what he needed to know. The compound was superbly effective against depression.

Kuhn reported his findings to the Second International Congress of Psychiatry in September 1967. Barely a dozen people turned up to hear his paper, and they scoffed. Nevertheless, imipramine won fast acceptance. More than five thousand scientific papers have since been written about it and untold millions of patients benefited by it.

A fine family of "tricyclic antidepressants" has grown from imipramine. The "tricyclic" name comes from their three-membered side chain. They seem to do the same sort of chemical job in the brain as do the MAO inhibitors, but by another mechanism.

Dr. Kuhn objects to all the stress that's been placed on chance in his discovery of imipramine. He made an emotional speech about it to a psychiatric symposium in Mexico.

"Chance admittedly had something to with the discovery of imipramine," he said. "Chance was not decisive, however, even though the discoverer was privileged to turn this chance to good account. Good fortune, too, played a part, but to this had to be added a measure of intellectual achievement that was able to 'invent' something completely new, something hitherto unknown. . . .

"The discovery of the antidepressive properties of imipramine thus appears not only as a unique event, as a lucky chance, but also an achievement of the progressively developing human intellect, with its manifold limitations and freedoms."

The lithium story took a few years longer to unfold, but the denouement was even more striking. Mankind got a drug that could prevent the highs and lows of manic depression from occurring. And the drug cost only pennies.

Lithium, the third of the chemical elements, has had an erratic history in medicine. Doctors first used it in 1859 for gout. Soon it was being administered for a variety of other conditions, and doing a lot more harm than good. A 1907 medical journal warned of cardiac depression ensuing from excessive consumption of lithium tablets. Lithium intoxication was another threat. By the 1920s, lithium had fallen into disuse. In the 1940s, it was employed again as a salt substitute for people with congestive heart failure, but it ended by killing some of them and badly poisoning others. In 1949, the U.S. Food and Drug Administration discouraged its use.

That was the year John Cade, an ebullient thirty-seven-year-old psychiatrist on the staff of the Repatriation Mental Hospital in Bundoora, a suburb of Melbourne, started on the pharmacological rehabilitation of lithium. The times couldn't have been worse for him or his lithium salts.

Dr. Cade believed that manic depression was caused by a chemical imbalance in the body. He assumed that "mania is a state of intoxication by a normal product in the body circulating in excess, while melancholia is the corresponding deprivative condition." If this thesis were correct, he reasoned, a manic depressive patient should excrete the guilty product in his urine.

He took uric acid excreted by manic patients and injected it into guinea pigs. The little animals went into wild convulsions and died inside of twelve to twenty-eight minutes. What would happen if he reduced the strength of the uric acid? Cade wondered. He couldn't add water to the uric acid; it is insoluble in water. So he mixed it with lithium salts.

He injected the new solution into his guinea pigs. This time, not one pig had a convulsion and died. Obviously, the lithium was protecting the guinea pigs against the very poisonous uric acid. But how? Cade injected lithium alone into the guinea pigs. Immediately, every guinea pig became wonderfully calm and relaxed.

When he placed the guinea pigs on their backs, they didn't try frantically to right themselves as they usually do.

"They merely lay there and gazed placidly back at me," he reported.

Fortune was at work again.

The intellectual leap that led Dr. Cade to try the lithium on manic depressive humans was, to use his phrase, "an express journey." On March 29, 1948, he gave lithium carbonate to a manic depressive patient at Bundoora. "This was a little wizened man of fifty-one who had been in a state of chronic manic excitement for five years," Dr. Cade said. "He was amiably restless, dirty, destructive, mischievous, and interfering." He was marooned in a back ward and seemed likely to remain there for the remainder of his miserable life.

On the fourth day, Cade felt sure that he was seeing a change for the better in the man. He admitted that it might merely be his imagination, though.

"The nursing staff was noncommittal but loyal," he remembers.

By the fifth day, there was no more doubt. The patient was definitely improving. Within three weeks, he was so much better that he could be moved from the hellish back ward into a pleasant convalescent ward. On July 9, 1948, he was discharged from the hospital and was soon working happily at his old job.

The patient was told to take a small dose of lithium carbonate three times a day to prevent his attacks from recurring. He did the same thing that most people do as soon as they think they're feeling better. He stopped taking his medicine. He relapsed and had to be brought back into the hospital. The lithium straightened him out again, and in two months he was released. This time, permanently.

Dr. Cade tested his lithium treatment on nine more manic depressives during their high spells. It succeeded with everyone.

In September 1949, he reported his findings, and the medical world scarcely heard a word he said. As Nate Kline later wrote, "Its modest proclamation in a journal of limited circulation in a remote country was to pass almost unnoticed."

Besides, who could trust lithium anymore?

The report wasn't completely ignored. Professor Erik Stroemgren, the director of the State Hospital for Psychiatric Research at Aarhus University in Risskov, Denmark, heard of Cade's affair with lithium, and in 1953 he assigned two of his researchers, Drs. Mogens Schou and Poul Baastrup, to look into it. Maybe lithium really could be as helpful as Cade said it was.

For thirty-five-year-old Dr. Schou, the time could not have been better for lithium research. He had a younger brother who was a diagnosed chronic manic depressive. Schou tried the lithium on him first, and it wholly eliminated the brother's symptoms.

"The discovery that a drug you have worked with can help one of your own is a gift in itself," Dr. Schou declared.

In a big experiment, Schou and Baastrup gave lithium to eighty-eight Danish women who had experienced two or more manic depressive attacks during the preceding two years. They received lithium continuously for a minimum of two years, and were closely observed for the next six and a half years. On lithium, the women went five to seven years without a relapse.

Nevertheless, corroboration came slowly for Dr. Cade and lithium. Research scientists started working with lithium in Europe and the Soviet Union in the late 1950s, but it was well into the 1960s before it gained any kind of acceptance. Lithium had too bad a reputation. The U.S. Food and Drug Administration didn't give lithium its official blessings until 1970.

Today, lithium is respectable. The psychiatric profession generally recognizes that it can contain manic behavior in five to ten days, and that a small maintenance dose will avert new attacks. If a patient should show indications of an oncoming episode, a quick increase in his lithium ration can ordinarily keep it off.

The substance is also proving effective against unipolar depression. Dr. Kline uses it as a prophylaxis against a recurrence of the disease. It has helped hundreds of his depressed patients.

John Cade is no longer an obscure Australian psychiatrist. Now he is president of the Australian and New Zealand College of Psychiatrists, and senior associate in psychiatry and examiner in psychological medicine at the University of Melbourne. A tall, well-built man, balding, with shell-rimmed glasses, Dr. Cade has lately been investigating another drug with a bad reputation: strontium. He likes to tackle the hard ones.

Anna Freud, Bender, Slavson
—*Innovators in Children's Psychotherapy*

Let's go back a way. We've been concentrating on psychotropic drugs and the men who developed them because that's the realm in which the greatest breakthroughs have been made in the treatment of mental illness. But there have been some interesting advances in the more traditional areas. And interesting people, too.

Anna Freud, daughter of the illustrious Sigmund Freud, was born in Vienna in 1895, schooled there, and became a psychoanalyst like her father. She fled the Nazis with him in 1938 and nursed him through his last cancer-tortured days in England. She wrote a book, *The Ego and Mechanisms of Defense*, in the mid-1930s that was a masterly explanation of the inner defense mechanisms that her father had discerned.

Anna Freud was to be more than a champion of her father's ideas. She originated her own school of child psychoanalysis. The orthodox child psychoanalysts insisted that they had to explore the deepest layers of a child's unconscious in order to help him, just as the classical Freudians did with adults. Anna Freud maintained that the child's ego structure was still building and that a psychoanalyst had more to do than merely interpret the child's unconscious. He had also to help educate the child. Furthermore, she said, child analysis was only "appropriate in the case of an infantile neurosis."

These were notable milestones in the evolution of child psychoanalysis. So was Anna Freud's recognition that a child psychoanalyst could not remain coolly aloof from his young patients. She felt that the child analyst's first job was to win the child's confidence. After all, the child is usually dragged by his parents to the analyst's office against his will. She devised a bagful of tricks with which to impress a child. She had one bratty patient who was interested in tying knots. She showed him that she could tie more complicated knots than he could, and the little imp began to cooperate in his analysis.

At eighty, Anna Freud was living in London and still digging determinedly into children's psyches.

Let's go back a bit again and meet another child psychiatrist, Dr.

Lauretta Bender. She created one of the world's most widely used psychological tests. It's known as the Bender Visual Motor Gestalt Test, and is an effective instrument for diagnosing functional and organic disorders of the mind.

You would have to go far to meet a more deliciously outspoken woman. She was born in 1897 in Butte, Montana. After working her way through the University of Iowa Medical School, she opted to be a neurologist. Not to practice, mind you, but to do research. She surprised herself by veering into child psychiatry. This, though she had said to herself, Of all the fields of medicine, psychiatry is the last thing I'll do because nobody knows anything about psychiatry; they're all talking a lot of foolishness.

While she was resident at Boston Psychopathic Hospital in Massachusetts, she became interested in Gestalt psychology, a German-born school of thought which believes that the whole is greater than its parts, especially when it comes to perception. As she tells it, she suddenly got an idea "out of the blue" for a personality test rooted in Gestalt thinking that would analyze the way a person copies nine geometrical forms—forms such as a diamond abutting a circle, a row of twelve unevenly spaced dots, and ten columns of three circles each that slanted slightly off from the vertical. The order in which the subject copies the various forms; the questions he asks; the random comments he makes; the resistance he puts up; and his ability to copy the angles, dots, and curves accurately, all enable a trained examiner to detect emotional instability, schizophrenia, brain damage, and maturational lags.

The U.S. Armed Forces made extensive use of the test on troubled G.I.s in World War II, and it has now been adopted throughout the world.

A friend calls the test Lauretta Bender's "out-of-wedlock but most beloved child," and Dr. Bender says, "That's really true because I don't know how I ever got into it."

She trained at Johns Hopkins with the distinguished Viennese psychiatrist Dr. Paul Schilder, followed him to Bellevue Hospital in New York, and married him. She headed the children's psychiatric division at Bellevue from 1934 until 1956, when she developed the children's unit at Creedmoor State Hospital, a mental institution on Long Island, New York.

Dr. Bender has been battling for years to convince her peers that child schizophrenia is inherited and is precipitated by brain damage either at birth or in the first two years of an infant's life. Therefore, it is incurable although patients can learn to cope with it, she says. It is a very arguable matter in psychiatric circles.

However, she concedes the effects of environment on all child psychoses. She says that children reared in institutions without a mother develop a psychopathic pattern.

"Children who don't have a relationship with a mother or a mother-substitute in the first year or two of their lives never get the capacity to relate to people," she declares. "Their personalities are warped. They become destructive to themselves and everybody around them."

She emphatically states that, "A bad mother is better than no mother at all."

Long before Dr. Benjamin M. Spock appeared on parental horizons, Lauretta Bender was prescribing permissive upbringing for children. "A child's behavior is never anything he should be punished for," she says. One would have to say that that is another arguable issue.

Dr. Schilder and she had three children. Eight days after the birth of the third, Schilder was killed in an automobile accident, leaving her to bring up the children by herself. One son is a physician, a second is a mathematician, and the younger child, a daughter, boasts two Master's degrees. In 1967, Dr. Bender was married again to Henry B. Parkes, a professor of history at N.Y.U. Four years later, Professor Parkes died of cancer.

When I talked with her at her New York City office, Dr. Bender was in her middle seventies, a little woman in a chic blue suit and blouse, her grey hair trimly done in pageboy style, with great gold earrings dangling.

She had been in psychiatry for nearly a half century, but she confessed, "I'm afraid of people. I don't know why I encouraged you to come. I usually chase off all journalists as fast as I can. On the other hand, I feel that my success in this field is because I can identify with the patients. Whenever I see children walking on tiptoes, I say, Why would one walk on tiptoes? So I try walking on tiptoes, and I realize that it increases the tone all over your body. That is one of the major problems a schizophrenic child has—the tone in his body is too poor. I try to think why a child would retire into autism. And I realize that the booming, blasting world is too noisy a place to live in. It often is for me because I'm a migraine sufferer. When I have a migraine attack, the world is just a godawful place. Then I realize that this is what these autistic children are suffering from."

"Do you really want to help these kids? Is that the reason you've done all this research."

"No," she said emphatically. "I don't think it's because I wanted to help the kids. I think it's because I wanted to understand schizophrenia. I don't know that one can even say I wanted to understand human beings. It's a little more pure than that."

Let's turn back once more to another person who has done much for the mental health of children. He is S. R. Slavson, who introduced group psychotherapy for children.

The "S. R." stands for Samuel Richard, but he dislikes both names. He asks people from age three to one hundred and three to call him Slavie. I talked with him in his tiny two-room-and-kitchenette apartment on the top floor of an old walk-up in a run-down section of New York City. A short, bald man, he was in his eighties and suffering severely from congestive heart failure, but he wasn't the least discouraged. He managed to live alone, climbing three flights of stairs and doing his own marketing, cooking, and cleaning. A very independent soul. He proudly showed me his fourteen published books and the manuscripts of two new ones.

Slavson was born in 1891 in Russia and emigrated to the United States with his parents in 1903 to escape the czarist pogroms. There were seven children and no money. He worked as an errand boy for $1 a week, tended a fruit stand, was a stock boy for a metal company, and felt like a millionaire when he got a job cleaning the gas street lamps. It paid him $7 a week.

He has no degree in child psychology or education. He says himself, "I'm the best-educated and least-schooled man I've met." Yet he has been an innovator in both fields.

He set out to teach. His way. "I want to dedicate my life to attacking education because it is destructive to children," he told the heads of New York's Walden School when they hired him to be a science teacher in the 1920s. He came up with the novel idea that children could teach themselves better than their teachers could. He let his seven- and eight-year-old pupils plan their own assignments and experiments. On an average day, he paid no attention to the class, and the class paid none to him.

He told me of a small boy who came up to him and asked, "Slavie, what's the heaviest thing in the world?"

Slavson said he handed a book to the lad. "Here, look it up for yourself," he said. "I forget."

The children flourished scholastically and psychologically, so much so that the renowned Maulding School in England asked Slavson to introduce the same program to a student body that included children and grandchildren of Nobel Prize winners.

Group psychotherapy for children grew directly out of these educational experiments. In 1934, Slavson went to work for the Jewish Board of Guardians, a child guidance center in New York City, to start a "creative recreational project" for small groups of socially maladjusted girls between the ages of eight and twelve. He gave arts and crafts materials to the girls and let them express themselves in any way they wished. He sat off in the corner.

"I insisted on only one thing from the board," Slavson said. "I demanded that the children should feel absolutely free, with no instruction, no correction, no criticism, and no help unless they asked for it. The children had to do whatever they wanted to do and discover the results for themselves."

The little girls reveled in their freedom and the chance for self-expression. Their hostility and antisocial behavior dwindled. They grew steadily more outgoing and friendly.

However, as he studied the girls' work, Slavson came to realize that it wasn't the creative factor that was helping them. It really was the inter-actions among the group. More groups of disturbed girls were formed, and groups of disturbed young boys, too. The results were as encouraging.

Slavson soon took the next vital step. Some children were too neurotic to be helped in this fashion, so he developed a new technique for them. These children merely worked at their arts and crafts part of the time. During their free periods, they sat together and openly discussed their problems among themselves. Their improvement was even more marked.

Initially, the Slavson program was called Therapeutics of Creative Activity. Then it got the more comfortable name of Group Therapy. Slavson put eight years into perfecting his methods before he published his findings in 1942. When he did, the technique was swept up by child guidance centers.

This was not the first use of group psychotherapy. A Boston internist, Dr. Joseph Hersey Pratt, employed it on adult tuberculosis patients in July 1905. He had large groups of them meet at his hospital to talk over their dreadful feelings of shame and discouragement. (Usually, the meetings turned into lectures by Dr. Pratt.) In 1921, E. W. Lazell ran group meetings (and lectures) for mental patients at St. Elizabeth's Hospital in Washington, D.C. Unquestionably, though, Slavson was the first to utilize group psychotherapy with children. The American Association of Group Psychotherapy has repeatedly hailed him as the progenitor.

Slavson says he has been motivated from his early years on by "an overwhelming compassion for mankind." Yet he confesses to a "an overpowering contempt for mankind because of the brutality and cruelty which are exercised by some people against others." He has been married and divorced twice and has had three children. Now that he is eighty-five years old, he says that if he had his life to live over, he wouldn't go into psychotherapy or education. He would be a choreographer.

Between them, this trio—Slavson, Bender and Anna Freud—has given disturbed children a lot better chance for able-minded lives.

Erikson and his "Identity Crisis"
—*Menninger, Psychiatric Iconoclast*

Now we come to another name in psychiatry, an even bigger one. Erik H. Erikson is certainly the most influential psychoanalyst living today. He has added broad new dimensions to Freudian theories and techniques. It was he who made the phrase "identity crisis" part of the psychiatric vocabulary. To cite one appraisal of him, "He has made psychoanalysis a viable, descriptive tool for the 'normal' as well as the 'sick' personality and opened new relationships between psychoanalysis and social science."

Erikson was born of Danish parents in Frankfurt, Germany, in 1902. His parents parted before he was born, and in 1905 his mother married Dr. Theodor Homburger, a Jewish pediatrician. For years his family practiced a "loving deceit" on him. They told him that he was Dr. Homburger's son. One can understand how he came to be so interested in the problem of identity.

He never went to college; he was too poor a student. He roamed around Europe in true bohemian fashion, studying painting here and there. He dropped in on Vienna in 1925 and got a job teaching in an experimental school. Sigmund and Anna Freud were intrigued by him and accepted him for training as a psychoanalyst. Anna analyzed him herself.

Erikson proved much wiser politically than his mentors. He didn't wait as they did. Immediately after the rise of Hitlerism, he emigrated to the United States. He was Boston's first child analyst. Although he had no M.D., Ph.D. or any other degree, he became a professor at the Yale medical school, then at the University of California at Berkeley. He quit his job at the University of California in 1950 to protest an idiotic ruling by a bigoted board of trustees ordering all faculty members to take an oath that they were not Communists. Erikson was not, nor had he ever been, a Communist, but on principle he objected to putting political handcuffs on teachers. He moved on to be medical director of the Austen Riggs Center at Stockbridge, Massachusetts, an institution for psychoanalytic treatment and research. In 1960, Harvard appointed him a full professor. His degreelessness didn't bother the folks in Cambridge, either.

Erikson has done some rare research. He investigated the way the Sioux Indians trained their children on a South Dakota reservation. He watched the upbringing that the children of Yurok Indians got in northern California. In World War II, he probed the psychology of Nazi U-boat crews. The war ended, he observed emotionally disturbed veterans in a San Francisco hospital. They really were not mentally ill, he decided. They just couldn't cope with the normal crises of postwar America. It reaffirmed his conviction that psychoanalysis should be an instrument for understanding the "vicissitudes of normal life."

His prime interest has always been identity. He spent years studying the internal psychodynamics of normal and abnormal children. He came to the conclusion that people could not be adequately explained in the old Freudian terms of id, ego, and superego. Each person is a whole, unique being.

To Erikson's mind, a person's sense of identity is the product of "a continuous progressive integrative process." Erikson says that identity flows from the interaction between body, mind, and milieu, with a number of distinct psychosocial stages occurring during each individual's life. One comes in infancy, when identity is related to the feeling of trust, or mistrust, that a baby develops in himself and his mother. At the age of two, when a baby discovers for the first time how to move his muscles, a feeling of autonomy or its antithesis—shame and doubt—is added to his earlier identities. Thus, a child's personality evolves, stage by stage, until he faces the traditional identity crisis in adolescence. Thereafter, the process continues, stage after stage, through adulthood.

This Erikson concept of identity has had a noted effect on psychoanalysts and others.

Erikson has written two heralded biographies, *Young Man Luther* and *Gandhi's Truth*. In them, he has shown that men can utilize their neurotic conflicts toward constructive social goals and in the process heal themselves. They led one writer to salute Erikson as "the most optimistic thinker the Freudian tradition has produced."

Erikson himself is not that sanguine. "Man is born only with the capacity to learn to hope," he says, "and then his milieu must offer him a convincing world view and within it, specific hopes."

In 1963, Erikson wrote an essay, "Womanhood and the Inner Space," in which he laid down the ironclad dictum that anatomy is destiny. A woman is "never not a woman," he declared.

The feminists cannot forgive him for that. It led to a feud between him and the "women's libbers." Many of them hate him.

A white-haired man with a white mustache, Erikson is now living in California in semiretirement with his Canadian-born wife, Joan Mowat Serson. They were married in Vienna in 1930 and have had three children: Kai, a sociologist, Jon, a photographer, and Sue, a social anthropologist.

Any discussion of present-day psychiatry must include the name of Karl Augustus Menninger, M.D. He hasn't contributed anything particularly original to psychiatry. But he has enlightened millions of people on the nature of psychiatry with his books, articles, and lectures, and he has probably trained more young psychiatrists than any other man.

Dr. Karl and his younger brother, Dr. William, both orthodox Freudians, won an international reputation for the Menninger Diagnostic Clinic in Topeka, Kansas, with the research and pioneering they sponsored. Dr. Karl directed the clinic for forty years. Now he and his second wife, Jeanette, spend a third of their time at the clinic in Topeka, another third in Chicago, where Dr. Karl does his writing, and the remainder on the road, where he busies himself consulting, teaching, and lecturing.

At eighty-three, old and wrinkled, Dr. Karl is a psychiatric iconoclast. He denounces "the pretentious, meaningless jargon" of psychiatrists. The use of words like "neurosis" and "psychosis" is misleading, he claims.

" 'Neurotic' means he's not as sensible as I am," he says. " 'Psychotic' means he's even worse than my brother-in-law."

He is campaigning for preventive psychiatry. "I've spent most of my time treating people and teaching young doctors to do so," he declares. "But more and more I see the still greater importance of something preventive. Psychiatrists should eventually work themselves out of business by preventing illness or disorganization."

He doubts that it will soon happen. "There's no money in prevention," he cynically notes.

The Retreat from Freud

Sigmund Freud wrote, "The poets and philosophers before me have discovered the unconscious; I have discovered the scientific method with which the unconscious can be studied."

No one can justly deny the imprint that Freud's "scientific method" made on the treatment of the mentally ill. There was a period when Freud's disciples reigned supreme in mental institutions throughout the world. Almost every medical school psychiatric department in the United States was controlled by Freudians who insisted on a lengthy analysis of each patient's unconscious, or at least a Freudian-type search for the very earliest origins of his illness. However, the Freudians are now in full retreat among the "talk" psychotherapists. Most Freud-oriented psychiatry departments cannot attract enough applicants to fill their annual vacancies for resident training.

Dr. Seymour R. Kaplan, a perceptive professior of psychiatry at the Albert Einstein College of Medicine in New York City, used to depend on

Freudian methods. No more. "During recent years," he said to me, "many psychotherapists have found that Freudian techniques did not meet the needs of patients affected by the turbulence of modern society. It can take months with classical Freudian techniques to analyze a patient's unconscious feelings, but the patient's problems can't wait months. The problems are real, and the patient is crying out for help with them now. So we psychotherapists have had to devise practical new techniques to help patients immediately to solve the problems of everyday living that are contributing to their symptoms."

Psychotherapists are more interested in solving current problems than digging into the patient's past, and they have introduced a variety of new techniques to replace the rigid Freudian approach. They are treating husbands and wives together as a couple. They are treating entire families at once. They are making wide use of group therapy. They are specializing in behavior therapy. They are working with hypnosis.

Skinner Uses "Behavior Therapy"

Behavior therapy is the one that's most worthy of note for two reasons: 1) its great and increasing usefulness; and 2) the fascinating Harvard psychologist who helped to develop it, Burrhus Frederic Skinner.

Behavior therapy is a method of modifying behavior patterns by a system of rewards and punishments, or by conditioning processes. Curing a woman of her paralyzing fear of thunder, for instance, by exposing her to other earsplitting sounds. Psychotherapists employ behavior therapy today to cure patients of their phobias, to remedy sexual dysfunctions, and—due to Skinner's activities—as a valid treatment in schizophrenia.

The foundations for behavior therapy were laid by the Russian psychologist Ivan Petrovich Pavlov when he made his laboratory dogs salivate on schedule. "Conditioned reflex" was the phrase. Fred Skinner went on from there. He discovered new and far-ranging principles of behavior therapy.

I met Dr. Skinner one morning in his sun-sprayed office at Harvard as he was hurriedly packing for a quick trip to London to talk over the BBC. He was tall and narrow, filled with youth, enthusiasm, and good humor.

He was born in Susquehanna, Pennsylvania, in 1904, and had a very normal boyhood. He read the funny papers on Sunday mornings and went to the movies on Saturday afternoons to watch Pearl White in "The Perils of Pauline." Summers he slept in rain-drenched pup tents at Boy Scout camps and got regularly sick on spoiled food.

"I was always building things," he said. "I built roller-skate scooters, steerable wagons, sleds, and rafts to be poled about on shallow ponds. I made seesaws, merry-go-rounds, and slides. I made slingshots, bows and arrows, blowguns and water pistols from lengths of bamboo, and from a discarded water boiler I made a steam cannon with which I could shoot plugs of potato and carrot over the houses of our neighbors."

He invented all sorts of Rube Goldberg-like contraptions. Once he created a flotation system for separating ripe elderberries from green ones. Another time he rigged up a sign on a pully in his bedroom to remind him to "Hang Up Your Pajamas."

At twenty-one, he graduated from Hamilton College in Clinton, New York, and started out to write fiction. A year and a half later, he "discovered the unhappy fact that I had nothing to say," and he began graduate studies in psychology, "trying to remedy that shortcoming." Human behavior always interested him. He obtained his Ph.D. in experimental psychology at Harvard, taught at the universities of Minnesota and Indiana, and returned to Harvard in 1947 for more experiments on pigeons, people, and other picturesque creatures.

Skinner contributed the basic concept of "operant conditioning" to behavior therapy: that you could make animals (and people) behave the way you wished by a system of rewards. He first proved the validity of the principle in the late 1930s by constructing a small box with a food dispenser and a lever in it. When rats were confined in this "Skinner box," they learned step by step that they could secure niblets of food for themselves by pressing on the lever with their paws.

Through his rewards system, Skinner taught one rat "to pull a string to get a marble from a rack, pick up the marble with its forepaws, carry it across the cage to a vertical tube rising two inches above the floor, lift the marble, and drop it into the tube."

During World War II, Skinner did some exotic research on his rewards system for the U.S. Navy. He trained pigeons to pilot Navy missiles and bombs by letting them peck at replicas of the targets. He employed the same rewards system in a classroom demonstration when he taught pigeons to play Ping-Pong. A pigeon got a grain of corn each time it made the right move.

Upon his return to Harvard, Skinner set out to prove that the rewards system would work with people. In conjunction with the Harvard medical school, he and a student, Ogden Lindsley, ran an experiment at the Metropolitan State Hospital in Waltham with schizophrenic patients who were so far gone that they scarcely moved all day. They were rewarded for doing as they were asked with food, cigarettes, or coins.

"They responded beautifully," Dr. Skinner said. "The rewards they got made life more interesting."

The same system was tested on a group of chronic schizophrenics—back ward "incurables"—at a Michigan mental hospital. A third of them improved so much that they could be discharged in a year. Not one patient in the control group got better. It was found that the system helped mentally retarded children, too.

So far we've barely touched the long list of Skinner accomplishments. It was John B. Watson, of Johns Hopkins, who changed psychology from the study of the mind to the study of behavior, but Skinner converted it into a science. "Skinner did what no one had done before," Dr. Richard Herrnstein, chairman of the Harvard psychology department, said. "He made the study of psychology objective. His contribution is gigantic—one of Copernican dimensions." Skinner has also had a vast impact on American schools. His system of "programmed education" has had great influence. And the man's inventions! A "teaching machine" that enables students to teach themselves. An "air crib" with glass walls in which a baby can sleep and play without clothes or blankets or a mother to watch over him.

In 1948, Skinner wrote a best-selling novel, *Walden Two*, the story of a Utopian community established on Skinner's principles of behavioral engineering. No private property; everything owned jointly; everyone happy. It continues to sell eighty thousand copies a year.

Dr. Skinner and Yvonne Blue have been married since 1936. They have two grown daughters, Julie and Deborah. The Skinners live in Cambridge, in a small modern house. He leads a very meticulous life, rising early, doing his exercises, walking to college, going to bed early. To relax, he plays the piano, the clavichord, and the electric organ. He does his writing in a basement study. He writes very slowly. It took him two minutes per word to write his Ph.D. thesis, and that remains his rate. From three to four hours of writing each day, he salvages about one hundred publishable words.

"I was taught to fear God, the police, and what people will think," Dr. Skinner says. "I usually do what I have to do with no great struggle. I try not to let any day 'slip useless away.' "

Behavior therapy has its vocal denunciators. Some psychotherapists feel that treating the behavioral symptom means that you're overlooking the underlying problem which caused the symptom in the first case. They say that "curing" the symptom merely tamps its cause deeper down, and it waits to flare up again in a different and possibly a more acute form.

Behaviorists like Skinner strongly dispute this. They hold that behavioral systems are conditioned emotional reactions from which patterns of behavior emerge. "If a symptom represents something learned, it can be unlearned," they declare.

The mass of psychiatric sentiment seems to be swinging toward the behaviorists. Behavior therapy is now employed in most mental hospitals and community mental health centers.

Lambo and Witch Doctors in Tribal Africa

The Nigerian psychiatrist Dr. Thomas Adeoye Lambo took the best of Western techniques—psychotropic drugs, electroshock, one-to-one psychotherapy, family therapy, group therpay, behavior therapy—and assigned them all to the treatment of the mentally ill of Black Africa.

But Dr. Lambo, who is surely among the world's most original psychotherapists, didn't call a halt there. He added some ideas of his own. He built a hospital for his mental patients that let them live in homelike village surroundings. He brought in traditional witch doctors to help him care for the patients.

It may sound bizarre, but the results don't. Lambo has achieved an unprecedented 80 percent cure rate with schizophrenics. He is lovingly known throughout Black Africa as the "physician of the soul."

A handsome African, tall and husky, he possesses a hoard of warmth and gentleness, plus a chuckling sense of humor. He is quite unaffected, more like a family physician than a leader of the international medical community. He was appointed assistant director-general of the World Health Organization in 1971 and deputy director-general in 1973.

We talked lengthily twice, once at the United Nations headquarters in New York City, another time in a motel room at Orangeburg, New York. Dr. Lambo had flown over from Geneva to address a conference sponsored by Rockland State Hospital. He and Nate Kline are pals.

Lambo was born in 1923 in Abeokuta, a city of eighty-five thousand in western Nigeria. His father was a very powerful tribal chief who had sixteen wives and somewhat more than thirty children. The father was Christianized, and he was anxious for all of his male children to get an education. (The girls didn't matter.) Lambo obtained his early schooling in Nigeria and his medical education at the University of Birmingham in England.

Why psychiatry?

"I've always been very gregarious," he said, "and I felt that biological medicine would not satisfy my innate desire to know people, to talk to people. I thought that psychiatry might bridge the gap."

He did his psychiatric training at the University of London, mostly in one-to-one therapy but with a little attention also to group therapy. No psychoanalysis.

"I've always been a bit antianalysis," he admitted.

When he returned to Nigeria in 1954, Dr. Lambo was the only black psychiatrist in Africa.

"Nobody even knew anything about psychiatry in Black Africa," he declared.

"Were they frightened of it?"

"Absolutely terrified. They didn't even realize that psychiatry had anything to do with medicine."

Lambo established the first mental hospital of its kind in Africa, the Aro Mental Hospital in Abeokuta. He told the Nigerian government, "I want to depart from the traditional type of mental hospital. I want a hospital that will have some meaning, some affinity for the African people."

Nigerian government officials were all for it until they found out what Lambo had in mind.

Most Africans live in villages in a collective, patriarchal society in which everyone knows exactly where he fits. When Africans become mentally ill, they feel miserably lost in an ordinary mental hospital and rarely benefit from the therapy.

Lambo's solution was to house most of his patients in an environment that was familiar to them. He went to four farming villages outside of Abeokuta and asked the inhabitants to take psychotic patients into their homes.

"I spoke to the *bale*—the head of the villages—and discussed the program with him. He then discussed it with the council of the villages. Of course, they were apprehensive. They said, 'You are our son. We would like to help you very much but what you are going to try has never been done before—to put mentally ill people to live in our homes. We are farmers and fishermen. We don't stay in our homes. We leave in the morning. We leave our wives and children to do the domestic work and the chores. Suppose these patients of yours attack our wives and children? What will happen?' "

Dr. Lambo gave the villagers his solemn pledge that no patient would ever do violence to their families.

"How could you be sure?" I asked.

"I had faith in my program," he said.

The villages agreed to try the plan for three months.

The Nigerian government was furious at Lambo. "We gave you £1,200,000 to start a mental hospital and you're sending violent patients out into the villages," a government official shouted. "If one patient kills someone, we'll disown you."

Lambo required a member of the patient's family—a mother, a wife, a sister—to go with the patient and live in the village with him. The relative did the patient's cooking and washing. Each morning, the patient went to the main hospital—a modern, well-equipped institution set on beautiful grounds—for his tranquilizing drugs, group therapy, occupational therapy, and, if need be, some one-to-one therapy with Lambo. The relative took part in the group therapy with him.

"The whole strategy was focused on normalcy," Dr. Lambo said. "The patients were living in normal homes, in a normal village, with members of their families doing their cooking and their washing, bringing them to the hospital. The patient was interacting day after day with normal people. That's what helped him."

Dr. Lambo recalls the first patient. It was at the end of November 1954. "He was a schizophrenic young farmer from a village one hundred and twenty miles away. He was accompanied by practically everybody in his village. His mother came, his father, his four aunts, six uncles. One hundred and eight people came with him in five lorries.

"They told me that this young man had not slept for several days. He refused to eat. He neglected his children and his farm. They thought he had malaria. After a week, they saw he was acting strangely and thought he'd been cursed by the God of Africa, so they gave him some native herbs. He slept, but not enough. About the eighth day, he started to attack people. They put him in handcuffs, tied his legs, and set out for Abeokuta.

"When they brought him to me, he was very excited and garrulous. I gave him an injection of chlorpromazine. Within half an hour he was fast asleep, and they couldn't believe their eyes. 'Look,' they said. 'Before, he was shouting. Now he is sleeping. Lambo is a magician.' The man slept for eighteen hours. Then we gave him a bit of electroshock and sent him out into a village with his mother. Both of them took group therapy. In a few weeks, he was doing fine."

When Dr. Lambo started his hospital, he had no staff for it. There wasn't a trained psychiatric nurse or attendant in Nigeria. He did something bold. He engaged twelve of the best witch doctors in western Nigeria, trained them in a few fundamentals of psychotherapy, and stationed them in his four villages. They cured patients that Lambo couldn't help with all his modern techniques.

Said Dr. Lambo, "Some superstititous patients were ill with hysteria. They thought they'd seen their great-great-grandfather in a dream and had forgotten to do some sort of ritual for him. I couldn't do anything for them because they didn't believe in me. The witch doctors would perform their rituals, the patients would believe in them, and recover."

The first three months convinced the villagers that they had nothing to fear. They let the program continue, and it was extended to eleven more villages.

In the seventeen years that Lambo directed this program, three thousand seriously ill schizophrenics, manic depressives, and other psychotics were housed in the satellite villages. Not one ever attacked a villager, not one committed suicide, and most of them got well. Lambo's 80 percent cure rate for schizophrenics was so high that the U.S. National Institute of Mental Health doubted his statistics. He had to prove to the NIMH that his records were accurate. The fact is that his satellite village program has worked so well that it has been adopted by five other African nations.

In 1966, Dr. Lambo was made dean of the faculty of medicine at the University of Ibadan, and in 1968 vice-chancellor of the university. In 1971, WHO wrote him, "You've done a lot for Africa. Now come to Geneva and be responsible for the health of the whole world." As deputy director-general of WHO, he supervises the training of new doctors and other medical personnel, research into new drugs, and all of WHO's efforts to combat noncommunicable diseases.

Dr. Lambo married Dinah Violet Adams, an Englishwoman, in 1945. They have three sons. The oldest is on the staff of the United Nations. The other two are twins who are identical in looks but in nothing else. One is a socialist, studying at the University of Manchester. The other is a very conservative psychologist in Ghana.

Back in Africa, Lambo used to work eighteen hours a day. In Geneva, he contents himself with a twelve-hour day. When he gets home in the evening, he has a beer or two ("I'm very addicted to beer," he says), eats dinner, listens to classical records for a while, and reads medical papers and/or a novel until his 12:45 A.M. bedtime. He is an avid collector of African religious art. He has more than three thousand pieces.

While he was working on his village program, Dr. Lambo says he found satisfaction "in blazing new trails." Now his satisfaction comes from training new young doctors for Black Africa, especially psychiatrists. "The need is so great," he declares.

A Tranquilizer for a Tiger—and a Mother-in-Law

A few last observations on the mental health scene.

Let there be no doubts—many hospitals are still snake pits. One day, I visited a disturbed ward at King's County Hospital Center in Brooklyn. Some thirty women were pacing the stark dayroom like caged animals.

Their faces were filthy, their hair uncombed. They were wearing dirty, ragged uniforms, often open to the waist with bare, flabby breasts dangling out. A half dozen of them were cruelly knotted into straitjackets.

I watched while burly men and women attendants forced a little white-haired old woman into a straitjacket. She was very frightened. Later, she called to the psychiatrist showing me around.

"Are you a doctor?" she said to him pleadingly. "I want to see a doctor."

The psychiatrist ignored her.

But most mental hospitals are not like that anymore. I went unannounced with Dr. Brill, the director at Pilgrim State Hospital, into a ward for the most agitated, violent women patients in the institution. About twenty of them, mostly in their fifties and sixties, were quietly sitting around a pleasantly furnished dayroom watching TV, reading, knitting. I could see that they were heavily medicated, but they all were neatly dressed in street clothes, with their hair combed.

One woman spoke to Dr. Brill. "When can I go home?"

"Soon," he genially promised her.

Outside, I asked, "Did you really mean soon?"

"Hell, yes," he said. "She's coming around fine."

Potted plants were hanging from the walls of every corridor in the hospital. "Do you see those flowerpots?" Dr. Brill said. "A few years ago, we wouldn't have dared put them there. The patients would have smashed the pots over each other's heads. And over ours."

It's wondrous what some psychotropic drugs can do. When Dr. Leo H. Sternbach, an enterprising Austrian-born chemist, first discovered the famous tranquilizer Librium, his superiors at Hoffmann-LaRoche were dubious about its effectiveness. To convince them, the new drug was flown out to the San Diego Zoo and fed to some of the most savage animals—Australian dingos, marmosets, and a big Sumatra tiger. The dingos were the most ferocious. With jaws like steel traps they attacked humans.

After Librium, the animals all became positively docile. The tiger was as coy as a kitten. The dingos wagged their tails like puppies.

A ranking physician at Hoffmann-LaRoche remained skeptical. This man had a cantankerous mother-in-law who came to dinner every Saturday evening and made his life miserable. One Saturday night, he slipped her some Librium. She was an angel all evening.

He reported, "Any drug that can tame that old witch is okay."

Librium went into production and became one of the most widely prescribed tranquilizers in the world.

Ask Joshua Logan, the director-playwright, about his manic depression. He'll say, "Many of our greatest people have had a touch of the manic in them. I think surely Edgar Allan Poe and Samuel Coleridge had some of it. Shakespeare must have had some. In between my illnesses, there must have been in me, as well as in some of my collaborators, a kind of a whirling current deep under the surface that was constantly fomenting, churning. At times in my life, I've worked with collaborators in the same room. We've exchanged ideas, and suddenly a chemical change took place in the room. We'd get higher and higher, the two of us or the three of us, and whirl in the air with ideas that went far into the ether. When we brought them back to earth and into the reality of a typewritten page, they were better, wilder, funnier than anything we could have done with a cold-blooded, calculated analysis of an idea.

"If only you could always be just a touch manic, just a soupçon manic. It's very stimulating. It's exciting. But being a little manic is like being a little pregnant. You can't stop there."

In 1969, a psychiatrist prescribed lithium for Logan to control his manic depression. It succeeded beautifully.

"Suddenly years were passing and I realized that I didn't have any problems anymore," Logan said.

Has the lithium hurt his creativity?

"No, thank God. It has made me know what my personality is. I can see myself."

Which is what mental health is all about.

9

COMES THE SEXUAL REVOLUTION

THE GREAT JEWISH PHILOSOPHER MOSES MAIMONIDES was one of the most eminent physicians of the twelfth century. Despite his religion, he was court physician to Saladin, the Moslem Sultan of Egypt. Indeed, his fame as a doctor was so broad that King Richard the Lion-Heart offered him a post as his personal physician. Maimonides declined because he preferred the civilized life of Egypt to the crudities of feudal England.

On many medical matters, Maimonides was a progressive, but it was a different situation with sex. He cherished as scientific fact almost every myth he had ever heard about the dangers of sexual intercourse. He constantly warned his royal patients to be chary of too much lovemaking.

"Effusion of semen represents the strength of the body and its life and the light of the eyes," he said. "Whenever it is emitted to excess, the body becomes consumed, its strength terminates, and its life perishes. . . . He who immerses himself in sexual intercourse will be assailed by [premature] aging. His strength will wane, his eyes will weaken, and a body odor will emit from mouth and his armpits. . . . His teeth will fall out and many maladies other than these will afflict him. The wise physicians have stated that one in a thousand dies from other illnesses and the [remaining] 999 from excessive sexual intercourse."

Seven hundred years later, the myths about sex were as farfetched, and as inhibiting. A Stanford University physician, Dr. Celia Duel Mosher, spent twenty-eight years, from 1892 on, studying the sexual habits of a group of forty-seven well-educated married women. The answers she got to her questionnaires would have made Maimonides happy.

One college-bred woman insisted that sex relations once a week was too frequent for good health. A Radcliffe graduate who had been married a year conceded that she "cared for" sex, but was convinced that it was "more wholesome to sleep alone and avoid the temptation of too frequent intercourse." A graduate of Ripon College stated that she and her husband "sleep together in the winter and apart in summer." A woman who had been married seven years by 1892 maintained that the proper sexual practice for married couples was "total abstinence with intercourse for reproduction only."

"Do you always have a venereal orgasm?" Dr. Mosher asked the forty-seven women.

Thirteen women replied, "Always"; thirteen said, "Sometimes"; and eleven said, "Never." The other ten were silent on this question.

Was sexual intercourse necessary for a man?

"Depends on early training in self-control," responded a woman who conscientiously restricted her own sexual intercourse to six or eight times a year.

The sexual scene was quite different by 1976.

A revolution in the sexual mores of America has taken place in the past few decades. It is not just that more people are making more love before marriage or out of marriage. It's that millions of people, of both sexes and all years, from adolescence to old age, have been manumitted from their sexual inhibitions. Sexual attitudes have become far freer.

Many factors have contributed to the transformation of our sex lives. The pill is one. It has metamorphosed contraceptive techniques and pregnancy fears. The advent of safe, inexpensive and legal abortions is a second. The birth of a new science of sex therapy for treating saddening sexual dysfunctions, such as impotence, premature ejaculations, and the inability of some women to achieve orgasms is a third. Perhaps the most important is the new understanding that we've gotten of ourselves as sexual beings. We've found that our sexual ideas and habits are not unique. Many guilt feelings that used to torment us have been banished by the discovery that most other men and women now do the same sexual things that we do.

The Kinsey Reports

Alfred Charles Kinsey, a professor of zoology at Indiana University, awakened us to this reassuring truth. He made the largest, most revelatory study of the sexual behavior of human beings that has ever been attempted. His findings changed the Western world's thinking about sex.

He was a stocky man with tawny hair, a square face, and lively grey-green eyes. His sartorial taste ran to rumpled clothing and an inevitable bow tie. To outsiders, Professor Kinsey was a man of "quiet dignity and correctness." To his associates, he was a driven man who worked sixteen, eighteen, and more hours a day at his sex research. There was so much to cover. Toward the end, his doctor warned him that he was killing himself with overwork, but he never let up.

Prok (a contraction of "Prof. K") was born in Hoboken, New Jersey, in 1894, the son of a professor at Stevens Institute of Technology. One day, his father brought home a book about flowers. The boy promptly found a flower which wasn't in the book. That interested him in nature. He graduated from Bowdoin College and went on to secure a Sc.D. from Harvard. In 1920, he joined the faculty of Indiana University. By 1929, he was a full professor of zoology and a nationally recognized authority on gall wasps. He collected 3,500,000 of them.

This was a very conservative young man insofar as sex was concerned. While he was in college, a friend asked him for help. The friend was guilt-ridden because he masturbated. On Kinsey's advice, the friend and he got on their knees together and prayed to God that the friend find the moral stamina to refrain from the evil practice.

In 1937, Indiana University decided to introduce a course in sex education, and, as a highly regarded zoologist and a husband and father of unimpeachable propriety, Dr. Kinsey was chosen to teach it. In preparing for it, he was surprised to find a dearth of scientific information on human sexual behavior, and he set out to remedy the lack. During the summer of 1938, he started to interview his campus friends about their sexual experiences.

Initially, Kinsey financed the project out of his own pocket. Later, he was able to get some money from the Rockefeller Foundation—until the political heat got too hot for the prudish foundation officials. Luckily for Kinsey and his finances, his reports on his sex research became best-sellers.

Kinsey and his three chief associates crisscrossed the nation looking for people who were willing to be interviewed on their sexual activities. Over the next ten years, they recorded the case histories of 11,240 men, women, and children. These people represented every social, economic, and educational class, the major religions, and all ages from two to ninety. They included such occupations as acrobat, archeologist, barmaid, clergyman, dice girl, housewife, missionary, politician, prostitute, prison inmate, riveter, and stick-up man.

The Kinsey interviews put as many as 521 questions on sex to each person. They asked people whether and how they masturbated; how old they were when they first had sexual intercourse, and with whom; if they had ever had homosexual or lesbian sex relations; if they had had sexual intercourse with an animal; how many extramarital experiences they had had. They inquired about male ejaculations and female orgasms.

Prok had a knack for getting people to divulge their innermost sexual secrets to him. He interviewed Cornelia Otis Skinner, the gifted actress-author, and she glowingly reported afterward, "He has the skill of a great actor. You forget your fears and have complete confidence in him."

When he took down the sex history of Dr. Wardell B. Pomeroy, the clinical psychologist who was later to be his chief associate, Pomeroy had a secret he wanted to keep to himself.

"I hesitated momentarily," he declared, "but it came right out."

Prok learned to talk the language of the streets as fluently as he did that of the campus. He didn't ask a whore, "How old were you when you were first paid as a prostitute?" He would say, "When did you turn your first trick?" There was no fooling him. Once he asked a prostitute how often she "rolled" her tricks—robbed them. She denied that she had ever robbed a "John." But she admitted that very few of her clients ever returned to her.

"Well, if you don't roll them," Prok shrewdly said, "why don't they come back?"

She confessed with a grin that she rolled her Johns on every possible occasion.

Prok always wanted more case histories. His goal was one hundred thousand by 1968. Traveling, Prok, Pomeroy, and Paul H. Gebhard, another associate, interviewed people from 8:00 A.M. or earlier till midnight and later. Some of the sex histories they recorded were spectacular. They encountered an important government official, sixty-three years old, who had carefully noted all his sex experiences in a diary. These included heterosexual relations with two hundred preadolescent females, homosexual relations with six hundred preadolescent males, and sexual intercourse with innumerable adults of both sexes and assorted animals. The man had plotted a family tree naming thirty-three relatives back to his grandparents. He had had sexual relations with seventeen of them. His first heterosexual experience had been with his grandmother. His first homosexual experience had been with his father.

The first Kinsey report came out in January 1948, and its reception was hard to believe. The scholarly 804-page report, entitled *Sexual Behavior in the Human Male*, sold 250,000 copies in the first two and a half months. The second Kinsey report followed in 1953. Entitled *Sexual Behavior in the Human Female*, it was 842 pages long, and its impact was almost as great. The word "Kinsey" became virtually synonymous with the word "sex" throughout the English-speaking world. The royalties from the sales of the two books helped to support the Institute of Sex Research that Kinsey had established in 1947.

The first study was based on interviews with 5,300 men and the second on the case histories of 5,940 women. Some critics claimed that Kinsey's samplings did not present a fair cross section of the American population. Nevertheless, nobody could gainsay the monumental dimensions of his investigation.

Kinsey found that most Americans had abandoned the traditional sexual rules. Science needed urgently to revise its categories of what was "normal" and "abnormal" in sexual behavior, Kinsey believed.

Kinsey found that most boys started sexual activity very early in life—immediately after adolescence, or even sooner. More than 99 percent of them began regular sex activity between the ages of thirteen and fifteen. But they peaked very quickly.

"The peak, with or without social control, comes between sixteen and eighteen, when the male is more active sexually than he ever again will be," Dr. Kinsey reported.

Most girls seemed to show little or no sexual response until they are twenty. The teen-age girl who did go "all the way" seemed to be motivated by social rather than sexual reasons. "She is interested because it means dates with boys, automobile rides, shows, and hilarious company," Dr. Kinsey wrote. "If intercourse is part of the tax, okay, so long as the other girls in her group are similarly involved."

However, the sexual roles reversed as the females grew older. Kinsey found that the average female's sexual appetites continued to rise until she was twenty-nine or thirty years old, and then remained on a high plateau until she was fifty or sixty. This often led to nasty marital complications inasmuch as the sexual needs of males generally ebbed from their early twenties on.

Virginity was going out of style. About 50 percent of the women who married by the time they were twenty-five had had premarital intercourse. So had 83 percent of all married men. Fidelity was falling out of fashion, too. Fifty percent of the married men and 26 percent of the married women reported that they had had extramarital sexual intercourse.

Sex was more satisfying for males than for females, Kinsey learned. Most married men had no difficulty arriving at orgasms. Almost all reached a climax in almost all their acts of coitus. However, one out of every four wives failed to experience a single orgasm throughout the entire first year of marriage. Over twenty years of marriage, less than half of the married females could say that they "always or almost always" experienced orgasms. Fifteen percent had never once had an orgasm during coitus.

For all their new sexual freedom, most people were still conventional in their lovemaking. The Kinsey group determined that practically every male used the "missionary" position in his lovemaking most or a large part of the time. That's the sexual situation in which the male stays on top of the female. Less than four out of ten married men with more than an elementary school education had ever made oral contact with their wives' genital organs, or had ever had their own genitals manipulated orally by their wives.

Sixty-two percent of the women and 92 percent of the men had masturbated at some time or other in their lives. In most cases, the women hadn't made a regular habit of it. Many men had.

One statistic was a real shock to the nation. Thirty-seven percent of American men had had at least one homosexual experience to the point of orgasm. Lesbian experiences were less widespread. The comparable statistic for women was 12 percent. Eight percent of the men and 3.5 percent of the women had performed sex acts with animals. That fact was another shocker.

Age was much harsher with men's sex lives than with women's, Kinsey found. Women could continue their sexual activity indefinitely, if they wished. Most men couldn't. Some 6.7 percent of the men in the study were impotent by the age of fifty-five, and 25 percent more by the age of sixty-five. By their mid-eighties, most men were impotent. Not all, of course.

Twenty-odd years later, I asked Kinsey's long-time collaborator, Wardell Pomeroy, by then one of the most respected sex therapists in New York City, which of the study's findings had most surprised the Kinsey group.

"We were very surprised by the amount of sexual responsiveness among women at the upper social levels," he said. "We had gotten the impression that the college-level females were not nearly as highly responsive as women in the lower levels were. We really had to shift our thinking a great deal."

He said that the Kinsey people were astonished by the sharp differences between upper- and lower-level men insofar as masturbation and premarital intercourse were concerned. Upper-level men engaged in much more masturbation before marriage. It also came as a big surprise to them that "the male breast, the male's nipple, was almost as erotic an organ as the female breast." Pomeroy said that 50 percent of the males in their study could be sexually aroused by having their nipples stimulated.

How do you happen to work with a man like Alfred Kinsey on sex research?

In Dr. Pomeroy's case, it was coincidental. He was born in 1913 in Kalamazoo, Michigan, and grew up in South Bend, Indiana, two of the most unlikely spots in the country to breed a broad-minded student of sexual conduct. He graduated from Indiana University and obtained a Ph.D. in clinical psychology at Columbia University. He was working for a mental hygiene clinic in South Bend in 1942 when Dr. Kinsey came to town to lecture. Pomeroy volunteered his sex history and, after the interview, they talked for hours in Kinsey's hotel room. Kinsey offered him a job the same night. The pay was only $300 a month, but Pomeroy accepted.

A handsome man of medium height with silvery hair, who wears turtleneck sweaters and perpetually smokes a pipe, Pomeroy regards his thirteen years with Kinsey as the top period of his life. He near-worshiped Kinsey. Still, he can be objective about him. He is the first to admit that Kinsey had his defects. To mention one, a touch of religious bigotry. Kinsey would hire only white, Anglo-Saxon, Protestant interviewers. Jews were *verboten*.

Dr. Pomeroy says frankly, "Prok rationalized this on the grounds that the subjects of the interviews would relate best to WASPs. I have a feeling, though, that deep down there was a little core of anti-Semitism."

Kinsey had a violent antipathy to facial hair, Pomeroy says; he loathed all mustaches and beards. "He would have had a terrible time with the long-haired hippies today," Pomeroy thinks. He concedes that Kinsey was a true male chauvinist. But, he points out, that was long before women's liberation.

"Prok had a great capacity for change," he declares. "My guess is that if he were living now, he'd be a pretty good women's libber."

Volcanic wrath poured down on Kinsey's head because of his undiluted sex reporting. Critics like Congressman Louis B. Heller of New York stridently denounced Kinsey's report on female sexual behavior as "the insult of the century against womanhood." Some bluenoses fretted that the publication of Kinsey's statistics might encourage immorality. A number of scientists took heated issue with his methods. Dr. Karl A. Menninger clamored that the Kinsey report did not truly represent American women, let alone the human female. Dr. Menninger said, "It should have been labeled 'What five or six thousand rather talkative ladies told me about sexual behavior of women in the United States under certain conditions.'"

The assaults by laymen didn't bother Kinsey because they didn't know any better. But criticisms by the scientific community stung him sorely.

These were attacks on his integrity. His colleagues begged him not to answer the critics, but he couldn't keep from striking back. Criticism of his methods was "careless reasoning or malicious misinterpretation," he snapped at Menninger.

Dr. Kinsey had a long, happy married life with Clara Bracken McMillan. They were wed in 1921 while she was a graduate student at Indiana University, and they raised two daughters and a son. A fourth child died in infancy. Before Kinsey went into sex research, they used to do a lot of hiking, gardening, and concert-going together. Not afterward. Once Mrs. Kinsey innocently complained, "I hardly ever see Prok at night any more since he took up sex."

Following several minor heart attacks, Kinsey's physician cautioned him in June 1956, to reduce his work schedule to four hours a day. If he did, he could live for two more years. Prok said, "I'll cut down to eight hours," He died that August.

Dr. Kinsey left a splendid memorial behind him. He built the greatest depository of truths about sexual conduct ever amassed. His study helped to free American sex mores from age-old shackles of misinformation, misjudgment, and superstition.

Dr. Pomeroy spent seven more years at Indiana University. In 1963, he came to New York City and went into private practice. He has been eminently successful.

He says he is very contented with the changes he has observed in sexual mores since the publication of the Kinsey reports. "When you look at young people today, the high school kids and the early college kids, you see that in many ways they are much more moral, if you'll let me use that word, than previous generations. They are not so much concerned with the penis and vagina, or an unbroken hymen, or any other kind of sexual behavior. They are more interested in relationships—real intimacy, companionship, concern for other people."

Dr. Kinsey would have been immensely pleased by the changes, he says.

Early Birth Control Methods

This, Kinsey and every other sex researcher knew: The dread of an unwanted pregnancy can do more than almost anything else to spoil sex relations.

Since the beginning of recorded time, men and women have searched for a safe, satisfying method of birth control. The first contraceptive measure was, certainly, *coitus interruptus*, or withdrawal of the penis before ejaculation, but it was soon followed by many others. Almost four thousand years ago, Egyptian women manufactured pessaries out of crocodile dung, a slightly alkaloid substance that may have had some spermicidal value. Early Indian women employed *coitus obstructus*, a technique for squeezing the penis to prevent ejaculation. The Jewish Talmud recommended a vaginal sponge. In Islamic countries, women made tampons of pomegranate pulp treated with alum and rock salt.

Ancient China had a "Thousand of Gold" formula which promised women that "the foetus will become like rice gruel and the mother will be without suffering." Japanese prostitutes rolled oiled bamboo tissue paper into a disk and covered the mouth of the uterus with it. Some Japanese men wore sheaths of tortoiseshell, horn, or leather. They were called *kyotai* (penis sack) or *kabutogata* (hard helmet).

During the Dark Ages in Europe, anal intercourse was a popular means of birth control. The condom was developed midway through the sixteenth century as a protection against venereal disease, but it also did contraceptive duty. When an eighteenth-century gallant had an amatory date with a girl, he often tied an "armor" of impervious lamb intestines on his penis with a ribbon. After one such dalliance, Samuel Boswell disgustedly diarized, "For the first time did I engage in armour, which I found but a dull satisfaction."

The poor people couldn't afford such luxuries. They resorted mostly to abortion and infanticide for birth control. "Infanticide is practised as extensively and as legally in England as it is on the banks of the Ganges," Benjamin Disraeli wrote in 1845.

The Industrial Revolution transformed birth control. The vulcanization of rubber in 1839 led straight to the rubber condom. Now birth control was no longer the exclusive province of the well-to-do; the lower classes could be careful, too. The diaphragm was devised in the 1880s, and women didn't have to rely on the caprices of their male lovers anymore. The diaphragm was introduced in America about the time a public health nurse named Margaret Higgins Sanger was establishing the first birth control clinic in a New York slum.

It was Mrs. Sanger who invented the expression "birth control." She wanted a catchier term than "conception" or "Malthusianism," the terms most widely used. She weighed such phrases as "population control," "race control," and "birth rate control." As she recounted the story, "Someone suggested 'Drop the rate.' 'Birth control' was the answer."

Nevertheless, birth control—family planning is the latest euphemism for it—remained a haphazard affair. Condoms broke. Diaphragms required more self-discipline than many couples could muster. The rhythm method—abstaining from sex relations on a woman's fertile days—which the Roman Catholic Church advocated, was a form of Russian roulette. Not until the development of the pill in the 1950s did women get a convenient, effective, and tasteful method of contraception.

The Pill

A covey of brilliant investigators did the research that created the pill: two biologists, Gregory Goodwin Pincus and Min Chuch Chang; a dauntless obstetrician-gynecologist, John Rock; and two chemists, Carl Djerassi and an eccentric fellow named Russell E. Marker.

The saga commences with Mrs. Sanger. (Most modern developments in the field of birth control do.) For decades, she sought an oral contraceptive that was dependable and safe. One day in 1950, the gynecologist Dr. Abraham Stone arranged a conference for her with Dr. Pincus. They hoped that he could find the oral contraceptive they wanted.

Dr. Pincus was an impressive-looking man with a mop of greying hair over a high forehead and piercing, deep-set eyes. He was born in Woodbine, New Jersey, secured a Sc.D. at Harvard, and had built a record of research feats in the reproductive sciences. Among them was the first fatherless mammalian birth. He had taken an ovum from a female rabbit, fertilized it with hormones and salt solutions at a high temperature, and implanted it in the rabbit's uterus. The developing egg grew to be an embryo and a fetus. Call it parthenogenesis.

In 1945, Pincus helped establish a new little laboratory, the Worcester Foundation for Experimental Research, in a barn in Shrewsbury, Massachusetts, and became its research director. Since the foundation didn't have much money, he continued teaching at Tufts medical school in Boston. With him at the Worcester Foundation was Dr. Chang, a thin, slightly stooped Chinese with an ever-present smile who was born in 1908 in Shansi Province and obtained his doctorate at Cambridge. He came to Worcester in 1945 for a year and was still there thirty years later. Chang loved everything about research. He was the kind of scientist who handled his own laboratory animals.

"I like to feel the experiments through my hands," he declared. "If your technicians do all the work, you lose the fun. Would you let someone else play tennis or chess for you?"

Mrs. Sanger was a true believer, so she was an excellent persuader. She got both Pincus and Chang interested in the search for an oral contraceptive. Then she raised hundreds of thousands of dollars to support their experiments. The two biologists started testing a female sex hormone, progesterone, for use as a contraceptive. It was known to inhibit ovulation in rabbits. Would it do as much for human females?

This much was sure. Working together, progesterone and the female sex hormone estrogen regulated the twenty-eight-day menstrual cycle of the human female and her entire child-bearing process. They made it possible for a mature ovum to come out of the ovary, be susceptible to fertilization by a male sperm, be lodged in the uterus, and grow into a baby.

Acting alone, estrogen could stop the ovum from leaving the ovary. In other words, it could prevent ovulation in a human female. But not always.

Dr. Pincus hoped that progesterone would give 100 percent protection to a woman.

One problem with progesterone was its exorbitant cost—$200 a gram. "You could only afford it for thoroughbred horses, not humans," Dr. Chang wryly noted.

That's where the two chemists, Drs. Marker and Djerassi, came into the picture. In 1939, Dr. Marker, a broad-shouldered professor at Pennsylvania State College, discovered a method of synthesizing progesterone in large amounts, using Mexican wild yams as his basic raw material. He tried in every way to get an American drug manufacturer to open a hormone plant in Mexico. None paid him any attention. Disgusted, he resigned from Penn State, moved to Mexico City, and set up a workshop in an abandoned pottery. He trudged through the Mexican jungles, machete in hand, with mules and a team of Indians, hunting for and collecting wild yam plants, which he synthesized into progesterone.

The sequel has become a legend in the pharmaceutical industry. In 1943, Marker walked unannounced and unknown into the offices of a miniscule Mexican company, Laboratorios Hormona, and asked if it wanted to purchase some progesterone. He set down on a desk two glass jars wrapped in newspapers that contained about four and a half pounds of synthesized progesterone valued at $160,000. They represented a sizable fraction of the world's total production of progesterone for a whole year.

When the two European refugees who owned the firm came out of shock, they asked Marker to join with them in launching a new company to manufacture synthetic progesterone. They named it Syntex S.A. Today, as Syntex Corporation, it is one of the leading manufacturers of the pill and other pharmaceuticals, with sales that have exceeded $160 million a year. Dr. Marker didn't wait around to see it grow, though. He got into a quarrel with the others and angrily exited from the new concern, leaving it with scarcely a clue to the extraction and refinement processes that turned wild yams into synthetic progesterone. They recreated it, and the price of progesterone tumbled precipitously to $3 a gram.

Now it was Carl Djerassi's turn to move stage center. A short, handsome man with modishly combed, longish grey hair and a carefully trimmed beard, he is not hesitant to tell you in a very cultivated voice that he is a great scientific genius. In fact, he is.

Dr. Djerassi was born in Vienna in 1923 of a Bulgarian father and Austrian mother. Both his parents were physicians, but he opted for research chemistry. He came to the United States in 1939 and graduated from Kenyon College in three years. He worked for a year for the Ciba pharmaceutical company, sharing in the discovery of the first antihistamine. Next came a Ph.D. at the University of Wisconsin; he was only twenty-one when he got it. He went to Syntex in Mexico City in 1949. It was shortly after the world had learned of the magical effect cortisone had had on the wretched arthritic patients at Mayo Clinic. An international race was underway to find a practical method of synthesizing cortisone from vegetable raw materials. Djerassi and his Mexican colleagues at Syntex won it.

When he began work with progesterone at Syntex, Djerassi didn't even have an oral contraceptive in mind. He was trying to develop a treatment for cancer of the cervix. He was also up against the scientific dogma of the time—nobody, this held, could alter the chemical structure of progesterone without lessening its potency. This belief had been very discouraging to the searchers of an oral contraceptive since progesterone was not fully effective by mouth.

Djerassi refused to accept the orthodox credo. He did a stellar reshuffling act with the progesterone molecules and succeeded in 1951 in synthesizing a new analog, or equivalent, of progesterone that was vastly more powerful than the hormone. Although Djerassi had only been looking for a cervical cancer cure, the Syntex people quickly sent the new progesterone product to Dr. Pincus.

The new substance, which came to be known as the 19-Norsteroids, proved to be an active progestational agent—that is, a substance that could modify a woman's reproductive system in the progestational, or pre-pregnancy, period, when ovulation takes place. As we shall see, when swallowed by a woman, it was even more active by mouth in inhibiting ovulation than progesterone was by injection.

Now we go to Dr. Rock's reproductive clinic in the rich Boston suburb of Brookline. John Rock had worked most of his professional life trying to cure infertility in women patients. Now he was about to help Pincus try to keep them from becoming pregnant. It called for a lot of spiritual grit from him, for he was a devout Roman Catholic, and he was inviting denunciation from the altar or grimmer ecclesiastic punishment.

A wonderfully friendly man, tall and thin, with twinkling Irish blue eyes and an enchanting sense of humor, Rock was born in Marlborough, Massachusetts, in 1890. He got his M.D. at Harvard medical school in 1918 after a circuitous route that led him through a brief, calamitous business career. He wasn't a businessman. He thought he would become a brain surgeon, but he switched to obstetrics-gynecology. Next to the brain, the reproductive system was the most important part of the body, he believed.

"There are two things that make society run: the activities of the brain and the activities of the gonads," he said smilingly, at the age of eighty-three. "If they work together, everything goes along nicely."

Infertility was a murky, unexplored area when Rock entered the field. "Any woman who came into Massachusetts General Hospital complaining of infertility was immediately sent over to surgery for a D&C (dilation and curettage)," he recalled. "If the husband could screw, that is. Nobody bothered to check whether he was infertile. All men were assumed to be fertile."

He located an unused laboratory in the basement of the Lying-In Hospital, swept it out, polished a big copper boiler until it glistened, and set to counting spermatazoa and examining human ova.

That first laboratory didn't last long. "I got married," Dr. Rock said.

"A different kind of research," I commented.

"But along the same lines," he grinned. "I was trying out the reproductive apparatus in another way."

By the mid-1920s, Rock had a fertility clinic at the Free Hospital for Women in Brookline and a lucrative ob-gyn practice. He was also doing outstanding research. In 1944, he accomplished the first fertilization of a human ovum in a glass dish.

In 1950, Rock came up with a fresh plan for curing infertility. He hypothesized that some women could not conceive because their Fallopian tubes and uteri were undeveloped. Perhaps the condition could be helped by treatment with female sex hormones. He assembled eighty women who had been infertile up to six years and dosed them for three months with increasing amounts of estrogen and progesterone. The hormones created pseudopregnancies in each of the women. They stopped menstruating, even had morning sickness, enlarged breasts, and more pigmentation in their nipples. After Rock halted the hormones, all eighty women lost their symptoms and resumed their normal menstrual cycles. Soon, many of them became pregnant, a phenomenon called the "Rock rebound reaction."

Drs. Rock and Pincus were old friends. At Pincus's suggestion, Rock devised a new experiment along similar lines, relying on progesterone alone. Instead of administering it continuously, he would give the progesterone from the fifth to the twenty-fifth day of the female cycle, then halt it to allow menstruation.

Rock used this new protocol with twenty-seven women who had each been infertile for more than two years. When they took the progesterone alone on a twenty-day cycle, ovulation ceased completely, menstruation followed, and the unpleasant pseudopregnancy symptoms did not appear. A number of women became pregnant later.

These Rock experiments fitted in neatly with the goings-on at the Worcester barn.

Drs. Pincus and Chang had assayed the value of hundreds of progesteronelike steroids on laboratory animals as oral contraceptives. Most were practically worthless. One was inactive orally. A second stirred up the uterus too much. Another behaved like a male sex hormone. It was rough sledding until Pincus and Chang came to Dr. Djerassi's progestational agent—the 19-Norsteroids. They showed themselves highly effective on animals in suppressing ovulation.

Rock and Pincus got together at a scientific conference in 1951 to mull over their respective investigations. Pincus proposed to Rock that he test the 19-Norsteroids in producing his "rebound" effect. At the same time, he could assess their effectiveness in inhibiting ovulation. Was it the birth control pill Pincus and Chang had been working toward?

Dr. Rock knew very well he would be challenging a most sacrosanct law of his church—he, a man whose marriage rites had been solemnized by a cardinal of the church.

Science prevailed over the outmoded tenets of the church. In December, Rock gathered fifty women who had been infertile for long stretches and started them on a regimen of 19-Norsteroids taken orally from the fifth to the twenty-fifth days of their cycles. In almost every case, the 19-Norsteroids completely suppressed ovulation during the experiment. Some of the women became pregnant soon after they ceased taking the drug. That gratified Rock—he was still anxious to cure infertility—but the paramount point was their success in preventing ovulation. *The pill worked!*

The three scientists immediately planned wider tests. Beginning in 1956, a series of trials of the oral contraceptive was inaugurated in Puerto Rico and Haiti. In San Juan, Dr. Edris Rice-Wray, the dogged little medical director of the Family Planning Association of Puerto Rico, toured a slum-clearance project looking for women volunteers who had already mothered children and wished no more.

They were poverty-stricken, uneducated women who had been taught by the church that birth control was a deadly sin. Yet as word got around of Dr. Rice-Wray's project, they deluged her with requests to take part. Many times more than the one hundred she had intended to use begged her to let them try her pill. It was the same in Haiti. All told, over sixteen hundred women in San Juan and Port-au-Prince went on the 19-Norsteroids and stayed on them for more than forty thousand ovarian cycles. Thousands more women participated in similar tests in the United States.

The pill was successful in every place it was tried. By the close of 1959, its effectiveness as a birth control measure was certain. Its failure rate was only one unwanted pregnancy in every one thousand cases, and as often as not those pregnancies were due more to forgetfulness on the part of the women than to any fallability of the pill. The Food and Drug Administration approved the pill for public use in 1961. The first to go on sale was the G.D. Searle Co.'s Enovid. Syntex and several other pharmaceutical manufacturers subsequently brought out their own pills.

These pills had more in them than the progestational agent. The field trials had shown that breakthrough bleeding occurred in some women when they depended on the progestational agent alone. To counter this, Rock and Pincus suggested that a few milligrams of estrogen be added to the progestational agent.

Dr. Rock embarked on a one-man campaign to win acceptance of the pill by Roman Catholics and the Roman Catholic Church. It was his duty to speak out, he felt, and talk out he did in lectures, articles and a passionately written book, *The Time Has Come: A Catholic Doctor's Proposal to End the Battle for Birth Control*. He had more success with Catholic people than he did with the Vatican.

For many centuries, the Roman Catholic Church prohibited all forms of birth control except abstinence. Pope Pius XII eased the church's stand in 1940, and authorized Catholics to employ the rhythm method for birth control. But they could use no other means of birth control. The Pope reiterated this ruling in 1958 with a statement banning the use of any drugs, pills, or medicines that "by preventing ovulation make fecundation impossible." Such birth control measures were immoral because they went against nature, he decreed.

Rock strongly protested that the pill could not be included in this category since its effects were physiological and maintained the integrity of the sexual act.

"The pill is not immoral," he stoutly stated. "Catholics can use the pill, and should use it, with an easy conscience."

How he was denounced! The Right Reverend Monseigneur Francis W.

Carney of Cleveland assailed him as a "moral rapist." Other epithets were even meaner. Some Roman Catholic physicians in Boston publicly snubbed him and stopped referring patients to him.

"It took real courage," Dr. Pincus told a friend. "Rock sacrificed a lot of his practice and the good opinion of many physicians."

The Holy See couldn't be budged. A new pope, Paul VI, issued an encyclical in July 1968, sternly reasserting the church's traditional approach to all artificial measures for preventing childbirth. But Rock's efforts and those of his fellow believers were not lost.

The 1970 National Fertility Study revealed that 68 percent of all married Catholics were employing contraceptive methods disapproved by the church.

Many honors were heaped upon Rock, Pincus, and Chang. Dr. Pincus had not much time left to savor them. He died in Boston in August 1967, leaving his wife, Elizabeth, and their two children. Dr. Chang has continued his research at the Worcester Foundation. He has been married to Isabelle Chin since 1948. They have had three children.

And Dr. Rock? He gave up the active practice of medicine in 1971 at the age of eighty-one.

One golden day in the autumn of 1973, I drove up to the town of Temple, New Hampshire (pop. 441), to a simple little house set deep in the crimson-streaked woods, where Dr. Rock was living in retirement with his son-in-law. He was the youngest eighty-three-year-old man I've ever encountered, still tall and erect, with good grey hair, dressed sprucely in grey slacks, a blue sports shirt, and a snappy green ascot. We ate a tasty lunch of Boston baked beans in his cozy living room sitting in front of a crackling fire.

His is a laughing, self-deprecatory but gentle sense of humor. When I remarked on how young he seemed, he chuckled. "Many people say I've never grown up."

Was he brought up in a religious household?

"Well, we said the Rosary during Lent and my father went to Mass at Christmas and Easter, having promised my mother that he'd be good and behave himself."

We talked about his struggle over the pill.

"You know, I've always been a very fervent, practicing Catholic," he declared. "Yet a lot of Catholics look askance at me. In fact, my very Catholic daughter still thinks I'm a renegade. I believe she prays for me every night."

He chuckled anew. "She's a great child."

Did the attacks on him by church leaders pain him?

"Well, they bothered me some, but my conscience was so damned clear. . . ."

"From a theological point of view?"

"It was a question of what was right and what was wrong. I wouldn't do anything that I thought was wrong. I was breaking some of the laws of the church, but to me the laws of the church are an artificial framework, a superstructure. The core of the edifice is in basic morality and basic values. The recognition of these is in one's own brain."

I said that he had spoken out bravely.

"Oh, no," he declared, "they couldn't do anything to me. There were some who objected to my receiving Communion, but I did just the same. I always went to confession first, but I wouldn't bother telling the priest that I was giving women pills for contraception because I felt that it was no sin. You don't confess things that are not sins.

"I remember I confessed something one time, and the priest said, 'Do you think that was a sin?' I said, 'No, Father,' and he said, 'Then why do you confess it?' If you can't decide in your own mind, you'd better take what the church says. If your own mind is clear and you're sure about it without any finagling, you obey your conscience."

Why did he get into research?

"To be of use. I figured out that the sources of the greatest happiness in humans were the brain and the gonads, and I was interested in human happiness and welfare."

Dr. Rock said that he had had thirty-six years of ideal married life with Anna Thorndike. They had five children. While he was a student at Harvard, he used to play squash, but after he got married he substituted social life for sports.

Now? "I read, read, read, and I smoke too much."

He has had four heart attacks. "I've gotten so used to them that they don't bother me."

"It must be true that God loves the Irish the best," I commented.

"I don't know if he does," Dr. Rock stated. "He certainly doesn't seem to have much interest in me. He hasn't yet brushed off any seat for me in Heaven, and I guess he doesn't want to send me to Hell. He just leaves me here."

And what of Carl Djerassi? He has done very well since those hectic days in Mexico City when he was reshuffling the progesterone molecules. He became a director of Syntex Corporation and president of Syntex Research. In 1969, he organized his own company, Zoecon Corporation, to produce a new kind of insecticide out of hormones. He is also a professor of chemistry at Stanford University. He has a big cattle ranch, and walks and climbs for hours every weekend despite a fused knee he got from a skiing accident. He still skis, too. He and his poet-wife, Norma Lundholm, live in a luxurious, modern home on a mountain near Palo Alto, California. They have two children.

Dr. Djerassi is quick to point out, "I'm a very civilized, cultivated man."

And a very realistic man when he talks about the elements that drive a research scientist. "To be the very first to discover something gives you a very considerable amount of personal satisfaction," he said. "But if it were only that, clearly you should be satisfied without telling anyone about it. You're not. It would be the same thing as someone climbing Mount Everest for the first time and keeping his mouth shut about it. An egotistical motive makes the mountain climber announce, 'I was the first to climb up there,' and it's the same with scientists. Sure, you get an enormous amount of satisfaction from bragging about it to other scientists. Not to the public! The public frequently couldn't care less. It doesn't even understand or appreciate the beauty of it. You're talking poetry to people who don't even know the basic vocabulary."

It was estimated that fifteen million women were using the pill for contraception in 1976. The authoritative *Medical Letter*, which evaluates drugs and treatments for nearly 70,000 American physicians, described the pill as "the most effective, convenient form" of birth control known. It said that the rate of accidental pregnancies is merely 0.1 to 1.5 per 100 woman-years of use.

Women who take the pill run risks, that's certain. British researchers have reported that the danger of death due to blood clots is seven to eight times as high among pill-users as nonusers. The risk of death due to heart attacks is said to be much higher, too, especially among women over forty; twice as many women over forty on the pill die of heart attacks as women in their thirties. In 1975, the FDA officially announced that women over forty would be wise to use other means of birth control.

There are some risks to most forms of contraception, of course. Childbirth itself can be hazardous.

IUDs

Some four million American women depend on intrauterine devices today to safeguard them against pregnancy. Most of these IUDs are fabricated of metals or inert plastics, and they come in an assortment of shapes: loops, coils, rings, shields. They are inserted semipermanently in the woman's uterus and, it is theorized, set off a mild inflammatory reaction that slays the sperm or does something to stop the implantation of the fertilized egg in the uterus. No one quite knows what.

The original notion for an IUD dawned on an acient Arab camel driver who inserted a smooth round stone in the womb of a camel to thwart pregnancy during a long desert trek. The idea was resurrected in the twentieth century by a German physician, Dr. R. Richter, who devised a ring-shaped IUD of silkworm gut in 1909. Dr. Karl Pust, another German, developed the first metallic IUD in 1923. He made it out of silver wire.

The IUD is not quite as effective as the pill. Its failure rate runs from 3 to 5 percent. Some dangerous complications are possible. Some women expel their IUDs spontaneously. Perforation of the uterus, pelvic infections, and excessive menstrual bleeding occur on occasion, and some physicians fear that the presence of a foreign device in the uterus for years conceivably might cause cancer. Nevertheless, the IUD has many advantages. Once it is inserted by a physician, the average woman usually has nothing more to do or worry about. Furthermore, the IUD is much cheaper than the pill. IUDs are especially useful in the developing countries where most women lack the education and the money to benefit from the pill.

Abortion
—Old and New

Abortion was a dirty word in most of America until January 22, 1973. On that date, the U.S. Supreme Court struck down the Texas statutes that made it a crime to seek an abortion or to attempt one unless a physician ordered it to save the life of a pregnant woman. The Supreme Court thereby nullified most criminal abortion laws in the United States.

The High Court laid down a set of careful guidelines governing abortions. It ruled that no state could interfere with any abortion during the first trimester. Through that period, it is exclusively up to each woman and her doctor whether she should have an abortion. During the last six months, a state may protect the mother's health by licensing and regulating persons and facilities doing abortions. Only during the last ten weeks of pregnancy can a state prohibit abortions.

The era of sneaky, back-alley abortions with desperate women dying under the dirty knives of illegal abortionists was ended. American women had the right not to have a child if they so desired.

Today, more than half of the people in the world live in nations that allow abortions for social as well as medical reasons. The U.S.S.R.

permits abortions practically without restrictions. India, China, and Japan have followed suit. In effect, the Japanese have substituted abortions for contraception. "Abortion has become a way of life," Professor T.S. Ueno of Nihon University in Tokyo declares. After a screaming debate, the French National Assembly voted in 1974 to legalize abortions on demand for the first ten weeks of pregnancy, at fixed prices. For the preceding fifty-four years, abortions for any reason had been a serious crime in France, punishable by a prison term not only for the abortionist but also for the woman.

WHO reports that fifty million abortions are now performed annually throughout the world.

Abortions have been known to womankind since earliest history. At times, they've been an abhorred practice; at times they've been socially palatable. Some primitive societies insisted that a woman be aborted if the father of her unborn child was unacceptable: a member of an unfriendly tribe, a slave or, possibly, someone possessed by a demon. In olden Greece, abortions were often advocated if the pregnant woman was too young or too old, or if the father of the unborn child was. Plato advised abortions whenever the father was past fifty-five or the woman over forty.

Ancient techniques of abortion were somewhat less than scientific. Women recited magical incantations, squatted over a magic plant, or rubbed a necromantic ointment on their bellies. Assorted herbs and medicinal concoctions were swallowed. Other techniques provided for punching a pregnant woman in the belly, making her jump repeatedly off a high rock, or inserting a pointed stick in her vagina.

Some of the techniques employed by present-day physicians are almost as savage—for example, D&Cs. In this procedure, the cervical canal is painfully dilated by metallic instruments until it is several times its normal size, and a razor-sharp steel curette is inserted through it to scrape the lining of the uterus and cut out the growing tissue of the embryo. Since the physician cannot see what he is doing, he easily can perforate the walls of the uterus.

Later in the pregnancy, physicians may inject a saline solution in an effort to make the uterus disgorge itself of the fetus. That can disrupt the woman's blood structure and central nervous system. She may go into convulsions.

These horrors are not mandatory anymore, though. A new suction technique has been created for performing early abortions safely in ten minutes or less on an outpatient basis. And the prostaglandins, the newest and most extraordinary of wonder drugs, are making late-term abortions more practical, too.

Karman Finds a Safe Suction Technique

Let us begin with early-stage abortions and Dr. Harvey L. Karman, the clinical psychologist who developed the technique that has humanized them. Karman is one of the most sincere, honest people in these pages, and by far the most controversial. He has already done time in prison for his abortion efforts. By the time this book appears, he could be behind bars again.

A lean, dark-haired man who talks very quietly, Karman was born in 1924 in Oregon. I met him in Los Angeles in the summer of 1975.

"I've been in trouble with authority all my life," he said. "My mother was a fundamentalist, so the only book you could read was the Bible. The Lord was coming any day, so it was a waste of time to read any other book. Mother was so rigid and so stern that it was easy to rebel. I was always being punished because I wouldn't conform. I was always being asked, 'Why can't you be like other people?' and I was saying to myself, God, the last thing I want to do is to be like other people."

He makes no bones about the fact that he was a juvenile delinquent. He said he stole a few cars when he was a teen-ager. He was never arrested for that, but he was placed on probation for traffic violations.

Years after, he worked with juvenile delinquents fresh out of reform school. "The first thing they wanted to do was to smoke dope in front of a police station to prove that those bastards hadn't gotten to them. My approach to them was; Look, I'm not going to tell you that the world is a wonderful place. It is a pretty stinking place. The question is, What are you going to do about it? You can bang your head against the wall. You can dare the police to arrest you, which they'll be happy to do. But if you really don't like the world, maybe you can do something to change it."

Dr. Karman has spent many years trying to change the world. However, he does not see himself as an outlaw any longer.

"Now I'm working inside the system to change it," he declares.

He graduated from U.C.L.A., got a master's, and started on a Ph.D. in clinical psychology. After he had completed his courses, he decided to finish his degree at the International University in Geneva. He said that it was because the Swiss institution gave him a $6,000 grant to do research on abortions. His critics, whose numbers are not small, question the worth of his Swiss degree. His friends, and they are many, claim that his Swiss doctorate is as good as any other.

Karman said that he first became interested in abortions as a psychology intern at U.C.L.A. "One of my semester projects was a study on the emotional aspects of abortions. I asked women who had had illegal abortions what they remembered of them. They all seemed to recall pretty much the same things: the indignity of the experience, the slimy way they were treated, the cloak and dagger atmosphere, the awful guilt they felt.''

Something had to be done to spare women this physical and spiritual degradation, he thought.

Because of his project, many U.C.L.A. students assumed that Karman was an expert in the field and begged his help in finding an abortionist.

As Dr. Karman says, ''It seemed like every guy who got a girl friend pregnant, everyone who had remotely heard about me, said, 'This guy knows about abortion.' I could have said, 'That's your problem.' That's what the system usually says to people who get into trouble. But I didn't see that I had any choice.''

He canvassed Los Angeles looking for doctors willing to perform illegal abortions. He was appalled by the exorbitant prices they demanded, $1,000 or more for an abortion, and the callousness they displayed.

''I'd say, 'But this little girl has only got $500,' and they'd say, 'Too bad. Tell her to call me when she's got the rest of the money.' ''

He finally found a few doctors who were reasonable, and he and his college friends organized a little underground to assist women to get abortions. In the spring of 1956, Karman was arrested by the Los Angeles police for allegedly performing an abortion himself that resulted in a woman's death. He denied then, and denies now, that he did anything more than take the woman to a motel to meet a physician who was to perform the abortion. Nonetheless, he was convicted of abortion and sentenced to two years in prison.

They were miserable years. ''I suffered very much because of my family. I had a wife and three infant children, and I felt very, very strongly about my need for being with them.''

He refused a parole. He said he would have had to admit that he had done something wrong and promise never again to help women have abortions. In 1964, several years after his release from prison, he was granted a full and unconditional pardon by Governor Edmund G. ''Pat'' Brown of California.

The more abortions Karman saw, the surer he was that doing D&Cs was the wrong way to perform them. ''The abortion itself wasn't dangerous. It was the procedure, the technology, the instruments, that were so dangerous. It seemed insane to risk sticking a rigid steel instrument up into a blind cavity.''

In 1958, three researchers in mainland China produced a new concept in abortion technique. Ts'ai-Kuang Wu-Tsung, Wu Yuang-T'ain and Wu Hsien-Chen drew oxygen out of a bottle, turning it into a vacuum. They attached a thin steel tube to the bottle, inserted the tube through the cervical canal into the uterus of a pregnant woman, and successfully sucked out most of the fetal contents. It was much quicker and less painful than the traditional D&C. Only a little work was left for the curette.

The Chinese suction technique—aspiration is its formal name—was taken up in Eastern Europe and spread to the West. To Karman's eye, the suction technique was still dangerous, though. That inflexible steel tube could perforate the delicate uterus.

Karman was determined to improve on the Chinese concept.

Forcing a woman's body to conform to the shape of a steel instrument was begging for trouble, he felt. The answer seemed clear to him: design a cannula that would conform to the shape of each woman's uterus. He took a piece of flexible polyethylene tubing, about seven inches long and 5-mm in diameter, and curved it gently to conform to the shape of the uterus. He cut little holes on opposite sides near the end, and gave the tube a blunt tip resembling the head of a crochet hook. The cannula was slim enough to pass through the cervical canal without the need for dilation. It was flexible enough so that it would bend if it were pushed hard against the wall of the uterus, "virtually eliminating the possibility of perforation."

Karman also decided to devise his own vacuum source that wouldn't rely on electricity for power. "When I began I didn't know what a vacuum was," he told me. "The only vacuum I knew was the goddamned vacuum cleaner."

He bought a vacuum gauge for $2 in a hardware store and began investigating all kinds of vacuums, even the vacuum a human mouth makes when it sucks on something. He finally designed his own vacuum device: a 50-mm syringe of plastic that had a locking arm to make sure no one using it could pump air into the uterus.

He took his two instruments, cannula and syringe, to the office of a friendly doctor in Los Angeles who was about to perform an abortion on a woman. The physician let Karman test the instruments. He passed the cannula into the uterus himself, attached the syringe to it, and aspirated the contents of the uterus. He got out 10 cc of fetal tissue with practically no discomfort to the woman. The entire procedure scarcely lasted three minutes.

The physician wasn't convinced that the woman had been aborted. He painfully dilated her cervix and went in with a steel curette. He needn't have scraped. Not a trace of fetal tissue was left.

That was in 1962.

Karman's published reports on his new technique were long ignored by the medical profession. "Because I had a Ph.D. instead of an M.D. at the end of my name," he ruefully says. By 1975, the situation was better. The Karman cannula was widely accepted in the United States, Europe, and

Asia for use in abortions through the seventh week of pregnancy. Dr. Edward M. Stim, a gynecologist on the staff of the Albert Einstein College of Medicine and director of a New York City abortion clinic, reported in 1975 on the results of twenty-five hundred abortions done with the Karman cannula technique up to the twelfth week of pregnancy. He and four other gynecologists had a 99.5 percent success rate and encountered serious complications in only 0.3 percent of their cases.

Dr. Christopher Tietze, senior consultant to the Population Council and the leading fertility-control statistician in the United States, if not the world, first saw an abortion done with the Karman cannula in 1970. It was a "revelation and a revolution," he said.

"The Karman cannula has contributed a lot to the acceptance of the suction method of abortion in the United States," he told me in 1975. He said 95 percent of all abortions in the United States are now done by suction.

Karman's syringe has not been as widely adopted as the cannula. Most physicians doing suction abortions in the United States prefer electric pumps.

One morning, I watched Dr. Stim perform an abortion with the Karman technique at his clinic in New York. The patient was a petite, twenty-two-year-old Puerto Rican girl who had come in on her lunch hour. Her boy friend was waiting nervously outside.

The girl was led into an immaculate cubicle where she removed her shoes, slacks, and underpants. She kept on her bra and her blouse. She climbed up on an examining table and put her feet in the stirrups. She was very frightened.

Dr. Stim softly reassured her. "It'll be over before you know it."

The atmosphere was informal. Stim, a slender man of forty-two who was wearing a white lab coat over sports shirt and slacks, sat on a small stool in front of the examining table. He gave the girl two mild injections of procaine in the cervix and waited a few moments for the shots to take effect. He made a digital examination of the uterus and measured it with a cannula to make certain that she really was the eight weeks pregnant she said she was.

"Wiggle your toes," he told her. She was still very tense and he wanted her to relax. She couldn't.

A nurse's aid who was standing alongside the table threatened her. "If you don't wiggle your toes, I'll tickle your feet."

The girl wiggled her toes.

Stim passed a 5-mm Karman cannula through the cervix to ease the passageway. Then he connected a 6-mm Karman cannula to a Karman syringe, inserted it into the uterus, and gently moved it back and forth. The syringe started to fill up with bloody, liquidy tissue. At one point, the girl felt a slight menstrual-like cramp, no more.

In nine minutes, the abortion was completed. "You're not pregnant anymore." Dr. Stim told the girl.

"*A Dios gracias,*" she murmured.

She lay on the table, resting, for ten minutes. After that, she dressed and left with her boy friend, hand in hand. The fee to the clinic for the abortion was $90. She paid it.

Through the years, Dr. Karman has continued his fight to change "the system." He has been arrested about ten times for his abortion activities. He has been convicted only once more, though, and then he was merely placed on probation.

The most sensational of the Karman cases involved another one of his inventions: the Supercoil. This is a device for aborting women in the second trimester of pregnancy. It rather resembles an IUD, consisting of a plastic strip, 40 cm long, wound up in a spiral. A physician inserts eight, ten, or twelve of these Supercoils in the uterus, as many as will fit. By the time they are removed twelve to twenty-four hours afterward, the uterus has pushed out the fetus. Karman claims that the Supercoil is much safer than saline induction. In 1971, he flew to Bangladesh at the request of the International Planned Parenthood Federation and successfully aborted 1,800 victims of mass rape with the Supercoil.

Karman got into trouble over his Supercoil in Philadelphia. In 1972 he was arrested on charges that he had used it in abortions on eleven young black women in their second trimester. Practicing medicine without a license, the indictment read, as usual. He was found guilty, but the conviction was quickly thrown out on appeal.

Dr. Karman has invented many other medical instruments. I asked him whether he wanted to make money out of them.

"Christ, no," he stated. "I'm not into money. I gave all the royalties from the cannula to a free abortion center in New York. The car I'm driving is twelve years old, my wife's car is eight years old. Our house cost us thirty-some thousands. I make some money giving lectures and workshops. My wife works."

Felice, his wife, went back to college in her forties and got a Ph.D. in clinical psychology. An attractive blonde, she just radiates warmth and charm. She and Karman were married in 1950 and have three children. Mrs. Karman and the children have lined up unequivocably with Karman in his battles with the authorities. The children risked prison to work with him in his abortion clinics.

"You're a psychologist," I said to Dr. Karman. "Diagnose yourself. What's the why of Harvey Karman?"

"I think if you don't do what you believe in, you'll hate yourself," he said.

Prostaglandins
—*The Newest Wonder Drugs*

Now let us take up the prostaglandins, and the two men who, more than any others, are turning these chemical mysteries into medical miracles. One is a taciturn Swedish physician-chemist, Dr. Sune Bergstrom, the other a cheerful Ugandan pharmacologist, Sultan M.M. Karim, who was expelled from his native country by its racist dictator, General Idi Amin, because he was of Indian extraction. The scientific distinction he had conferred on Uganda meant nothing to the egomaniac dictator.

First, what are prostaglandins?

They are hormonelike chemical substances that are found in microscopic amounts in almost every cell in the human body, from the scalp to the toes. So far, fourteen different prostaglandins have been identified, and they are an odd lot. At times, they behave like hormones, at other times like vitamins, and they actually are neither. One prostaglandin can have a diametrically opposite effect from another. PGE_1 acts to deter blood clots; PGE_2 helps blood clots to form.

The functions of the prostaglandins are a complete mystery. We do know that they are incredibly powerful. As little as a billionth of a gram can have an enormous impact upon any human organ. A solitary ounce of one prostaglandin is sufficient to induce abortions in fifteen thousand women.

Medicinally, they offer wonders galore. Early research indicates that they can lower dangerously high blood pressure to a healthy level in a matter of moments without hazardous side effects. They can relieve the suffocating grasp of asthma. They can bolster the kidneys by increasing urine volume and sodium excretion. They can turn off gastric acids that eat into the stomach lining and cause ulcers. They can alleviate the pain of gastric ulcers.

Physicians in one California hospital recently tested prostaglandins on a score of male patients with duodenal ulcers, the most recalcitrant of all ulcers. The prostaglandins cut the level of their irritating stomach acids by 90 percent and kept it that low for hours.

The prostaglandins may also be invaluable in the treatment of arthritis, obstructive lung disease, fever, glaucoma, bone resorptions, and sickle cell anemia.

They promise to do more for abortion and contraception than anything we've seen to date. In some cases, they are already doing it.

Prostaglandins were discovered in 1930 by a couple of New York gynecologists, Drs. Ralph Kurzrok and C.C. Lieb. Something in human semen made strips of human uterus contract and relax, they noted. In 1935, a Swedish physiologist at the Karolinska Institute, Ulf von Euler, detected the same mysterious substance in the semen of sheep. He assumed that it derived entirely from the prostate gland and gave it the name prostaglandin. In 1946, Dr. von Euler persuaded a young assistant in the biochemistry department at the Karolinska to follow up on his investigations of the semen. He was Sune Bergstrom.

Dr. Bergstrom is a tall, very thin, balding man whose English is rendered with a lilting Swedish accent. I talked with him at an international symposium on prostaglandins in Augusta, Michigan, sponsored by the Upjohn Company, the pharmaceutical manufacturer that has financed much of the research. Sixty of the world's principal experts on prostaglandins were there. Bergstrom was No. 1 among them.

He said that he was born in Stockholm in 1916, got his M.D. at the Karolinska in 1943, and went straight off into research. "Already in my first year at medical school I got hooked into research on heparin," he declared, "and I stayed in research."

He found that prostaglandins were active in many biological systems. "Anything occurring in the body that is so active in so many ways must have some regulatory functions," he decided.

His research went at an excruciatingly slow pace because he had such infinitesimally small amounts of prostaglandins to work with. Tons of sheep glands were needed to produce a millionth of a gram of prostaglandin. The cost was towering.

The first great advance came in 1949 when Bergstrom discovered that prostaglandins were not one individual compound, but a group of compounds. Still, nobody but Bergstrom and von Euler was very elated by the news.

"The scientific people didn't believe that these were new compounds," Dr. Bergstrom said.

In 1957, Bergstrom proved it to them conclusively. He isolated a prostaglandin, PGF$_1$-alpha, in pure crystal form. By 1959, he had isolated another prostaglandin and deciphered the prostaglandins' molecular structure.

"The stuff Nobel prizes are made of," Dr. John A. Hogg, director of experimental chemistry and biology for Upjohn, has called Bergstrom's achievements.

Dr. Karim took Bergstrom's basic research, and with amazing energy and daring, demonstrated its practical value to hundreds of patients for abortions, for inducing labor, and in contraception.

I met Dr. Karim at the Upjohn symposium on prostaglandins. He was a very different sort of man from Bergstrom, slim, dark-skinned with curly black hair, bubbling over with zeal and boyish humor. He was born in 1935 in a small village about one hundred miles from the capital city of Kampala in Uganda. His father was a businessman, like most Indians, and he wanted Sultan to join his three brothers in the family's thriving coffee business.

Karim was no more cut out for a business career than was John Rock. "Academically, I came out of high school with a miserable record," he declared. "I failed my exams."

His father sent him to England in 1953 to train as an accountant. When he got to London, Karim decided that this was not at all what he wanted. But in an Indian family one does not lightly rebel against one's father.

"I picked up some courage and broached the idea to the family of changing the field of education," he said. "I wanted to do medicine and the family that was supporting me wanted me to be an accountant. Eventually, we came to a compromise. I would enter the University of London and study pharmacy with the expectation that I would go back to Uganda someday to start a drugstore."

One of his professors turned Karim's attention to research, and he took a Ph.D. in pharmacology at the University of London in 1964. His principal interest was obstetrics, and he started research in the chemistry of childbirth. Why did the umbilical cord spontaneously stop bleeding after childbirth? Was there some substance in the cord that caused the artery in it to close down? He had read about Bergstrom's prostaglandins. Were they implicated?

It developed that they were. Karim discovered that the substance that stopped the umbilical cord from bleeding was a mixture of four prostaglandins. But where did they originate? He tracked them down to the amniotic fluid that surrounds the fetus in the mother's womb. He was able to report in 1966 that prostaglandins probably had a lot to do with the start of labor as well as spontaneous abortion.

By 1967, Dr. Karim had been away from Uganda for fourteen years, and he and his Ugandan wife were "hungering for home." His father had forgiven him for becoming a scientist instead of a solid businessman, so the Karims returned home with their three small children. He was invited to join the faculty of Makerere University medical school in Kampala. He would be working for the same hospital in which, ten years before, Denis Burkitt had first seen his lymphoma and cured it. It was a much more modern hospital now, with one thousand beds and a maternity service that handled twenty thousand deliveries a year.

Karim set out to investigate the role of prostaglandins in inducing and/or preventing childbirth. He did it by "trying to mimic the processes of nature."

He injected prostaglandins into baboons and human volunteers to establish the safe dosages. Next, he administered prostaglandins to women with dead fetuses. It made them deliver them. In February 1968, he administered a prostaglandin, PGF$_2$-alpha, to one hundred women with live fetuses who were at term or near it. These were Bantu women, mainly, who needed help in getting labor started because they were overdue, their membranes had broken prematurely, or they had other pregnancy complications. As a control, Karim gave oxytocin, a conventional labor-inducing drug, to one hundred other African women with similar pregnancy problems.

The oxytocin failed completely to bring on labor in forty-four of the hundred women. But ninety-one of the hundred women who received the PGF$_2$-alpha went into labor within seventeen hours on an average.

"There were no side effects, and all infants at birth were in good condition," Dr. Karim recorded.

The Karim findings were cold-shouldered even more brusquely than Dr. Bergstrom's. His first paper on the subject was rejected by six medical journals.

"I finally found a way of presenting it at a joint pharmacological conference between British and Italian medical societies," Dr. Karim said. "I was supposed to give a paper on something else, and I slipped this in."

After that, a British medical journal accepted the Karim paper for publication, and the prostaglandin parade commenced. By 1972, prostaglandins had been used to induce labor in five thousand women throughout the world.

Could prostaglandins do as much for abortions as they do for delivery? It seemed likely to Dr. Karim, and he resolved to give the idea a try. "When a neighbor's prize Siamese cat became pregnant by the ginger tom next door, much to her owner's distress, I gave the Siamese PGF$_2$-alpha, and that solved that."

In 1969, Karim effectively aborted fourteen of fifteen women in their second trimesters with a single intravenous injection of PGF$_2$-alpha. This time he had no difficulty getting his news to the medical world. The best British medical journal, *Lancet*, published his paper happily. During the following year, Karim used prostaglandins successfully in nearly three hundred second-trimester abortions. Some disturbing side effects— diarrhea, nausea, and vomiting—were experienced. Karim controlled them by administering the prostaglandins directly into the amniotic fluid via the vagina.

The prostaglandins are far safer than saline induction for late abortions. They eliminate the risk of damage to the blood structure and the central nervous system.

I asked Dr. Karim whether his prostaglandins might also be of use in early abortions. He said no. "They can't compete with the suction method," he declared. "No drug can compare with the suction method in early abortions. But prostaglandins will be very, very valuable in late pregnancies."

The FDA gave its official approval in 1974 to the use of one prostaglandin—Karim's pet, PGF$_2$-alpha—for inducing labor and abortion under controlled conditions in hospitals and clinics. The British government has licensed two prostaglandins for the same purposes.

The prostaglandins promise to be even more useful as contraceptives. In fact, they may be the most valuable contraceptives ever developed. They may be the "morning after" pills that women have yearned for. In fact, women won't even have to take them on the morning after they've had unprotected intercourse. They can safely wait until the following month.

Dr. Karim has demonstrated experimentally that a woman whose menstruation is delayed need not worry. She can let seven to ten days go by after her period is due, and then take a prostaglandin. In most instances, it will induce menstruation in two to seven hours.

"A woman wouldn't have to take the prostaglandins every month," Dr. Karim explained. "Even if a woman has intercourse thirty days a month, she isn't going to get pregnant every month. She would only have to take the prostaglandins when her period is late."

The advances that have been recorded with prostaglandins were made possible by some fine research at Harvard University and the Upjohn Company. Chemists at both places synthesized prostaglandins in 1968. Enough material became available for researchers to work on, and the researchers leapt to it. At last tally, between four hundred and five hundred laboratories were investigating the effects of prostaglandins on all manner of diseases as well as contraception, abortion, and childbirth.

Scientists in the pharmaceutical industry like to call the decades of the forties and the fifties, which produced the antibiotics and the steroid hormones, the golden age of drug discovery. They say that the coming age of prostaglandins bodes well to eclipse it.

Dr. Bergstrom may never win a Nobel Prize for his work with prostaglandins for an unusual reason. He may disqualify himself because he is chairman of the nominating committee for the Nobel Prize in physiology or medicine. It would be a pity.

Bergstrom has climbed high since the days when he was a lowly assistant at the Karolinska Institute. In 1969, he was chosen to be rector of the Karolinska. He doesn't like to talk about himself. He admits merely that he has been married to Maj Gernandt since 1943, that he works seven days a week from eight to six, and that he plays golf only on his vacation.

Motivation? He said, "Basically, curiosity, I guess; understanding what's around us."

When we met, Sultan Karim was still living in Kampala with his wife, Pitu, who is a speech therapist, and their son and two daughters. His routine then was to drive the children to school and continue on to the hospital, arriving by 8:00 A.M. and staying until his work was done. Sometimes that came at five in the afternoon, often at five in the morning. He never took work home with him, though.

"My work is completely cut off when I leave the hospital," he said.

Dr. Karim has certain self-destructive instincts. "The thing that has always interested me is motorcycle and motorcar racing," he stated. "I would have liked to be a racing-car driver. Unfortunately, it is too late now." But, and he grinned, "I race around a lot on a motorcycle."

"Fast?"

"Very fast."

Unlike Dr. Bergstrom, Dr. Karim does not mind revealing himself. "I must be honest with you and say that helping people wasn't my intention. I didn't start out to be a do-gooder. The research itself was its own reason. However, helping people has become very important to me. I consider that any woman who has become pregnant and doesn't want to continue with the pregnancy is going through hell. She has to be helped."

Soon after Amin seized power in Uganda in 1971, he expelled every person of Asian extraction from the country, including people like Karim, whose families had lived there for generations. Thereby, the Amin regime cut Uganda off from scientific and all other freedoms. It also littered the countryside with corpses of dissenters.

After some harrowing experiences in Uganda, Karim and his family made their way in 1973 to Singapore and the medical faculty of the University of Singapore. He is continuing his research on prostaglandins at the Kandang Kerbau Hospital.*

Uganda's loss was Singapore's gain. And the world's.

---

*Dr. Karim wrote me from Singapore at the end of November 1975, "The work is progressing satisfactorily in many areas, apart from reproduction—in ulcer healing, treatment of nasal congestion, bronchial asthma, and high blood pressure. In all these areas we are now conducting clinical trials in Singapore.

"We enjoy living in Singapore. Life is more relaxed and the pace a bit slower. I have had to settle for a smaller (and not so fast) motorcycle, but I still enjoy riding."

Masters and Johnson
—*Pioneers in Sex Therapy*

In the spring of 1975, the Family Services Association of America conducted the first nationwide survey of sex therapy ever made in the United States. F.S.A. experts checked on the sex therapy situation in fifty-seven cities in twenty-six states, from New York to California. They did it at my request.

The results of the study were consternating. In the average American community, 50 percent or more of all married couples were dissatisfied with their sex lives. In some cities, as many as 85 percent of married couples considered their sex lives inadequate.

The causes of this epidemic of sexual disenchantment were a puzzlement. Could all the newly found truths about sex, the newly available techniques of contraception, and the freshly evolved sexual mores be producing more problems than they caused? Or was it possible, as seemed likely, that the current sexual revolution had at last made American men and women face up honestly to their troubled sexual equations? No one knew.

What to do about it?

Until recently, there was very little that a married (or unmarried) couple could do about their sexual difficulties. A woman who did not attain orgasms usually accepted the lack as a sexual fact of life. Orgasms weren't very ladylike anyway. A man who discovered himself prematurely impotent felt that his case was probably hopeless. The family physicians told both of them so. The state of medical ignorance on the subject of sex was unbelievable.

Dr. Harvey W. Caplan, a psychiatrist at the University of California medical school sex clinic, told me of a fifty-three-year-old man in San Francisco who was having minor sexual difficulties—a temporary episode of impotence. The man went to his family physician for help.

"You're past fifty years of age, why don't you just forget about sex?" the physician said. "You're over the hill, so you'd better reconcile yourself to it."

It almost broke up the man's marriage. Fortunately, his wife persuaded him to go to a trained sex therapist, and he was functioning well again sexually in a few weeks.

Sex therapists are a new breed of specialists who have come on the scene in the past few years. They are helping thousands of troubled people today to attain better sex lives.

A St. Louis gynecologist started this new specialty with the help of a woman assistant. Their joint names have come to connote sex therapy to the world—Masters and Johnson.

William Howell Masters is a husky bald-headed man with powerful eyes that lock onto you. There is little warmth or humor to him, just intense concentration. A churchgoing Episcopalian, a registered Republican who cast two votes for Nixon, he is, obviously, a very conservative man, which is probably all to the good in as unorthodox a field as sex research.

I talked with Dr. Masters in his small, dark office at the Foundation for Reproductive Biology that he established in St. Louis. He said that he was born in 1915 in Cleveland of a lower-middle-class family. A wealthy aunt put him through Hamilton College and the University of Rochester medical school. He became interested in sex research during his third year of medical school because there was a vacuum in the field. No one knew anything about the mechanics of sexual functioning.

"Do you realize that the very first course in human sexual functioning ever given in any medical school anywhere was taught here in St. Louis in 1960?" he said. "Until then, no medical school had ever allowed a formalized discussion of natural sex functioning to be part of the curriculum."

Why such diffidence?

"Sex was a taboo subject in medicine as elsewhere," Dr. Masters declared.

Two of Masters' professors advised him that he needed three things if he planned to do sex research: 1) some chronological academic seniority; 2) a definite reputation for research in a different field; and 3) the sponsorship of a medical school.

Kinsey had the first two, not the third. Masters wanted all three. He took a residency in gynecology and joined the staff of the Washington University medical school in St. Louis. He did some outstanding research there in hormone replacement in the menopausal and postmenopausal years. In 1953, he figured that he was ready. He applied to the chancellor of Washington University for permission to do research in sexual inadequacy in both sexes.

"It's professional suicide," the chancellor warned him, but he gave his permission.

"I was gambling," Dr. Masters said to me. "The gamble was very simple. One had to win. One had to be productive. If you do research in a controversial area, you must succeed or you'll be hooted out of the profession."

The university provided some of the research funds; most of them Masters raised himself. When he ran out of funds, he laid out his own money. In July 1954, he set up a laboratory with a bed in it, electrocardiographs, electroencephalographs, biochemical gear, a color movie camera, and floodlights.

For the first twenty months, Masters worked with prostitutes. "They had a great deal to teach me. I didn't know anything about sexual functioning. I learned from them, by interrogation, observation, by practically living with the prostitutes."

It was a prostitute who convinced him that he needed a female collaborator. "One particular girl who was very pretty and well educated—she had a Ph.D. in sociology and was supplementing her income in this manner—had been trying to get a certain female sexual concept over to me. It wasn't that I wasn't buying it, I just didn't understand it. Finally, she said, 'I don't think you're ever going to know anything about female sexual functioning. What you need is an interpreter.' "

He asked the university placement bureau to find the right woman assistant for him for sexual research. In January 1957, the bureau sent him thirty-two-year-old Mrs. Virginia Eshelman Johnson.

"What does Mrs. Johnson look like?" I asked Dr. Masters.

"She's five feet five and a half, slender, and most attractive."

"Blonde or brunette?"

"She varies," he said in his only joke of the day. When I met Mrs. Johnson, she had light brown hair.

Although she is world-famous as a social scientist, Mrs. Johnson never got a college degree. "She wouldn't stand still to go through a university," Dr. Masters said. "She only took the courses that interested her."

She was born on a farm in the Missouri Ozarks. Originally, she studied music at Drury College (she has a rich mezzo-soprano voice), and she sang over the St. Louis radio regularly. After that she explored sociology and psychology at the University of Missouri. In 1951, while she was taking courses at Washington University, she married a young student, George Johnson, who led his own band. She sang with the band until their divorce in 1956.

"Ginny has the finest intellect of any woman I've ever encountered," Dr. Masters declared. "She's so much superior to me intellectually that there's no comparison. She's responsible for more than sixty percent of our new concepts in sex therapy."

Masters wanted to learn how the sexual organs—the breasts, clitoris, labia, vagina, cervix, penis, testes—as well as other parts of the human body, responded to stimulation during coitus and masturbation. He was determined to measure their responses scientifically during all stages of intercourse and masturbation.

He got eight female and three male prostitutes to engage in sexual activity and let him assess their responses. This experiment didn't work well. Many of the women prostitutes had pelvic infections, probably the aftermath of constant sexual arousal unsatisfied by orgasms, that distorted their sexual reactions. Moreover, prostitutes were a migratory group, here tonight and somewhere else tomorrow night.

There was only one alternative. In 1957, Dr. Masters and Mrs. Johnson switched to "respectable" people. They looked for volunteers in the St. Louis area and got a flood of them—694 men and women, blacks and whites, Protestants, Catholics, Jews, and atheists. They numbered among them 276 married couples and a diverse assortment of unmarried persons, divorced people, widows, and widowers. The youngest man was twenty-one; the oldest eighty-nine. The women's ages spanned eighteen to seventy-eight.

All the volunteers—including the men in their eighties—had to be capable of having an orgasm during intercourse and masturbation in the laboratory. Any applicant who couldn't achieve these orgasms under observation was dropped from the project.

Volunteers came to the laboratory day and night, whenever they could. They were asked to do such basic things as masturbate with their hands or fingers; masturbate with an electric vibrator; have their breasts stimulated erotically without genital contact; engage in sexual intercourse with the woman on her back; have intercourse with the man on his back. The women were also asked to use a transparent plastic tube shaped like a penis for intercourse. This artificial phallus had electronic apparatus in it which recorded everything that happened to the vagina and the cervix during coitus and masturbation.

In the course of their research, Masters and Johnson observed ten thousand male and female organs. They discovered many things about sex acts that no one had ever before noted.

The sexual cycle had four stages, they found. The first phase is excitement. For the male, the first sign of this is the erection. In the female, the first sign is lubrication of the lining of the vagina. It occurs within ten to thirty seconds. Most researchers had presumed that the lubricating fluid came from various glands or the uterus. Masters and Johnson discovered with the artificial penis that the lubricating fluid originates in the vaginal walls themselves. The woman's breasts swell and her nipples have erections during this excitement phase.

The second stage is called the plateau. The male testes enlarge by 50 percent and are drawn high up into the scrotum. The tissues in the outer third of the vagina swell greatly. The diameter of this portion of the vagina is reduced by as much as 50 percent, which enables the vagina to grip the penis tightly, heightening the pleasurable friction for the male. The inner two-thirds of the vagina does exactly the opposite. It swells into a vast cavity.

By the end of this stage, men and women are both on the verge of orgasms.

The third stage is the orgasmic. The outer third of the vagina and the tissues embracing them—Masters and Johnson describe this area as "the orgasmic platform"—are convulsed by a spasm, followed by a series of rhythmic muscular contractions. In a particularly intense orgasm, there may be as many as eight to twelve. The uterus and many muscles may also have rhythmic contractions. The male has much the same thrilling experience. His penis contracts throbbingly until he ejaculates.

In both men and women, the pulse races, so does the respiratory rate, and the blood pressure climbs. Often their entire bodies are flushed.

The fourth stage is the resolution. Both men and women feel a gladsome release from the sexual tensions that have been gripping them.

Masters and Johnson were able to solve two sex mysteries. Freud claimed that a clitoral orgasm was immature, even male-like. A vaginal orgasm was much to be preferred, he decreed, because it was more mature and satisfying. Other students of sex disagreed. They maintained that women enjoyed clitoral orgasms much more than vaginal orgasms. Ergo, masturbation was superior to coitus. Arguments raged over this matter for generations until Masters and Johnson settled it. They proved with the artificial penis that from a physiological point of view, a clitoral orgasm and a vaginal orgasm could not be told apart.

The other mystery concerned the stimulation of the clitoris during intercourse. Most sex researchers had posited as irrefutable law that the penis rubs against the clitoris, arousing it. Hence, some female frigidity was ascribed to the fact that in some women the clitoris was situated too high, out of reach of the penis. Masters and Johnson showed that neither the penis nor the pubis, the region at the base of the penis, ever comes in contact with the clitoris during coitus. The clitoris stimulates itself by rubbing against its hood.

As part of foreplay, some men attempt to stimulate women by stroking the clitoral glans. Masters and Johnson learned that many women find this distinctly unpleasant. Rhythmically stroking the whole mons area above the clitoris or the areas along the sides of the clitoris was said to be more pleasurable.

In 1959, Dr. Masters and Mrs. Johnson made their big move. They accepted people with sexual dysfunctions as patients. The pair of them worked as a team with the theory that it takes a female therapist to understand a woman's sexual hang-ups, and a male therapist to grasp a man's sexual problems. They insisted that both husband and wife had to participate in the therapy. There is no such thing as an uninvolved partner in a sexual dysfunction situation, they said.

They recognized that most sexual dysfunctions are psychological in origin and must be treated by psychological means.

"We just don't treat sexual dysfunctions. We treat relationships," Dr. Masters repeated to me again and again. "The two partners are resolving their difficulties within the marriage at the same time as their sexual function is being reconstituted."

He added, "Sex is a natural function. We are well aware that there is no way to teach a man to achieve an erection, or a woman to be orgasmic. We just try to create an opportunity for Mother Nature to take over."

Each couple receives two weeks of intensive, seven-day-a-week therapy. They stay at a nearby hotel, reporting each day for treatment and returning to the hotel to practice what they've learned. The first morning, each partner is given a thorough medical examination. (Masters and Johnson well know that diabetes can cause impotence and a vaginal infection can make intercourse unbearably painful.) After that, Masters and Johnson take complete medical, psychological, and sexual histories on the couple. On the third day, the two patients and the two therapists sit around a table and discuss the couple's sexual difficulties.

Each day thereafter, Masters and Johnson show the patients functional new techniques they've developed for curing sexual dysfunctions. To cite a few . . .

If it's a matter of premature ejaculation, the therapists explain the "squeeze" technique. The male's penis is stimulated until it is about to ejaculate. At that moment, the woman pinches the man's penis just hard enough to turn him off sexually. This technique is repeated time after time until the man learns to control his ejaculations.

With impotence, Masters and Johnson help the couple to overcome the man's pervasive "fear of performance." It's the most common cause of the problem. They show the woman how to keep the man relaxed and undisturbed while they engage in sex play. If he fails to achieve an erection, the woman learns to assure him not to worry. He'll get one tomorrow. Or the day after.

A couple concerned about female frigidity—the inability to have orgasms—are also taught how to create a relaxed and undemanding atmosphere. The husband is given specific ways to stimulate his wife. The wife is shown techniques for overcoming her compulsions and fears. A woman who, deep down, is afraid of losing control of herself, may be told to keep her hand over her husband's hand while he stimulates her mons. In that fashion, she keeps control of the lovemaking.

Masters and Johnson urge their patients each time they make love to try to forget their sexual failures, their hostilities, and their guilt feelings, and to concentrate totally on the sexual experience they're having. They call this "sensate focus." Above all, they encourage each couple to communicate with each other—to tell each other what they like and dislike about their sexual interplay. Masters and Johnson say that most couples have never learned to talk openly to each other on sexual matters.

This is an expensive form of therapy: $2,500 per couple for the two weeks. But it has proven highly effective. Masters and Johnson have reported a success rate of 74.5 percent.

Human Sexual Response, a scholarly tome by Masters and Johnson reporting the results of their early research, was published in 1966. It was as big a hit as the first Kinsey report. It sold 250,000 copies and was translated into nine languages. A second report, *Human Sexual Inadequacy*, came out in 1970 and also galloped onto the best-seller lists.

As was Kinsey, Masters and Johnson were very controversial people in the beginning. The New York psychoanalyst Dr. Natalie Shainess denounced their therapy, for instance, as "oversimplistic and naïve." She charged that it glossed over symptoms without delving into their complex psychosexual causes. Other critics excoriated their activities as obscene. But they and their work have been honored by the American Medical Association and many other professional groups.

"Aren't you becoming too respectable?" I quipped to Dr. Masters.

He took me seriously. "I think you have a very real point," he replied. "There's nothing controversial about us anymore. We're sort of becoming grandpa and grandma to the field now."

How did they win acceptance so readily?

"Ginny has always said that we're existing because of our times, not in spite of them, and I think she's right," he declared.

Intellectual curiosity was also the motivating force behind his research. "This was an area that needed investigation, I felt, and I'm sure that Ginny felt essentially the same way."

Masters and his first wife, Elisabeth Ellis, were divorced in August 1970. He and Mrs. Johnson were married in January 1971. It was actually Mrs. Johnson's fourth marriage. "The first I was only nineteen, and that lasted two days," she said. "He was a political figure, and a nineteen-year-old bride was clearly not for him." Her second marriage was to a much older lawyer. "I assume we married to have a family. When I realized he had no intention whatsoever of taking that responsibility, I got a divorce.'' She has two children by her third marriage and Dr. Masters has two children by his earlier marriage.

The two of them appear much in love. His eyes rejoice when he speaks of her. "I couldn't have done it without her," he glowed. "I let down after work just by being with her, just by her physical presence."

"When I was without him, I was restless," she purred. "It took him to make me whole."

They are with patients or do research six and a half days a week, plus three or four nights. He gets to work by seven-thirty, she arrives about nine. They take Sunday afternoon off for pro football or baseball. "I suffer or cheer, usually suffer, for the St. Louis Cardinals," he said. Thursday and Saturday evenings they are at the St. Louis Symphony. When they are tired of it all, they just go to bed, "hold tight, and go to sleep."

They live well in a $100,000 home with a swimming pool on the outskirts of St. Louis. Dr. Masters draws a salary of $50,000 a year from their practice. Mrs. Johnson gets $47,500, and they earn many thousands more from their books and other writings.

As late as 1966, only a few sex clinics were in operation. There, a handful of psychiatrists, psychologists, and gynecologists tried as best they could to treat sexual dysfunctions. Masters and Johnson showed that sexual dysfunctions were curable and brought an aura of respectability to sex counseling. Since then, hundreds of thousands of people, married and single, have turned to sex therapists for aid.

"It is a vast field, sexual dysfunction," Dr. Masters said. "It affects every branch of medicine. It affects every area of theology. There is no form of counseling, from behavioral to marital, that it doesn't affect. It is the greatest single cause for divorce.

"Before, we couldn't do anything about it. Now we can."

Masters is deeply conscious of the sexual revolution that has taken place these past decades. Like John Rock, Wardell Pomeroy, Harvey Karman, and Sultan Karim, he thinks we will be the happier for it.

10

THESE MIRACLE FINDERS

A FEW DAYS AFTER DR. George Cotzias, the unconquerable Greek-born physician who discovered the miraculous effects of L-dopa in the treatment of Parkinson's disease, was himself operated on for lung cancer, he received a long-distance telephone call in his hospital bed from a Harvard scientist with whom he was collaborating on a research project.

"With this cancer bit of yours, George, I don't know how long you're going to be around," the Harvard man cold-bloodedly said. "So, let's try to get our problems settled now."

The remark shocked me, but not Dr. Cotzias. "How did you react to it?" I asked him when he told me about it.

"It pleased me," he said simply.

Most of the men and women researchers who staff the laboratories and the hospital wards seeking cures for disease are a genre apart. The great ones seem to have different reactions, hungers, and dreams from those of other people. They live in a world of their own design by laws they've enacted themselves. They know what they want to do with their lives, and they won't let anything deflect them.

You ask yourself what makes these medical investigators tick. To find an answer, you must begin by examining their motivations.

Intellectual curiosity heads the list. I've talked with scores upon scores of eminent medical researchers. I've watched them peer into microscopes, mix chemicals, transplant cancers into frightened white mice. I've stood beside them in operating rooms while they tried new surgical procedures on patients with ailing hearts. I've seen them inject new drug combinations into leukemic children and tensely pace a hospital corridor waiting to see how bad the side effects would be. I've observed them as they sought to interest withdrawn schizophrenic patients in new types of psychodramas. I've sat in their homes and talked the night through about their experiments. Every one cited intellectual curiosity as a cardinal reason for going into research.

Curiosity about what?

About anything and everything. "I have a kind of obsessive curiosity about everything," said Dr. Nathan Kline, the vibrant psychopharmacologist who transformed the treatment of mental depression. "I find it difficult ever to be bored because no matter what I do I'm always curious about all kinds of people and things.

"A lot of people are extremely interesting if you ask them the right questions," he added.

At eighty-three, Selman Waksman was still bursting with youthfulness and curiosity. When I visited him in his New Haven apartment, he wanted to hear the latest scientific, academic, and political gossip. Every morsel of it.

As a boy in Russia, Dr. Waksman started out to be a Talmudic scholar, but he was too curious about the fundamental facts of life to shut himself into an ivory tower.

"I grew up in a little Russian village where I could see the peasants' crops coming up out of the ground. I could see the chickens, the cows, the horses, the pigs, and the other animals growing. I would go anxiously and look at them on market days, and I would ask myself questions. What is this life I feel vibrating around me? How does it operate?"

It made a microbiologist of him instead of a Talmudist, and a Nobel Prize winner for finding streptomycin.

Then there is the challenge of the unknown. The real medical investigator is acutely aware of it. For him, research is a fierce struggle to solve the mysteries of nature, a struggle in which he must match his acuity and resourcefulness against nature. He is deeply determined to vanquish nature and unriddle its tightly held secrets.

Most medical investigators are also genuinely moved by a desire to help people. "I have a personal battle against sickness," Dr. Heinz Lehmann said. "I hate suffering. As soon as I see suffering, I am personally enraged."

Dr. Lehmann is the gentle German physician who escaped the Nazis to become the leading psychiatrist in Canada. It was he who introduced chlorpromazine (CPZ), the best of the tranquilizing drugs, to North America.

Of course, I've met researchers who don't give a damn about people, sick or well. Pure science is all that matters to them. I suspect that they are not as fortunate as the Heinz Lehmanns. They don't know the delight that comes to a researcher when a patient suddenly says, "Doctor, I feel better."

A creative impulse stimulates many researchers. It is surprising how many medical scientists view themselves as artists. Dr. Edward Freis, the cardiologist who first awakened medicine to the fact that moderate hypertension can kill, believes that his thirty years of research have intrinsically been an expression of his artistic temperament. "If I were a peon in Mexico," he said, "I'd probably be doing handicrafts, making silver ornaments."

"If I weren't doing surgery, I'd be a composer or a writer," declared Dr. Irving Cooper, the rogatory brain surgeon. He was quite wistful about it.

Some researchers are consciously seeking places for themselves in eternity. Dr. Phil Gold, the young Canadian physiologist who discovered the promising CEA blood test for detecting cancer at the earliest moment, voiced it vividly. "It's a matter of trying to leave a scratch on the rock."

A hunger for present-day fame, and the public adulation that can go with it, drives many medical investigators. Other investigators want only the recognition of their scientific peers. However, they all dream of winning a Nobel Prize, which affords both. Many do more than dream. They campaign for a Nobel as strenuously as any candidate running for political office, with newspaper publicity, influence-swapping and backslapping. (I haven't seen any baby-kissing by scientists yet, but I don't doubt that it is coming.) A very human wish for a bigger, better-paid position impels many researchers, and a yearning for power in their professional field. Power can mean a lot to a researcher. It can garner support, financial or otherwise, for his investigations, and deny it to his rivals.

Riches?

No. Very few investigators have money on their minds. Only one, a heart surgeon, even mentioned it as a goal. Some physicians do make fortunes from their professional activities. Certainly, Dr. Michael DeBakey's annual income soars into the millions, and Dr. Denton Cooley's isn't far behind. But they are exceptions, and they earn their millions more by their surgical skill and speed than their research ability. The average laboratory researcher draws a limited salary that rarely is enough to purchase many luxuries for his family. Most physicians who do clinical research don't make plutocratic incomes, either. They usually think more of their patients' pocketbooks than their own.

Dr. Edmund Klein, the dermatologist who found the cure for skin cancer, has some of the wealthiest people in the world among his private patients, as well as some of the poorest. Still, he has to be badgered into sending out bills.

"Honest to God, I have nothing against money," Dr. Klein says. "I just happen to be more interested in curing cancer than in becoming rich."

To proceed with our analysis of the great medical investigators and their characteristics . . .

The vast majority are imaginative, resourceful, and daring persons. Daring, particularly. Many investigators hate that word "daring," I know. They think it connotes recklessness and a cavalier disregard of the patient's life and comfort. I imply no such things. To me, a daring investigator is one willing to try an original and nonconformist approach in his research even if he must jeopardize his reputation and livelihood to do it.

I'm thinking of Dr. Min Chiu Li, the Chinese who dared to try highly toxic methotrexate on a twenty-four-year-old woman dying of cancer of the womb. It was the first time that methotrexate had ever been pitted against a solid tumor. Even though the woman was merely hours away from death, Li would have been blamed had she died. It could have ruined his professional career. He did it because it was the woman's only chance for life. Happily, she was completely cured of her cancer.

I'm thinking of Dr. Isaac Djerassi, probably the boldest medical research worker alive, who dared to administer methorexate in doses two hundred times the normal strength to children with acute leukemia. When he saw that it helped them, he raised the dosages to one thousand times the regular potency. He did it gradually—"hurrying slowly," he calls it—but it still meant bucking the medical establishment. He was condemned in every power center of the cancer world until he proved that his method not only could safely cure childhood leukemia but also lymphosarcoma, reticulum cell sarcoma, and bone cancer, and that it could even give patients with terminal lung cancer several extra years of life and health.

Which poses a crucial question: When does a physician have a right to try an experiment on a very ill patient?

The consensus seems to be this: First, the physician must try every kind of therapy of proven value on the patient. Only after the physician has nothing left in his arsenal of known value that can help the patient may he try experimental techniques. But then the physician is obligated to try every experimental treatment that can conceivably help the patient, assuming that the risks to his life and comfort don't outweigh the possible benefits. And provided that the patient consents.

Perhaps the most important attribute that great medical researchers share is what Pasteur called a "prepared mind"—a mind that is trained to expect the unexpected. Pasteur's trenchant statement here was, "Fortune favors the prepared mind." Another Frenchman, Dr. Charles J. Nicolle, who won the Nobel Prize for his work on typhus, went further. "Fortune favors only those who know how to court her," he said.

You'll understand the worth of a prepared mind when you think of the many medical advances in which serendipity has played a key role: The accidental discovery of penicillin by Alexander Fleming. Karl Folkers and the lucky route that led him to vitamin B12, the remedy for pernicious anemia. John Cade and the coincidental way he found that Lithium could relieve manic depressives. Henri-Marie Laborit and the tranquilizers. Nathan Kline and the antidepressants. Robert A. Good and the two-component immune system. Edmond Klein and his chance finding that immunotherapy could cure cancers. Min Chiu Li and the cure for choriocarcinoma. Samuel Rosen and the surgical treatment for deafness. Irving Cooper and the fortuitous fashion in which he converted an operating table catastrophe into an effective surgical technique for counteracting a whole parcel of crippling brain disorders. The list could go on and on.

The one trait, more almost than any other, that distinguishes the great investigator from the mediocre one is the ability to recognize that the irrelevant may have immense relevance. This capacity for taking advantage of good luck has contributed enormously to medical progress.

"Pasteur's statement is really true," Dr. Good remarked to me. "For years, I have been trying to teach my students that opportunism is a real way of science. . . . If you pay attention to the things that don't fit, you are much more likely to make discoveries than if you try to find out things that fit. It's the things that don't fit that really count. Very often nature's experiments are better than the experiments we can do in the laboratory."

A liking for hard work—a compulsion for it, I would say—is another characteristic of outstanding medical researchers. Dr. Oscar Auerbach, the pathologist who taught dogs to smoke in order to demonstrate that cigarettes cause lung cancer, gets to his laboratory in a V.A. hospital in New Jersey at 4:15 A.M. He works there for twelve hours, and goes home to work seven and a half more hours at his microscope. That's a seven-day-a-week schedule. Dr. Good, Dr. DeBakey, Dr. Klein, and Dr. Philip Sawyer, the heart surgeon who devised the gas endarterectomy procedure, are others who contentedly put in 120-hour work weeks.

Recently, I met a seventy-two-year-old woman who had been cured of a squamous cell carcinoma by Dr. Klein. Late one night in 1970, she was brought into Roswell Park Memorial Institute in Buffalo, New York, with a horrible tumor eighteen inches square and five inches high that sprawled over her shoulder, chest and breast. I saw color photos of the tumor. It was oozing rivulets of blood. At the time, this cancer was considered incurable, but Dr. Klein pulled the woman through with a combination of chemotherapy and his new immunotherapy.

"That Dr. Klein, he never sleeps," the woman said. "I'd wake up at two o'clock in the morning and I'd see him standing there watching over me."

She hasn't a trace of cancer today.

Most great medical researchers have a dogged persistence. They need it to overcome the opposition and obstacles they have inevitably to meet. Think of the biochemist Murray Shear, who had to bootleg his experiments at the National Cancer Institute because his myopic superiors couldn't see any possible use for chemotherapy in cancer. Think of Dr. Waksman, who was about to be fired, and Dr. Kendall, who was faced with early retirement. Neither of them lost heart. Think of Dr. Choh Hao Li, who surmounted anti-Oriental discrimination at the University of California and went ahead to isolate the human growth hormone.

Think of Dr. Folkers. His associates at Merck & Co. urged Folkers to halt his long search for a treatment for pernicious anemia. They argued at him, "You can't succeed, and even if you do, there's no money in it. Why don't you forget about it?"

He wouldn't. "Some people say of me that when I get locked in on a problem, I don't give up easily," Dr. Folkers said. "They are quite right."

Drs. André Cournand and Dickinson Richards, who won the Nobel Prize for perfecting cardiac catheterization, drew up a five-point code of personal characteristics that they thought every medical scientist should have. Dr. Cournand let me see a copy of it.

First, the pair called for intellectual integrity; second, objectivity; third, the doubt of certainty.

"You must doubt even what you have said previously," Dr. Cournand declared. "You must doubt your own authority."

Fourth, the two Nobel laureates called for tolerance; and fifth, a commitment to service.

"You belong to science and that should commit you to serve society, to be a real participant in social life," Dr. Cournand stated. "A true scientist is one who doesn't look for personal advantage but is motivated by the desire to serve. That's fundamental."

I asked Dr. Cournand whether most of the research scientists he has known followed his code. He smiled indulgently, "The good ones have."

I fear that these great medical investigators are beginning to sound like demigods. I hope not. Most are very human men and women who become overly enthusiastic when their research is going well, miserably dejected when their experiments founder or their applications for research funds are rebuffed. They have the same dread of pain and death as any nonmedical persons. Dr. C. Walton Lillehei, who pioneered in open-heart surgery, went into an emotional tailspin that lasted for days when he was told that he faced death from cancer.

"I was scared stiff," he declared.

Some superb surgery saved him, and, he said, "I felt as though I'd been reborn."

Actually, doctors have more fear of death than lay persons. An interesting study in this connection was conducted in Chicago. A group of eighty-one physicians, another group of ninety-two severely ill patients, and a third group of ninety-five normal, healthy patients were closely questioned about their feelings on death. It was discovered that the physicians were "substantially" more afraid of dying than either the healthy people or the seriously sick ones.

As a group, the great medical investigators are insecure, self-centered, and often very selfish. Their work takes precedence over their families, their friends, and everything else. They can be intolerably abrasive. Their conceit can be colossal.

Somebody once asked Dr. Jonas Salk, who developed the killed-virus vaccine for polio, why he had devoted his life to research.

"Why does Mozart compose music?" Dr. Salk unabashedly replied.

By the same token, Michael DeBakey has no hesitancy in saying that he is the greatest heart surgeon alive, and Robert Good can talk unblushingly about the "genius" he has displayed in his immunity research.

Almost all have an insatiable appetite for publicity, and the more they receive the more they want. They hate to have this called to their (or the public's) attention, though. One physician threatened to take legal action to prevent an author from publishing a book that mentioned how much this doctor liked to see his name in public print.

The competitiveness of these medical researchers cannot be ignored. Some will go to extreme lengths to deprecate the work of others. A number of years ago, Dr. Lillehei presented a delightful series of slides at a symposium on heart disease in Philadelphia depicting his satiric version of "the seven stages in the evolution of an idea," with particular reference to the rivalry that goes on in medical research. His slides purportedly quoted the reactions of one researcher to the accomplishments of another.

1. Idea stage: "Won't work. Been tried before."
2. Successful experiments in animals: "Won't work in man."

3. After one successfully treated patient: "Very lucky. Doubt if patient really needed treatment. Too bad, a tragedy really, because now they'll continue."

4. After four or five clinical successes: "Highly experimental, too risky, immoral, unethical. I understand they've had a number of deaths they're not reporting."

5. After ten to fifteen patients: "May succeed occasionally in carefully selected cases, but most patients with the defect don't need operation anyway."

6. After a large series of successes: "So-and-so in Shangri-La has been unable to duplicate their results. I hear that a number of their patients are now dying late deaths."

7. Final stage: "You know, this is a fine contribution. A straightforward solution to a difficult problem. I predicted this. In fact, in 1929 I had the same idea. Of course, we didn't publish anything, nor did we have penicillin, cortisone, and fine anesthesia in those days."

Heaven knows, an allergy to new ideas is nothing new in the annals of medical research. When Dr. Jenner reported his discovery of a smallpox vaccine to the Royal Society in London, the society bigwigs didn't believe a word of it. They mailed back his report to him with a letter urging him to terminate his absurd research lest he permanently injure his reputation. The Hungarian obstetrician Dr. Ignaz Semmelweis had his life ruined because of his discovery that multitudes of women were dying in childbirth from infections spread by unsterile hospital practices. He demanded that physicians wash their hands before they examined patients and that the wards be cleaned with an antiseptic. For that, he was discharged from his post in a Vienna hospital and run out of Vienna. It wasn't until after his death (insane, at the age of forty-seven) that his theories were accepted, and a statue of him erected in Budapest, not Vienna.

Many modern investigators have known the same harsh treatment. To single out a few—Albert Sabin with his years of tussling to prove the merit of a live-virus vaccine against polio, Nathan Kline with his avant-garde psychotropic drugs, Samuel Rosen with his ear operation, and Irving Cooper with his controversial operations on the brain. Each of them can testify to the rock-ribbed opposition that can greet new medical thinkers and thinking.

They can also testify, if they will, to the dirty politics that are rife in the medical research community. Some investigators and administrators can teach the sachems of Tammany Hall cards and spades about cutting throats, wrecking reputations, and deliberately frustrating the work of their adversaries while parceling out patronage and kudos to their pals. I know a distinguished cancer researcher whose supplies of research drugs were abruptly cut off by Washington administrators with whom he was feuding. It didn't count an iota to them that they were endangering the lives of cancer patients.

There are subtle ways officials can disparage the work of a researcher who belongs to a rival camp when he applies for government funds. The word is spread that "He's an anecdotalist." Or they say, "He's an enthusiast." The inference is that the investigator never has enough data to support his research claims. When his applications for research funds come up for approval, he hasn't a chance.

The politics can be savage at the local level, too. "I have, as everyone does in a teaching hospital, a lot of political problems persuading people to let me work in their areas," Dr. Philip Sawyer lamented. "All doctors tend to be very jealous of their prerogatives. If they're academic doctors, they have four times as much jealousy and competitiveness about their prerogatives."

Clinical investigators may have to play politics in order to get patients to treat. The average physician doesn't like to let a patient out of his hands. He may not be able to do anything more for a sick man, but he won't refer him to a researcher who has a new treatment that might save him. That would be an admission of failure on his part. To bribe him, a clinical investigator may have to sign the physician's name as a coauthor of his study.

I asked Dr. Min Chiu Li, "Do you mean to say that a physician would accept credit for a study to which he contributed nothing?"

"Well, he contributes the one thing a clinical investigator can't do without—a patient," Dr. Li declared.

He sighed and said, "A good investigator must also be a good politician."

Some mediocre investigators try to get ahead by pirating the work of others. An epidemic of this kind of scientific piracy has been underway. According to one eminent cancer researcher, whose own research findings have been stolen, the thievery operates like this:

"Let's say that someone else has published the first report of an important discovery. The best way for you to steal it is to redo the experiment yourself with a slight variation. In your first report, you refer very briefly to the original experiment. But from then on you ignore it. You flood the scientific literature with a mass of papers reporting on the same phenomenon and you make absolutely no mention of the original paper. After a while, everyone forgets the first report and considers you to be the original discoverer."

"What can the original investigator do about it?" I wanted to know.

"Not much," I was told. "Many fine scientists have been edged out of Nobel prizes that way."

Who gets credit, and for what, is one of the prime sources of strife in medical research, even when the disputants have legitimate claims. The angry arguments between Drs. Min Chiu Li and Roy Hertz over which of them contributed most to the choriocarcinoma cure have continued for more than twenty years. The Texas heart kings, DeBakey and Cooley, have been hotly wrangling that long over who performed the first operation for removing an aneurism from the thoracic aorta. No researcher ever seems to get enough credit to suit him.

Except Denis Burkitt.

Mr. Burkitt, the admirable British surgeon who discovered Burkitt's lymphoma, the dreadful cancer of the jaw in children, has some apostatic ideas on the subject of credit. He thinks that credit should not be restricted; instead, that it should be spread around more widely. As an example, he spoke to me of the remarkable achievement of the virologist Dr. Anthony Epstein in isolating the EB virus in Burkitt's lymphoma. This is the nearest medical science has yet arrived to establishing a viral cause for a human cancer. Mr. Burkitt then talked about other virologists who went to Africa and found other viruses.

"The point I want to make is this," Mr. Burkitt declared. "Several excellent people looked for viruses. Some found one virus, some found another. It just happened that the virus found by Tony Epstein and his group would now appear to be the right virus, and all honor and praise and glory to them. But let us remember the fellows who did the same amount of work but found something else. Their work was also valuable. We tend to give the plaudits to the fellow who is successful. But the fellow who isn't successful deserves commendation because that work has to be done, too.

"If I may digress a little, because I've gotten a lot of undue credit myself in a way: Once I asked an artist to make a drawing for me for lecture purposes of some fingers trying to undo a very tight knot. Then I had him do several other drawings. These show people pulling and pulling until they've gotten the knot a bit loose. Then somebody comes along and pulls out the last strand and it's quite easy. Everybody claps and says, 'Marvelous, old chap, you've got the knot undone.' But he'd never have done it unless the other chaps had loosened it.

"The credit must be shared between workers. It's never a one-man show."

I cannot say that Mr. Burkitt's proposal was received with much enthusiasm. The general feeling among Mr. Burkitt's peers was that the race goes to the swiftest in science as everywhere else.

The Women's Role

You may have noticed how few women are to be found among the medical researchers whose work is described in these pages. Just four women are included: Dr. Helen Taussig, the determined pediatrician who had the original concept for the blue baby operation; Anna Freud, the daughter of Sigmund Freud, who went on from being her father's daughter to establish her own influential school of child psychoanalysis; Dr. Laurette Bender, the psychiatrist who created the Bender Visual Motor Gestalt Test for diagnosing emotional instability, maturational lags, schizophrenia, and brain damage in patients; and the winsome Virginia Johnson, who collaborated with her husband, Dr. William Masters, in developing an exceptional new system of therapy for helping people with sexual dysfunctions.

Why so few women researchers here?

Why, for that matter, has only one woman ever won the Nobel Prize in medicine—Dr. Gerty T. Cori, who was awarded the 1947 prize together with her husband, Dr. Carl F. Cori, for basic research on carbohydrate metabolism?

The answers lie in the history of medicine. Until lately, few women were admitted into the hallowed realms of the medical profession. Most medical schools wouldn't accept them as students. Dr. Taussig still seethes when she recalls how she was turned away by Harvard medical school.

Traditionally, it was permissible for women to become nurses, but not physicians. Doctoring wasn't ladylike. It was immoral. Queen Victoria once wrote an outraged letter to Prime Minister William E. Gladstone suggesting that Sir. William Jenner would inform him of something that appalled her: "What an *awful* idea this is—of allowing *young girls* and young men to *enter* dissecting rooms together."

The prime minister agreed with Her Majesty and Sir William that coeducation would be "repulsive" in medical schools.

Today women are finally being welcomed into all medical schools, hospital staffs, and medical research laboratories. Ten years hence, even five years hence, women will be far better represented in the ranks of great medical discoverers. They'll be seen in every medical specialty.

Women also have a pivotal role in medical research as wives. Sometimes, it is a helpful one; at other times, it can be notoriously destructive. And the same truths hold for the roles played by husbands in the careers of women researchers.

Some very successful collaborations in medical research have been recorded by husbands and wives. The Coris, for instance, and Masters and

Johnson. Those two work together exquisitely. Up to his accidental death, the psychiatrist Dr. Paul Schilder and his psychiatrist-wife, Laurette Bender, made fine research partners. Some wives have aided in different ways. Mary Gibbon helped her husband, John, wire the first heart-lung machine. Helen Rosen assisted her husband perform his ear operation all over the world, from Cairo to Tokyo. Rose Shear learned to speak Russian and Japanese fluently so she could act as an interpreter for her husband, Murray, at international cancer conferences. Tika Djerassi worked as a nurse for years to support her husband, Isaac, while he was a penniless research fellow.

Most of the wives are intently concerned with their husbands' research. They discuss their experiments with them and weigh the results for them. You can apply to them Emile Roux's charming statement about Mme. Pasteur. He said she loved her husband "to the point of understanding his work."

There have been some long-lived, tender love affairs between medical researchers and their wives. Following his retirement from surgery in 1967, Dr. Gibbon used to spend every minute of every day with his wife, Mary. That was after thirty-six years of marriage. Selman Waksman declined many lucrative invitations to lecture when his wife, Deborah, fell ill.

"I wouldn't leave her," he said. "I couldn't leave her."

That was after more than a half century of marriage.

But it is not all rose petals and bliss. Many well-known researchers have placed unbearable strains on their marriages by the long hours they put in and their utter absorption in their work.

"What does a work schedule like yours do to a marriage?" I asked Dr. Malcolm Artenstein, the U.S. Army virologist who helped to develop the first effective vaccines against spinal meningitis.

You'll remember his poignant answer: "It's hell."

By the same token, some wives have turned the lives of their researcher-husbands into horrors with their calls for more money and status. They have stridently demanded that their husbands quit research altogether and go into private practice where the financial returns are so much richer.

The broken marriages have been many. Robert Good, Jonas Salk, Albert Sabin, Harry Meyer, F. Mason Sones, Jr., Samuel Slavson, and William Masters are just some whose marriages have come to real grief.

Very early in their married lives, most medical researchers and their wives have to make a judgment as to which will get precedence, the research or the marriage. Almost invariably, the research wins.

Selye Sees the Drastic Effects of Stress

With a few exceptions, I've been talking about applied scientists, the medical investigators who've sought cures for particular diseases or methods of preventing them. This is not to say that they mean more to mankind than the basic scientists who are interested in knowledge solely for knowledge's sake. Both groups are vital. The applied scientist cannot go far without the fundamental information provided him by basic research, and the basic researcher usually needs the help of applied scientists to transmute his pure knowledge into something of tangible use.

The decision to concentrate on applied scientists was made because they have been the ones most intimately involved with the advances of modern medicine. I grant you that some applied scientists are little more than technicians who merely test the data of the basic scientists without adding any original thinking of their own. However, the truly great applied scientists modify the basic data, supplement it with their own ideas, and convert it into new ways of combatting disease.

Some basic scientists could not be passed by. John Enders's isolation of the polio virus was strictly basic research, but his activities were so closely interwoven with the development of the polio vaccine that its story could not be honestly told without including the entire Enders chronicle. The finding of the antibiotics was basic science, the discovery of cortisone, too, but the three men most responsible—Fleming, Waksman, and Kendall—had such an immediate and far-reaching impact on medical practice that they assuredly belonged here.

One other basic scientist must be reckoned with. He is Dr. Hans Selye, whose theory of stress has had such influence on twentieth-century medical thinking.

Today, Dr. Selye is a jovial man of sixty-nine, tall and thin, with white hair and happy hazel eyes. I talked with him at the University of Montreal where he directs the Institute of Experimental Medicine and Surgery. He told me that he was born in Vienna and obtained his M.D. at the German University of Prague. In 1931, he won a Rockefeller research fellowship. It brought him to Baltimore and Johns Hopkins University, and from there to Montreal.

He got interested in stress in 1936 by accident. (Page Professor Pasteur again!) Studying hormones, Selye injected some ovarian and placental extracts into rats. When he autopsied the rats, he discovered that their organs had changed. In each rat, the adrenal cortex was sizably enlarged, the thymus had atrophied, and the gastrointestinal tract was riddled with ulcers. Selye thought he was on the track of an unknown hormone, but quickly realized that the damage was due to stress. His injections of tissue extracts had placed such a strain on the rats' bodies that they couldn't bear it.

In the next few years, Selye subjected fifteen thousand laboratory animals to different types of stress. He put them next to shrieking air-raid sirens, made them run in whirling cages until they dropped from exhaustion, dosed them with hormones and other chemicals, deliberately frightened them.

Out of the experiments came Selye's theory, the general adaptation syndrome, which explains what happens when the human body tries to adapt itself to stress of any sort. There are three stages to the syndrome. First comes the "alarm" stage; second, the "adaptation" stage; and third, the "exhaustion" stage, in which the hormonal defense system collapses and the body is left in a condition of dangerous chemical imbalance.

In its efforts to adapt to stress, Selye showed, the body may do itself serious injury.

The Selye theory gave medicine a unifying concept for hypertension, rheumatoid arthritis, stomach ulcers, and a variety of other stress-tinged diseases. It placed the adrenal glands in their proper physiological perspective, and it called the attention of researchers to the importance of steroids.

I asked Dr. Selye what prompted him to do research. He pondered my question for several weeks. Then he wrote me, quoting a sentence of the British philosopher Bertrand Russell: "Three passions, simple but overwhelmingly strong, have governed my life: the longing for love, the search for knowledge, and unbearable pity for the suffering of mankind."

Tomorrow's Miracles

What is next?

What is medical science likely to achieve in the near future? In the coming quarter of a century, say?

Some of the biggest advances in the history of medicine, I anticipate. There is high optimism among medical researchers today. They see another golden age of discovery ahead.

One can safely predict cures for, or, better yet, effective ways of preventing, many of the worst forms of cancer. By the year 2001, cancer will no longer be a major threat. We'll be able to prevent most cardiovascular disease; those twin devils, coronaries and strokes, will terrorize us no more. We'll have cures for rheumatoid arthritis and osteoarthritis. We should be able to prevent or cure most infectious diseases by immunotherapy. (The other day, Dr. Klein reported a cure for one of man's most ancient scourges, leprosy. He used immunotherapy against it.) We'll cure schizophrenia with drugs, just as we now do depression. We'll be able to diagnose many genetic and congenital disorders before a baby is born and correct them while the baby is still in the mother's womb. We'll be able to select the sex we want for our babies. We'll be able to transplant lungs, livers, intestines, and other organs as a routine matter. We'll have artificial hearts that will be more efficient than the natural ones. They will be as commonplace as cardiac pacemakers are now.

A "cure" for aging is highly possible. That is to say, people may regularly live to be one hundred years old, and they won't look it. They won't feel it either. The ugly processes of aging—the greying, the wrinkling, the slowing down physically and mentally—are biochemical in origin, and they can be controlled biochemically. Learning to enjoy these extra decades of youth may be a bit more difficult.

Some problems will continue to defy us. Millions of people will go on killing themeslves each year with cigarettes, environmental pollutants, and other suicidal devices. Millions more will die of the consequences of malnutrition, for overpopulation will continue to be a grim menace. A new Orwellian-type spectre will be haunting us, too—the dangers implicit in human engineering. By the century's end, scientists will be able to tamper with human genes. One can only pray that they will use this power wisely.

Overall, medical scientists have done nobly for mankind. Now it remains to be seen whether all of the wonders they have wrought can be made available to all people everywhere. In medicine, a miracle is a poor miracle indeed if it benefits only the rich and the powerful. The real miracles are those that help all people, regardless of nationality, wealth, and accidents of geography, to better health and more happiness.

BIBLIOGRAPHY

Alexander, Franz G., and Selesnick, Sheldon T., *The History of Psychiatry*. New York, Harper & Row, 1966.

Asimov, Isaac, *A Guide to Science*. New York, Basic Books, 1960, 1965, 1972.
——*The Human Body*. Boston, Houghton Mifflin, 1963
——*Asimov's Biographical Encyclopedia of Science and Technology*. Garden City, New York, Doubleday, 1964.

Ayd, Frank J., and Blackwell, Barry, eds., *Discoveries in Biological Psychiatry*. Philadelphia, Lippincott, 1970.

Barnard, Christaan, and Pepper, Curtis Bill, *One Life*. New York, Macmillan, 1969.

Benson, P.B. and McDermott, W., eds., *Textbook of Medicine*, twelfth ed. Philadelphia, Saunders, 1967.

Berg, Roland H., *The Challenge of Polio*. New York, Dial, 1946.

Blaiberg, Philip, *Looking at My Heart*. London, Heinemann, 1969.

Blakeslee, Alton, and Stamler, Jeremiah, *Your Heart Has Nine Lives*. Englewood Cliffs, New Jersey, Prentice-Hall, 1963.

Brecher, Edward M., *The Sex Reseachers*. Boston, Little, Brown, 1969.

Brecher, Ruth, and Edward M., eds., *An Analysis of Human Sexual Response*. Boston, Little, Brown, 1966.

Boorde. A., *The Breviary of Healthe*. London, Thomas East, 1575.

Brain, W.R., and Walton, J.N., *Brain's Diseases of the Nervous System*, seventh ed. London, Oxford University Press, 1969.

Brown, Bertram S., and Torrey, E. Fuller, eds., *International Collaboration in Mental Health*. National Institute of Mental Health, Washington, D.C., U.S. Government Printing Office, 1973.

Calabro, John J., and Wykert, John, *The Truth About Arthritis Care*. New York, David McKay, 1971.

Calder, Nigel, *The Mind of Man*. New York, Viking, 1971.

Calder, Ritchie, *Medicine and Man*. London, George Allen & Unwin, 1958.

Caldwell, Anne E., *Origins of Psychopharmacology From CPZ to LSD*. Springfield, Illinois, Charles C. Thomas, 1970.

Camerson, Charles S., *The Truth About Cancer*. Englewood Cliffs, New Jersey, Prentice-Hall, 1956.

Carter, Richard, *Breakthrough: The Saga of Jonas Salk*. New York, Simon & Schuster, 1966.

Cartwright, F.F., *The Development of Modern Surgery*. London, Arthur Barker, 1967.

Castiglioni, Arturo, *A History of Medicine*, trans. by E.B. Krumbhaar. New York, Knopf, 1958.

Celsus, A.C., *Of Medicine*, trans. by James Grieve. London, Printed for D. Wilson and T. Durham, 1756.

Clark, Marguerite, *Medicine on the March*. New York, Funk & Wagnalls, 1949
——*Medicine Today*. New York, Funk & Wagnalls, 1960.

Coelho, George V., and Rubenstein, Eli A., eds., *Social Change and Human Behavior*. National Institute of Mental Health, Washington, D.C. U.S. Government Printing Office, 1972.

Conference on Future Directions in Health Care; The Dimensions of Medicine. New York, Blue Cross Association, Rockefeller Foundation, and University of California School of Medicine, San Francisco, 1975.

Conn, Howard F., ed., *Current Therapy—1965*. Philadelphia, Saunders, 1965.

Cook, J. Gordon, *Virus in the Cell*. New York, Dial, 1957.

Cooley, Denton A., and Hallman, G.L., *Surgical Treatment of Congenital Heart Disease*. Philadelphia, Lea and Febiger, 1966.

Cooley, Donald G., *The Science Book of Wonder Drugs*. New York, Franklin Watts, 1954.

Cooper, Irving S., *Involuntary Movement Disorders*. New York, Hoeber, 1969.

Cooper, Joseph D., *The Economics of Drug Innovation*. Washington, American University, 1969.

Cope, Sir Zachary, *The Royal College of Surgeons of England: A History*. London, Anthony Bland, 1959.

Copeman, W.S.C., *A Short History of the Gout*. Berkeley, University of California Press, 1964.

Cotzias, George C., and McDowell, Fletcher H., eds., *Parkinson's Disease*. New York, Medcom, 1971.

Coxe, J.R., *The Writings of Hippocrates and Galen*, epitomized from the original Latin translations by J.R. Coxe. Philadelphia, Lindsay and Blakiston, 1846.

Crichton, Michael, *Five Patients, the Hospital Explained*. New York, Knopf, 1970.

Debus, Allen G., ed., *World Who's Who in Science*. Chicago, Marquis-Who's Who, 1968.

Delgado, José R., *Physical Control of the Mind*. New York, Harper & Row, 1969.

De Kruif, Paul, *Microbe Hunters*. New York, Harcourt, Brace, 1926.

Diehl, Harold S. *Tobacco and Your Health*. New York, McGraw-Hill, 1969.

Eckstein, Gustav, *The Body Has a Head*. New York, Harper & Row, 1970.

Engel, Leonard, *Medicine Makers of Kalamazoo*. New York, McGraw-Hill, 1961.

Epstein, Samuel, and Williams, Beryl, *Miracles from Microbes—The Road to Streptomycin*. New Brunswick, New Jersey, Rutgers University Press, 1946.

Erikson, Erik H., *Childhood and Society*. New York, Norton, 1950.
——*Young Man Luther*. New York, Norton, 1958.
——*Ghandi's Truth*. New York, Norton, 1969.
——*Life History and the Historical Moment*. New York, Norton, 1975.

Fishbein, Morris, ed., *The New Illustrated Medical and Health Encyclopedia*. New York, Stuttman, 1966.

Flugel, J.C., *A Hundred Years of Psychology*. London, Gerald Duckworth, 1933, 1951.

Freud, Anna, *The Ego and Mechanisms of Defense*. London, Woolf, 1937.

Freud, Sigmund, *An Autobiographic Study*, trans. by James Strachey. New York, Norton, 1935.
——*An Outline of Psychoanalysis*, trans. by James Strachey. New York, Norton, 1940.

Fromm, E., *Man For Himself*. New York, Holt, 1947.

Garrison, F.H., *Introduction to the History of Medicine*. Philadelphia, Saunders, 1917.

Gebhard, Paul H., Pomeroy, Wardell B., Martin, Clyde E., and Christenson, Cornelia V., *Pregnancy, Birth and Abortion*. New York, Harper, 1958.

Gerber, Alex, *The Gerber Report*. New York, McKay, 1971.

Glemser, Bernard, *Man Against Cancer*. New York, Funk & Wagnalls, 1969.
——*Mr. Burkitt and Africa*. New York, World, 1970.

Goldenson, Robert M., *The Encyclopedia of Human Behavior*. Garden City, New York, Doubleday, 1970.

Gomez, Joan, *A Dictionary of Symptoms*, Marvin J. Gersh, ed. New York, Stein & Day, 1968.

Goshen, Charles E., ed., *Documentary History of Psychiatry*. New York, Philosophical Library, 1967.

Graham, H., *Surgeons All*. London, Rich and Cowan, 1956.

Gutman, Alexander B., ed., *Gout - A Clinical Comprehensive*. New York, Medcom, 1971.

Haggard, Howard W., *Devils, Drugs and Doctors*. New York, Harper & Row, 1929.

Harper, Robert A., *Psychoanalysis and Psychotherapy*. Englewood Cliffs, New Jersey, Prentice-Hall, 1959.

Harris, Maureen, ed., *Early Diagnosis of Human Genetic Defects*. National Institutes of Health, Washington, D.C., U.S. Government Printing Office, 1972.

Havemann, Ernest. *The Age of Psychology*. New York, Grove, 1957.

Hippocrates, *The Genuine Works*, trans. by Francis Adams. London, The Sydenham Society, 1849.

Hoehling, A.A., *The Great Epidemic*. Boston, Little, Brown, 1961.

Holvey, David N., ed., *The Merck Manual of Diagnosis and Therapy*, twelfth edition. Rahway, New Jersey, Merck, Sharp & Dohme Research Laboratories, 1972.

Huff, Barbara B., ed., *Physicians' Desk Reference*, twenty-eighth ed. Oradell, New Jersey, Medical Economics, 1974.

Institute of Medicine, *Legalized Abortion and the Public Health - Report of a Study*. Washington, National Academy of Sciences, 1975.

Jones, Ernest, *The Life and Work of Sigmund Freud*. New York, Basic Books, 1953-1957.

Kalinowsky, L.B., and Hoch, P.H., *Shock Treatments, Psychosurgery and Other Somatic Procedures in Psychiatry*. New York, Grune & Stratton, 1952.

Kaplan, Seymour R., and Roman, Melvin, *The Organization and Delivery of Mental Health Services in the Ghetto - The Lincoln Hospital Experience*. New York, Praeger, 1973.

Katchadourian, Herant A., and Lunde, Donald T., *Fundamentals of Human Sexuality*. New York, Holt, Rinehart & Winston, 1972.

Kendall, Edward C., *Cortisone*. New York, Scribner's, 1971.

Kennedy, Edward M., *In Critical Condition*. New York, Simon & Schuster, 1972.

Kinsey, Alfred C., Pomeroy, Wardell B., and Martin, Clyde E., *Sexual Behavior In the Human Male*. Philadelphia, Saunders, 1948.

Kinsey, Alfred C., Pomeroy, Wardell B., Martin, Clyde E., and Gebhard, Paul H. *Sexual Behavior in the Human Female*. Philadelphia, Saunders, 1953.

Kistner, Robert W., *The Pill*. New York, Delacorte, 1969.

Knowles, John H., ed., *The Teaching Hospital*. Cambridge, Massachusetts, Harvard University Press, 1966.

Krevans, Julius R., and Condliffe, Peter G., eds., *Reform of Medical Education - The Effect of Student Unrest*. Washington, National Academy of Sciences, 1970.

Lambo, T. Adeoye, ed., *First Pan-African Psychiatric Conference*. Ibadan, Nigeria, Government Printer, 1962.

Lewis, Howard and Martha, *The Medical Offenders*. New York, Simon & Schuster, 1970.

Lindman, Frank T., and McIntyre, Donald M., Jr., eds., *The Mentally Disabled and the Law*. Chicago, University of Chicago Press, 1961.

Lloyd, Wyndham E.B., *A Hundred Years of Medicine*. London, Gerald Duckworth, 1936, 1968.

Maisel, Albert Q., *The Hormone Quest*. New York, Random House, 1965.

Margotta, Roberto, *The Story of Medicine*. New York, Golden Press, 1968.

Masters, William H., and Johnson, Virginia E., *Human Sexual Response*. Boston, Little, Brown, 1966.
——*Human Sexual Inadequacy*. Boston, Little, Brown, 1970.

Meade. R., *An Introduction to the History of General Surgery*. Philadelphia, Saunders, 1968.

Mello, Nancy K., and Mendelson, Jack H., eds., *Recent Advances in Studies of Alcoholism*. Washington, U.S. Government Printing Office, 1971.

Melzack, Ronald, *The Puzzle of Pain*. New York, Basic Books, 1973.

Menninger, Karl A., *Man Against Himself*. New York, Harcourt, Brace, 1938.
—— *The Human Mind*. New York, Knopf, 1945
—— *Whatever Became of Sin?* New York, Hawthorn, 1973.

Miller, Stuart, and Remen, Naomi, eds., *Dimensions of Humanistic Medicine*. San Francisco, Institute for the Study of Humanistic Medicine, 1975.

Moore, Francis D., *Transplant - The Give and Take of Tissue Transplantation*. New York, Simon & Schuster, 1972.

Morton, L.T., *Garrison and Morton's Medical Bibliography*, second ed. London, Grafton, 1954.

National Program for the Conquest of Cancer, Report of the National Panel of Consultants on the Conquest of Cancer to the United States Senate Committee on Labor and Public Welfare. Washington, D.C., U.S. Government Printing Office, 1971.

Newman, James R., ed., *The Harper Encyclopedia of Science*. New York, Harper & Row, 1963.

Nobel Foundation, ed., *Nobel, The Man and His Prizes*. Amsterdam, Elsevier, 1962.

Nourse, Alan E., *The Body*. New York, Time-Life Books, 1964.

Packard, Vance. *The Sexual Wilderness*. New York, McKay, 1968.

Paul, John R., *A History of Poliomyelitis*. New Haven, Yale University Press, 1971.

Pauling, Linus, *Vitamin C and the Common Cold*. San Francisco, Freeman, 1970.

Pearson, Michael. *The Million Dollar Bugs*. New York, Putnam's, 1969.

Pomeroy, Wardell B., *Dr. Kinsey and the Institute for Sex Research*. New York, Harper & Row, 1972.

Rapaport, Roger, *The Super-Doctors*. Chicago, Playboy Press, 1975.

Richardson, Robert G., *Surgery: Old and New Frontiers*. London, George Allen & Unwin, 1958, 1968.
—— *The Scalpel and the Heart*. New York, Scribner's, 1970.

Riesman, D., *The Story of Medicine in the Middle Ages*. New York, Hoeber, 1935.

Roback, A.A., *A History of American Psychology*. New York, Crowell-Collier, 1952, 1964.

Robinson, Donald, *The 100 Most Important People in the World Today*. Boston, Little, Brown, 1952.
—— *The 100 Most Important People in the World Today*. New York, Putnam's, 1970.

Robinson, Victor, *The Story of Medicine*. New York, Albert & Charles Boni, 1931.

Rogow, Arnold A., *The Psychiatrists*. New York, Putnam's, 1970.

Ross, Walter Sanford, *The Climate Is Hope*. Englewood Cliffs, New Jersey, Prentice-Hall, 1965.

Rothenberg, Robert E., ed., *Understanding Surgery*. New York, Trident, 1965.
—— *The New Illustrated Medical Encyclopedia for Home Use*. New York, Abradale, 1970.

Rothgeb, Carrie Lee, *Abstracts of the Standard Edition of the Complete Psychological Works of Sigmund Freud*. National Institute of Mental Health, Washington, D.C., U.S. Government Printing Office, 1971.

Rusk, Howard A., *A World To Care For*. New York, Random House, 1972.

Rusk, Howard, and Taylor, Eugene J., *New Hope for the Handicapped*. New York, Harper, 1949.

Salisbury, Harrison E., ed., *The Soviet Union: The Fifty Years*. New York, Harcourt, Brace & World, 1968.

Schwartz, Harry, *The Case for American Medicine*. New York, McKay, 1972.

Seiler, Paula, *The New Handbook of Modern Birth Control*. New York, Dell, 1963.

Selikoff, Irving J., ed., *The Management of Tuberculosis*. Baltimore, Waverly Press, 1956.

Selye, Hans, *The Stress of Life*. New York, McGraw-Hill, 1956.

—— *From Dream to Discovery*. New York, McGraw-Hill, 1964.
—— *Stress Without Distress*. Philadelphia, Lippincott, 1974.

Selzer, Arthur, *The Heart: Its Function in Health and Disease*. Berkeley, University of California Press, 1966.

Shimkin, Michael B., *Science and Cancer*. Washington, D.C., U.S. Government Printing Office, 1973.

Shippen, Katherine B., *Men of Medicine*. New York, Viking, 1957.

Skinner, B.F., *Walden II*. New York, Macmillan, 1948.
—— *Verbal Behavior*. New York, Appleton-Century-Crofts, 1957.
—— *Beyond Freedom and Dignity*. New York, Knopf, 1971.
—— *About Behaviorism*. New York, Knopf, 1974.
—— *Particulars of My Life*. New York, Knopf, 1976.

Slavson, S.R., *An Introduction to Group Therapy*. New York, Commonwealth Fund, 1943.
—— *Analytic Group Psychotherapy*. New York, Columbia University Press, 1950.

Smith, Richart T., and Landy, Maurice, eds., *Immune Surveillance*. New York, Academic Press, 1970.

Starzl, Thomas E., *Experience in Renal Transplantation*. Philadelphia, Saunders, 1964.

Starzl, Thomas E., with Putnam, Charles W., *Experience in Hapatic Transplantation*. Philadelphia, Saunders, 1969.

Stecher, Paul G., *The Merck Index - An Encyclopedia of Chemicals and Drugs*. eighth ed., Rahway, New Jersey, Merck & Co., 1968.

Stedman's Medical Dictionary, twenty-first ed. Baltimore, Williams & Williams, 1966.

Sydenham, Thomas, *The Whole Works of That Excellent Physician, Dr. Thomas Sydenham*, seventh ed., trans. by J. Pechey. London, Feales, 1717.

Thompson, Thomas, *Hearts*. New York, McCall, 1971.

Torrey, E. Fuller, *The Mind Game*. New York, Emerson Hall, 1972.

Tunley, Roul, *The American Health Scandal*. New York, Harper & Row, 1966.

Uhr, Jonathan W., and Landy, Maurice, eds., *Immunologic Intervention*. New York, Academic Press, 1971.

Viscott, David S., *The Making of a Psychiatrist*. New York, Arbor House, 1972.

Von Leden, Hans, and Cahan, William G., *Cryogenics in Surgery*. New York, Medical Examination Publishing Co, 1971.

Walker, Kenneth, *The Story of Medicine*. New York, Oxford University Press, 1955.

Walpole, Horace, *The Letters of Horace Walpole, fourth earl of Oxford*, P. Cunningham, ed. London, Bentley, 1891.

Watson, James D., *The Double Helix*. New York, Atheneum, 1968.

Welch, Claude E., ed. *Advances in Surgery*. Chicago, Year Book Medical Publishers, 1966.

Williams, Greer, *Virus Hunters*. New York, Knopf, 1960.

Wilson, J.L., *Handbook of Surgery*, fourth ed. Los Altos, Lange Medical Publications, 1969.

Wilson, John Rowan, *Margin of Safety*. Garden City, New York, Doubleday, 1963.

Wittels, Fritz, *Freud and His Time*. New York, Liveright, 1931.

Wrenshall, G.A., Hetenyi, G., and Feasby, W.R., *The Story of Insulin*. Bloomington, Indiana, Indiana University Press, 1962.

Wright, Helen, and Rapport, Samuel, eds., *The Amazing World of Medicine*. New York, Harper & Row, 1961.

Zimmerman, L.M., and Veith, I., *Great Ideas in the History of Surgery*, second ed. New York, Dover Publications, 1967.

Zinsser, Hans, *Rats, Lice and History*. Boston, Little, Brown, 1935.

INDEX

Abortion, 264, 274–286; ancient techniques of, 275; suction technique, 276–281; Supreme Court and, 274

Academy of Medical Sciences (USSR), 144

ACTH (hormone), 18, 28

Actinomycin, 6, 8

Actionomycin D, 8, 111, 117–118

Acupuncture, 99

Addison's disease, 14, 16, 17

Adenoviruses, 50

Adler, Alfred, 221

Adrenal cortex, regulation of, 28

Air pollution, 107

Alexander the Great, 23

Allopurinol, 76

Alsop, Stewart, 123

American Association of Group Psychotherapy, 243

American Cancer Society, 105, 155, 156, 158, 179

American Heart Association, 187

American Laryngological, Rhinological and Otological Society, 94

American Medical Association, 45, 222, 293

American Psychoanalytic Association, 231

Amin, Idi, 281, 286

Amoebic dysentery, 9

Anchkov, Nikolai, 179

Anthrax, 4

Antibiotics, *see* names of antibiotics

Antidepressant drugs, 228–235

Antilymphocyte globulin (ALG), 77, 82

Aristotle, 161

Arsumi, Kazuhiko, 209

Artenstein, Malcolm S., 56, 60–63, 306

Artenstein, Mrs. Malcolm S., 63

Arthritis, xi, 14, 16, 281

Artificial heart, 169, 209–212

Artificial hip, 96–99

Artificial kidney, 68–73

Artsenkamer (Nazi organization), 69, 70

Asbestos, link with cancer, 12

Ascheim, Selmar, 13

Asian flu, 50, 66

Aspirin, 2

Assyria (ancient), 1

Atomic Energy Commission, 30

A2 flu virus of 1968, 52

Auerbach, Oscar, 158–159, 160, 299

Auerbach, Mrs. Oscar, 159

Augustine, St., xi

Australian and New Zealand College of Psychiatrists, 239

Ayd, Frank J., 219

Azathioprine, 25, 76

Baastrup, Poul, 238
Babylon (ancient), 1
Bacon, Francis, 23
Baer, John E., 183–185
Bailey, Charles, 169
Bakk, Earl, 176
Bankhead, Tallulah, 52
Banting, Frederick G., 13
Barbiturates, 2
Barnard, Christiaan, 197, 198, 202, 203–206, 207–208, 210
Barnard, Mrs. Christiaan, 206
Barr, Yvonne, 138
Bavolek, Cecilia, 172
Bayliss, William M., 13
Bealer, Greg, 105–106
Beattie, Edward J., Jr., 129
Behavior therapy, 247–250
Bein, Hugo J., 183
Belzer, Folkert O., 77
Ben Gurion, David, 94
Bender, Lauretta, 239–243, 305, 306
Bender Visual Motor Gestalt Test, 240, 305
Bergstrom, Sune, 281–286
Bergstrom, Mrs. Sune, 286
Bernard, Claude, 235
Best, Charles H., 13
Beyer, Karl H., Jr., 183–185
Bicêtre Prison (France), 219
Biggs, Peter, 143
Billroth, Theodor, 67
Bini, Lucio, 221–222
Birth control, 263–286; abortion, 274–286; in history, 263–265; IUDs, 273–274; the pill, 265–273; prostaglandins, 281–286
Bismarck, Otto von, 104
Blaiberg, Philip, 205
Blalock, Alfred, 164–168, 171, 199
Blalock, Mrs. Alfred, 168
Blokhin, Nikolai N., 145
Blood poisoning, 4
Blue babies (cyanotic), 164–168
Bonadonna, Gianni, 128
Bone transplants, 84

Borremans, Jean-Baptiste, 83
Boswell, Samuel, 264
Bovet, Daniel, 2
Brain pacemaker, 90
Brain surgery, 84–91
Brain transplants, 84
Breast cancer, 17, 68, 104
Briggs, George, 21
Brill, Henry, 217, 227, 234–235, 254
Brink, Dr. Norman, 22
Brodie, Maurice, 39–40, 41
Broome, John D., 115
Brown, Bertram D., 216
Brown, Edmund G. "Pat," 277
Brucella, 66
Brunhilde virus, 40
Bruton, Ogden C., 149
Buescher, Edward L., 56
Burchenal, Joseph H., 114, 128, 139
Burkitt, Denis P., 135–141, 151, 304
Burkitt, Mrs. Denis P., 140
Burkitt's lymphoma, 128, 135–141, 144, 304
Burmester, Ben R., 142–144
Burmester, Mrs. Ben R., 143
Burnet, Frank Macfarlane, 37–38, 74
Burroughs Wellcome Company, 24, 25, 113

Cabrol, Dr., 206
Cade, John F. J., 235–239, 299
Callender, George, 162
Calne, Roy Y., 76, 82
Campbell, McFie, 229
Cancer, xi, 8, 10, 12, 13, 46, 67, 68, 83, 304, 308; blood test for, 153–154; chemotherapy, 105, 106–112, 116–120, 135–141; and cigarettes, 12; drugs combating, 112–115; immunotherapy, 146–153; as a killer, 103–106; medical advances and research in, 101–160; search for viruses in, 141–146; sex and, 104–105; surgical advances in, 129–130. *See also* types of cancer
Candicidin, 8

Candidin, 8
Caplan, Harvey W., 287
Carcino-embryonic antigen (CEA), 154
Carrel, Alexis, 74, 193, 201–202
Cerletti, Ugo, 221–222
Cervical cancer, 105, 155
Chain, Ernst B., 3, 4
Chang, Min Chuch, 265, 269, 271
Chang, Mrs. Min Chuch, 271
Chang, Timothy S., 149
Charlemagne, 23
Charles I, King, 1
Charnley, John, 96–99
Charnley, Mrs. John, 98
Chemical Warfare Service, 109
Chemopallidectomy, 88
Chemothalamectomy, 88
Chemotherapy, 102, 105, 106–112, 116–120, 135–141; for Burkitt's lymphoma, 135–141; first total cure with, 116–120
Chiarugi, Vincenzio, 218–219
Children's psychotherapy, 239–243
China (ancient), 1
Chloramphenicol, 9
Chlorothiazide, 182, 183, 185
Chlorpromazine (CPZ), 224–228, 230, 231, 235, 296–297
Cholera, 49, 182, 230
Cholesterol level, 179
Choriocarcinoma, 115
Churchill, Edward D., 68, 170
Ciba Pharmaceutical Company, 183, 230–231, 267
Cigarette smoking, 12, 122–123, 179–180
Cioppa, Joseph, 86–87
Clarke, Cyril A., 66
Cleave, T. I., 140
Coitus interruptus, 264
Coitus obstructus, 264
Coleridge, Samuel, 255
Colonoscopy, 99–100
Colon-rectum cancer, 104, 140
Conjunctivitis, 145
Conolly, John, 219
Contraception, *see* Birth control

Cooley, Denton A., 190, 197–201, 202, 206–207, 208, 209–212, 297, 304
Cooley, Mrs. Denton A., 201
Cooper, Irving S., 30, 84–91, 94, 130, 299, 302
Cooper, Mrs. Irving S., 90
Cooper, Max, 150
Cori, Carl F., 305
Cori, Gerty T., 305
Coronary arteriography, 176–178
Corticosteroids, 14
Cortisone, 2, 13–19, 28, 267; risks and beneficial aspects of, 17–18
Cortisone (Kendall), 18–19
Cotzias, Constantin, 34
Cotzias, George C., 29–34, 295
Cotzias, Mrs. George C., 34
Cournand, André F., 162–164, 177, 178, 300
Cowpox, 35–36
Cox, Herald R., 44
Crafoord, Clarence, 169
Crick, Francis H. C., 113–114
Cryosurgery, 88–90
Curie, Pierre, xiii
Cushing, Harvey W., 68
Cutter Laboratories, 42
Cyclophosphamide, 128

Dameshek, W., 76
Daraprim, 25
Darrow, Clarence, 50
Darvall, Denise Ann, 204, 205
Darvall, Edward G., 204
Darwin, Charles, 23
Daunomycin, 115
DeBakey, Michael Ellis, 155, 189–201, 202, 207, 209, 210, 211, 214, 297, 299, 301, 304
DeBakey, Mrs. Michael Ellis, 197
De humani corporis fabrica (Vesalius), xii
Dehydrocorticosterone, 17
DeKruif, Paul, 43, 55
Delay, Jean, 226
Dementia praecox, *see* Schizophrenia

Demikhov, Vladamir, 169, 202, 209
Dengue fever, 43
Deniker, Pierre G., 226, 227, 228
Deniker, Mrs. Pierre G., 227
Deoxyribonucleic acid (DNA), 113–114
Depression, 217–218, 220–221
Derom, Fritz, 83
DeRudder, Michael, 193–194
DeWall, Richard A., 174
Diabetes, 2, 13
Dibenazepine, 235
Diphtheria, 66, 109
Disney, Walt, 103
Disraeli, Benjamin, 264
Dix, Dorothea Lynde, 219
Djerassi, Carl, 265, 266, 267, 269, 272–273
Djerassi, Mrs. Carl, 273
Djerassi, Isaac, 101–102, 107, 112, 123–129, 135, 153, 298, 306
Djerassi, Mrs. Isaac, 124
Djerassi, Rami, 127
Djerassi, Mrs. Tika, 306
Dmchowski, Leon, 144
Doll, Richard, 157
Domagk, Dr. Gerhard, 2, 8
Dos Santos, J. C., 192
Dubos, Dr. René, 6
Dulles, John Foster, 103
Duschinsky, Robert, 115
Dwarfism, control of, 26–29
Dystonia, 89
Dystonia musculorum deformans, 84–85

Eagleton, Thomas F., 223
Echo II virus, 56
Eddy, Bernice, 141
Egypt (ancient), 1, 264
Ehrlich, Paul, 2
Eisenhower, Dwight D., 169
Electric shock therapy, 221–224
Eliot, T. S., 103
Emphysema, 158
Enders, John Franklin, 36–49, 57
Enders, Mrs. John Franklin, 49
Enders vaccine, 47–49, 53

Engerset, Arne Kaare, 132
Epilepsy, 90, 182, 230
Epstein, Anthony, 138, 304
Epstein-Barr (EB) viruses, 138
Erikson, Erik H., 244–245
Erikson, Jon, Kai, and Sue, 245
Erikson, Mrs. Erik, 245
Estrogen (hormone), 108, 270
Ether, xiii
Euler, Ulf von, 282
Eustace, Dorothy, 174

Family Planning Association of Puerto Rico, 269–270
Family Services Association of America, 287
Farber, Sidney, 107, 109–112, 121, 123, 153
Farber, Mrs. Sidney, 112
Favoloro, René, 213
Fermi, Enrico, 103
Fernandel, 103
Filatov, Nils Feodorovich, 99
Filatov Institute (USSR), 99
Finn, Ronald, 66
5-Fluorouracil (5-FU), 115
Fleming, Alexander, 3–4, 5, 9, 34, 224, 299, 307
Fleming, Lady Alexander, 4
Florey, Howard W., 3, 4
Flu, 49–54; types of viruses, 51
Fluphenazine enanthate, 216
Folkers, Karl, 19–23, 34, 299, 300
Folkers, Mrs. Karl, 23
Forssmann, Werner Theodor Otto, 162, 164
Fortner, Joseph, 129
Foundation for Reproductive Biology, 288
406th Medical General Laboratory (U.S. Army), 51
Fox, Dr. Herbert H., 10, 12
Francis, Thomas, Jr., 40, 41–42
Freda, Vincent J., 64
Freedman, Samuel O., 154
Frei, Emil, III, 128
Freis, Edward R., 180–182
Freis, Mrs. Edward R., 182

Freud, Anna, 239–243, 244, 305
Freud, Sigmund, 200, 220–221, 228, 244, 246, 291, 305
Furth, Jacob, 113

Galen of Pergamum, xii
Gallstones, xi
Gandhi's Truth (Erikson), 245
Garattini, Silvio, 107
Garney, Rev. Francis W., 270–271
Gastric ulcers, 67
Gebhard, Paul H., 259
George III, King, 219
George VI, King, 103
Gerecke, William B., 196
German measles, 66; vaccine against, 54–59
Gestational choriocarcinoma, 116
Gibbon, John, 192, 306
Gibbon, Mrs. John, 306
Gibbon, John H., Jr., 170–171
Gibbon, Mrs. John H., Jr., 170
Gilbert, René, 131
Gilman, Alfred, 108–109
Gilot, Françoise, 47
Gladstone, William E., 305
Glaucoma, 281
Glick, Bruce, 149
Glidden, Gregory, 174
Goethe, Johann Wolfgang von, 23
Gold, Phil, 153–154, 297
Goldschneider, Emil, 62–63
Goldschneider, Irving, 59–60
Gonorrhea, 4, 8, 218
Good, Robert A., 147–153, 160, 299, 301, 306
Good, Mrs. Robert A., 151
Gorman, John G., 64, 65
Gorman, Katherine, 65
Gotschlich, Emil C., 60, 62
Gout, 14, 113; preventing dangerous consequences of, 23–26
Gramicidin, 6
Great Epidemic, The (Hoehling), 50
Gregg, Norman, 54–55
Grigsby, William, 81–82
Gross, Ludwik, 141
Gross, Robert E., 164–165, 166, 169

Grunberg, Emanuel, 10, 12
Guthrie, Charles, 201–202

Halsted, William Stewart, 68
Hamburger, Jean, 75, 80
Hammond, Edward Cuyler, 155–160
Hammond, Mrs. Edward Cuyler, 157
Hansen, Hans, 154
Hardy, James D., 202
Harl, J. M., 226
Hartman, Frank, 13–14, 15
Harvey, William, xii
Hearing, restored, 91–95
Heart and cardiovascular disease, 161–215; arteriography, 176–178; artificial heart, 209–212; blue babies and, 164–168; catheter exploration, 162–164; coronary prevention, 185–188; hypertension, 180–185; to open plugged arteries, 213–215; risk factors involved in, 178–180; surgery, 189–215; transplants, 189–215
Heartbreak (Barnard), 206
Heart-lung machine, 72, 170–172, 193–194, 210, 306
Heidelberger, Charles, 114–115
Heller, Louis B., 262
Helm, Fred, 152
Hench, Philip S., 16, 17, 18
Henle, Gertrude, 138
Henry VI, King, 23
Hepatitis, 102
Herpes virus, 46, 143
Herrick, Ronald and Richard, 76
Herrnstein, Richard, 249
Hertz, Roy, 117, 119–120, 304
Hertz, Mrs. Roy, 119
Hess, W., 104
Hewitson, Rodney, 204, 205
HGH (hormone), 26–29
Hill, A. Bradford, 157
Hilleman, Jeryl Lynn, 53
Hilleman, Kirsten, 53
Hilleman, Maurice R., 49–53, 59, 141, 143

Hilleman, Mrs. Maurice R., 54
Hiller, Salomon, 115
Hippocrates, xi–xii, 1, 103
Hirschkowitz, Basil I., 100
Hitchcock, François, 204
Hitchings, George H., 23–26, 76, 113–114
Hitler, Adolf, 2
Hodgkin, Thomas, 103–104
Hodgkin's disease, 8, 102, 103–104, 115, 128, 149; stages of, 132; X-ray treatment of, 130–134
Hoehling, A. A., 50
Hoffman-LaRoche Inc., 10, 11, 12, 115, 154, 232, 254
Hogg, John A., 282
Homburger, Theodore, 244
Homosexuality, 259, 261
Hong Kong flu, 51–52
Hormones, secretion of, 13
Hornykiewicz, O., 32
Huebner, Robert Joseph, 50, 141, 145–146
Huebner, Mrs. Robert Joseph, 146
Hufnagel, Charles A., 169, 175
Huggins, Charles B., 108
Human Sexual Inadequacy (Masters and Johnson), 293
Human Sexual Response (Masters and Johnson), 293
Hürting, F. H., 104
Huxley, Aldous, 103
Hypertension, 308; drug control of, 180–185
Hypothermia, 130

Ichikawa, K., 107
I.G. Farbenindustrie, 2
Imipramime, 235, 236
Immunology, 35–66
Immunotherapy, 102, 107, 146–153
Inca Indians, 1–2
Infanticide, 264
Inflammatory eye diseases, 17
Insanity, 182
Insulin, xiii, 2, 13, 28
International Congress of Psychiatry, 236

International Planned Parenthood Federation, 280
Intra-aortic balloon pump, 72–73
Intrauterine devices (IUDs), 273–274, 280
Iproniazid (Marsalid), 11–12, 232
Isoniazid, 8, 10–13
Isonicotinic acid hydrazide, 10

Japanese B encephalitis, 43
Jarrett, Arthur, 141
Jenner, Edward, xiii, 35–36, 143, 302
Jenner, William, 305
Jewish Board of Guardians, 242
Jews, 104, 105, 262
Joboulay, Mathieu, 74
John E. Harvey (ship), 109
Johns, Richard, 45
Johnson, George, 289
Johnson, Lyndon B., 168, 208–209
Johnson, Mrs. Virginia Eshelman, 287–294, 305–306
Johnson, W. Dudley, 213
Johnson and Johnson Company, 64
Journal of the American Medical Association, 187
Jung, Carl Gustav, 200, 221
Juvenelle, André, 170

Kahn, Julius, 113
Kalinowsky, Lothar B., 221–224
Kalinowsky, Mrs. Lothar B., 223
Kantrowitz, Adrian, 206, 209–210
Kaplan, Barry, 203
Kaplan, Henry S., 103, 130–134
Kaplan, Mrs. Henry S., 133
Kaplan, Seymour R., 246–247
Kaplitt, Martin, 214
Karim, Sultan M. M., 281–286, 294
Karim, Mrs. Sultan M. M., 286
Karman, Harvey L., 276–281, 294
Karman, Mrs. Harvey L., 280
Karp, Haskell, 210–211
Kasperak, Michael, 206
Katz, Samuel L., 48
Kelman, Charles, 99
Kendall, Edward C., 14–19, 34, 300, 307

Kendall, Mrs. Edward C., 18
Kennaway, Sir Ernest, 107
Kennedy, Charles, 129
Kennedy, Edward M., 127
Kennedy, Edward M., Jr., 127
Kidd, John G., 115
Kidneys, 68–71; artificial, 68–73; cancer of, 111
Kidney transplants, 13, 25, 74–81
Kinmouth, John B., 132
Kinsey, Alfred C., 257–263, 288
Kinsey, Mrs. Alfred C., 263
Kinsey Report, 257–263, 293; criticism of, 262–263
Klee, Professor, 10
Klein, Edmund, 102–103, 107, 120–123, 124, 125, 147, 152, 153, 297–298, 299–300, 309
Klein, Mrs. Edmund, 122
Klein, George, 136
Kline, Marna, 234
Kline, Nathan S., 12, 228–235, 238, 250, 296, 299, 302
Kline, Mrs. Nathan S., 234
Koch, Robert, xiii
Kocher, Theodor, 68
Kolff, Willem J., 68–73, 75, 97, 209
Kolff, Mrs. Willem J., 73
Kolmer, John A., 40
Koprowski, Hilary, 44
Kountz, Samuel L., 77–80, 83
Kountz, Mrs. Samuel L., 80
Krasno, Dr. Louis R., 185–188
Krugman, Saul, 57
Kuhn, Roland, 235–239
Kunkel, Henry, 148–149
Kurzrok, Ralph, 282
Küss, R., 75

Laborit, Henri-Marie, 224–226, 227, 228, 299
Laborit, Mrs. Henri-Marie, 227
Lactobacillus lactis lactis, 21
Laënnec, René Théophile, xiii
Lambo, Thomas Adeoye, 250–253
Lambo, Mrs. Thomas Adeoye, 253
Lancet (journal), 284
Landsteiner, Karl, 37, 68

Langan, John, 154
Lansing virus, 40
Lasker, Mary, 155
Lasker Foundation, 136
L-asparaginase, 115
Lawler, Richard H., 75
Lazell, E. W., 243
L-dopa (drug), 29–34, 295
Lederle Laboratories, 44, 110
Leeuwenhoek, Antony van, xii, xiii
Lehmann, Heinz E., 227–228, 231, 296–297
Lehmann, Mrs. Heinz E., 228
Lempert, Julius, 93
Leon virus, 40
Leopow, Martha, 62
Leprosy, 218, 309
Leukemia, 25, 53, 76, 101, 102, 104, 105–106, 109–110, 112–113, 114, 115, 296; treatment for, 123–129
Li, Choh Hao, 26–29, 300
Li, Min Chiu, 116–120, 128, 298, 299, 303–304
Li, Mrs. Min Chiu, 118–119
Librium, 253–254
Lieb, C. C., 282
Life (magazine), 88
Liley, A. William, 64
Lillehei, Clarence Walton, 172–176, 202, 203, 207, 301–302
Lillehei, Mrs. Clarence Walton, 176
Lind, James, xii–xiii
Liotta, Domingo, 211, 212
Lipman, Jacob, 5, 7
Lister, Joseph, xiii
Lithium, 236–239
Liver transplants, 81–84
Lobo, Lionel, 81
Lobotomy, 221
Logan, Joshua, 223, 255
Long, Crawford, xiii
Longoria, Peggy, 116–117
Lower, Richard R., 202, 207
Lung cancer, 12, 34, 102, 104, 126, 295; cigarettes and, 155–160; mortality rate, 104
Luther, Martin, 23
Lymphosarcoma, 109, 127

Mackay, Gordon, 67
McQuarrie, Irving, 148
Magic, xi
Maimonides, Moses, 256
Malaria, 25
Mally, Josef, 10
Manganese poisoning, 31-32, 33
March of Dimes, 40
Marek's disease, 142-144
Margaret of Anjou, 23
Marker, Russell E., 265, 266-267
Masters, William Howell, 287-294, 305-306
Masturbation, 261, 291
Mathé, Georges, 115, 152-153
Measles, 39, 66; Enders vaccine against, 47-49; epidemics of, 47-48
Medawar, Peter Brian, 74-75, 77, 80
Medawar, Mrs. Peter Brian, 74-75
Medical Letter, 273
Medical research: against cardiovascular disease, 161-215; in cancer, 101-160; historical background, xi-xiii; immunology, 35-66; mental illness, 216-255; miracle drugs and, 1-34; motives for, 295-309; and rebuilding the body, 67-100; role of women in, 305-306; sexual revolution, 256-294
Medical World News, 126-127
Medicine men, xi
Meduna, Lazlo von, 221
Meningitis, 8, 60
Menninger, Karl A., 245-246, 262, 263
Menninger, Mrs. Karl A., 246
Menninger, William, 246
Mental illness, 216-255; behavior therapy, 247-250; children's psychotherapy, 239-243; drug therapy for, 253-255; drug treatment, 224-239; in history, 218-219; research in, 216-255; shock therapy, 221-224
Mercaptopurine, 25
Merck & Company, 8, 16, 18, 20, 21, 22, 50, 53, 54, 184, 300

Merrill, John P., 75, 76
Methotrexate, 110, 113, 117, 125-126, 127, 128, 298
Metrazol (drug), 221
Meyer, Hans, 10
Meyer, Harry M., Jr., 54-59, 306
Meyer, Mrs. Harry M., Jr., 58
Microbe Hunters (DeKruif), 43, 55
Milton, John, 23
Minot, George, 19-20
Mitchell, Joe, 200
Moniz, Egas, 221
Montague, Lady Mary Wortley, 35
Moore, Dan, 144
Morello, Aldo, 87
Morse, Wayne, 73
Morton, William T. G., xiii
Mosher, Celia Duel, 256, 257
MSH (hormone), 32
Muller, J. M., 183
Mumps, 52-53, 66, 146
Murphy, William P., 20
Murray, Gordon, 169
Murray, Joseph E., 76
Murrow, Edward R., 103
Mustard gas poisoning, 109

Napoleon I, xiii, 217
Nasser, Gamal Abdel, 94
National Cancer Institute, 105, 115, 116, 128, 141, 155, 300
National Fertility Study, 271
National Foundation for Infantile Paralysis, 40, 41, 44, 45, 46
National Heart Institute, 178, 212
National Institutes of Health, 46, 50, 55, 58, 107, 116, 216-217, 253
Navajo Indians, 12
Nazi Party, 2, 3, 30, 68, 69-70, 71, 96, 121, 123, 162, 164, 193, 220, 222, 223, 227, 228, 244
Neomycin, 8
Neville, Philip, 176
New England Journal of Medicine, 29
Newsweek (magazine), 206
Newton, Sir Isaac, 23
New York College of Medicine, 119

New York Times, The, 40, 47, 51, 157
Nicolle, Charles J., 299
Nicotinic acid, 19, 23
Novello, Frederick C., 183–185

Ochsner, Alton, 155
O'Connor, Basil, 39, 40, 41, 42, 45, 46
O'Donovan, Terry, 204
Oettlé, A. G., 137
Olitsky, Peter K., 43
One Life (Barnard), 206
Open-heart surgery, 172–176
Orchitis, 52–53
Ormandy, Eugene, 96
Ortho-Research Foundation, 64
Osler, Sir William, 14
Osteoarthritis, 14
Otosclerosis, 92

Pacemakers, 175–176, 210
Page, Irvine, 187
Para-aminhippuric acid, 184
Paracelsus, xii
Paré, Ambroise, xii
Parkes, Henry B., 241
Parkinson, James, 29
Parkinson's disease, 86–90, 130, 295; control of, 29–34
Parkman, Dr. Paul D., 54–59
Parkman, Mrs. Paul D., 59
Pasternak, Boris, 103
Pasteur, Louis, xiii, 5, 34, 299, 306, 307
Pasteur Institute of Epidemiology and Microbiology (USSR), 59
Paul, John R., 38, 42–43
Paul VI, Pope, 271
Pauling, Dr. Linus, 23
Pavlov, Ivan Petrovich, 247
Pearl, Raymond, 155
Peebles, Thomas, 48
Pellagra, 19
Penfield, Wilder G., 68
Penicillin, 7, 28, 184, 224; discovery of, 3–4
Penicillium notatum, 3

Pernicious anemia, 19–23, 300
Perry, Seymour, 129
Peters, M. Vera, 131
Petrovsky, Boris Vasilevich, 84
Phenylalanine, 33
Picasso, Pablo, 47
Pien Ch'iao, 201
Pill, the, 265–273
Pincus, Gregory G., 265, 266, 267, 269, 270, 271
Pincus, Mrs. Gregory G., 271
Pinel, Philippe, 219
Pinkel, Donald, 128
Pithecanthropus erectus, xi
Pius XII, Pope, 270
Plague, 66
Plato, 275
Platt, Sir Harry, 97
Pneumonia, 2, 4, 48
Poe, Edgar Allan, 255
Poliomyelitis, 36–47, 57, 66, 301, 302; doctrinal controversy about, 39–42; vaccines against, 41–47; virus in a test tube, 36–47
Pollack, William, 64, 65
Pomeroy, Wardell B., 259, 261, 262, 263, 294
Population Council, 279
Pott, Percival, 103
Poultry Research Laboratory (Department of Agriculture), 142
Poultry Science (publication), 149–150
Pratt, Joseph Hersey, 243
Progesterone, 266–267
Prostaglandins, 281–286
Prostate, cancer of the, 104, 108
Psychotherapy, for children, 239–243
Pust, Karl, 274
Putchkivskaya, Nadeja, 99

Q_{10} (vitamin), 22–23
Quinine, 1–2, 25

Rabies, 66
Radical mastectomy, 68
Rauscher, Frank J., 128
Rauwolfia serpentina, 182–183, 230

Rayburn, Sam, 103
Reed, Major Walter, xiii
Rehn, L., 104
Reichstein, Tadeus, 14, 15, 17
Repatriation Mental Hospital (Australia), 237–238
Reserpine, 182, 183
Reticulum cell sarcoma, 127
Retinal blastoma, 132
Revere, Paul, 96
Rhazes (physician), 47
Rh disease (erythroblastosis fetalis), 63–66
Rheumatic fever, 14, 43
Rheumatoid arthritis, 13, 14, 17, 18, 43, 308
RhoGAM vaccine, 65
Ribonucleic acid (RNA), 113–114, 145
Rice-Wray, Edris, 269–270
Richard I, King, 256
Richards, Dickinson W., 162–164, 177, 178, 300
Richards, Gordon, 131
Richter, R., 274
Rickettsiapox, 145
Rivers, Dr., 44
Rivers, Thomas, 41
Robbins, Frederick C., 38–39
Robitzek, Edward H., 10, 11, 12
Rock, John, 265, 267–272, 294
Rock, Mrs. John, 272
Rocky Mountain spotted fever, 145
Rodriguez, Julie, 82
Roentgen, Wilhelm, xiii
Roosevelt, Franklin D., 36, 40
Rosen, Mrs. Helen, 306
Rosen, Samuel, 91–95, 99, 299, 302
Rosenberg, Saul, 133
Rosenthal, Alfred, 122
Ross, Donald N., 207
Rous, Francis Peyton, 106, 141
Roux, Emile, 306
Rowe, Wallace P., 50
Royal Society, 302
Rubella, 54–59, 66
Rundles, R. Wayne, 25–26
Rush, Benjamin, 227
Russell, Bertrand, 308

Russell, Louis, 207
Rutgers, Carol, 66
Ruth, Babe, 103
Ruttman, Robert J., 114

Sabin, Albert B., 38, 39, 41, 42–47, 302, 306
Sabin, Mrs. Albert B., 47
Sabin vaccine, 42–47
Sakel, Manfred, 221
Saladin, Sultan, 256
Salk, Jonas E., 39, 41–42, 44, 301, 306
Salk vaccine, 41–42, 44, 45, 47
Salvarsan (arsenic compound), 2
Sanger, Martha Higgins, 264, 265–266
Sarett, Lewis H., 16, 17, 18
Sawyer, Philip N., 190–191, 213–215, 299, 303
Scarlet fever, 109
Schafstadt, Mevrouw Sofia, 71
Schilder, Paul, 240, 306
Schizophrenia, 23, 220–221, 305; behavior therapy for, 247–250
Schlitter, Emil, 183
Schnitzer, Robert, 10, 12
Schou, Mogens, 238
Schwartz, Robert, 76
Scott, A. C., 67
Scott, Charles P., 232
Scribner, Belding, 71
Scurvy, xii–xiii, 19
Searle Company (G.D.), 270
Selikoff, Irving J., 10–13
Selye, Hans, 307–308
Semmelweis, Ignaz, 302
Sen, P. K., 206
Septicemia, 3
Sexual Behavior in the Human Female (Kinsey), 259–260
Sexual Behavior in the Human Male (Kinsey), 259–260
Sexual revolution, 256–294; birth control, 263–286; Kinsey Report, 257–263; Masters and Johnson studies, 287–294
Seyss-Inquart, Artur von, 69
Shainess, Natalie, 293

Shakespeare, William, 255
Shannon, James A., 58
Sharp & Dohme Research Laboratories, 183
Shear, Murray J., 107–108, 300
Shear, Mrs. Rose, 306
Shinya, Hiromi, 99–100
Shirey, Earl, 178
Shope, Richard E., 141
Shorb, Mary, 21
Shumway, Norman, 201–202, 203, 204, 206, 207, 208
Sickle cell anemia, 281
6-mercaptopurine (6-MP), 25, 76, 114
Skin cancer, 120–123, 152
Skinner, Burrhus Frederic, 247–250
Skinner, Mrs. Burrhus Frederic, 249
Skinner, Cornelia Otis, 259
Skinner, Deborah, 249
Skinner, Julie, 249
Sklodowska, Marie, xiii, 103
Slavson, S. R., 242–243
Sloan-Kettering Institute for Cancer Research, 102, 114, 118, 120, 147
Smallpox, xiii, 143; immunity against, 35–36
Smorodintsev, Anatoly A., 59
Snakebite, 182
Snyder, Eugene R., 91
Sobel, Sol, 214
Sones, F. Mason, Jr., 176–178, 213, 306
Spanish influenza of 1918–1919, 49–50, 51
Spiegelman, Sol, 144
Spinal meningitis, 4, 66, 306; bacterial organisms of, 60; immunity against, 59–63
Spock, Benjamin M., 241
Sprague, James M., 183–185
Squibb & Son Laboratories (E.R.), 10, 50, 230
Staphylococci, 3
Starzl, Thomas E., 77, 80, 81–83
Starzl, Mrs. Thomas E., 83
Stein, Gertrude, 103
Sternbach, Leo H., 254
Stewart, Sarah, 141

Stim, Edward M., 279–280
Stomach cancer, 104
Stone, Abraham, 265
Streptococci, 2
Streptomyces griseus, 6, 7
Streptomycin, 4–9, 28
Stress, effects of, 307–308
SubbaRow, Yellapragada, 110
Sulfa drugs, 2, 60
Sulfanilamide, 2
Sumer (ancient), 1
Supercoils, 280
Svenson, Evert, 232
Swingle, Wilbur W., 13–14, 15
Syntex Corporation, 266, 267, 270, 272
Syphilis, 2, 4, 8, 218

Taft, Robert A., 103, 128
Talmud, 264
Taussig, Helen, 164–168, 207, 209, 305
Terasaki, Paul I., 77
Tetanus, 66
Tetracycline, 9
Thiosemicarbazones, 10
Thomas, Everett, 207
Thomas, Vivian, 166
Thorp, J. M., 186
Thyroxin, 15
Tietze, Christopher, 279
Time (magazine), 88
Time Has Come, The: A Catholic Doctor's Proposal to End the Battle for Birth Control (Rock), 270
Tofranil, 235
Tranquilizers, 224–229, 296–297
Transplants: heart, 189–215; kidney, 74–81; liver, 81–84
Trapeznikov, Nikolai N., 84
Trask, James D., 38
Trimethoprim, 26
Trois Frères cave, xi
Ts'ai-Kuang Wu-Tsung, 277–278
Tuberculosis, xi, 7–8, 66, 149; streptomycin defeat of, 7–8; treatment of, 9–13
Tucker, Mrs. Howard, 75
Typhoid fever, 9, 66

Typhus, 9, 66, 299

Ueno, T. S., 275
Ullman, E., 74
Ultrasonic frequencies, 99–100
Undulant fever, 9
U.S. Department of Agriculture, 21, 142
U.S. Food and Drug Administration, 58, 237, 238, 270, 273
U.S. Public Health Service, 42, 45, 51, 108
Upjohn Corporation, 282–283, 285
Uracil, 114, 115
Uric acid, 23

Vaccination, purpose of, 36
Vakil, Rustom Jal, 183
Vereecken, Alois, 83
Vesalius, Andreas, xii
Victim Is Always the Same, The (Cooper), 90–91
Victoria, Queen, 305
Vineberg, Arthur, 213
Virchow, Rudolf, xiii, 104
Vitamin A, 2, 19
Vitamin B, 2
Vitamin B$_3$, 19
Vitamin B$_{12}$, 19, 22; isolation of, 19–20
Vitamin C, xii–xiii, 17, 18, 19, 23
Vitamin D, 19
Vitamin E, 23
Vorondy, U., 74

Waksman, Byron, 5
Waksman, Mr. and Mrs. Jacob, 5
Waksman, Selman A., 4, 5–9, 21, 34, 111, 296, 300, 307
Waksman, Mrs. Selman, 5, 6, 9, 306
Walden Two (Skinner), 249
Wangensteen, Owen H., 173
Ward, Claire, 169
Warner-Chilcott Laboratories, 232

Warren, John C., xiii
Washansky, Louis, 203–205, 206
Watson, James D., 113–114
Watson, John B., 249
Weaver, Arthur W., 130
Weller, Thomas H., 38–39, 57
West, Randolf, 22
White, Paul Dudley, 169
White, Pearl, 247
Wiener, Alexander, 64
Wilkins, Robert W., 183
Wilm's tumor, 8, 111
Windsor, Duke of, 103, 191
Witch doctors, xi
Witter, Richard L., 143
Wooden legs, 96
Worchester Foundation for Experimental Research, 265, 271
World Health Organization (WHO), 31, 32, 51, 52, 62, 229, 250, 253, 275
World War I, 109
World War II, 3, 21, 43, 68, 74, 96, 109, 173, 224, 244, 248
Wu Hsien-Chen, 277–278
Wu Yuang-T'ain, 277–278

Xanthine oxydase, 25
X-rays, xiii, 11, 65, 85, 99, 102, 112, 113, 127, 177; for treating Hodgkin's disease, 130–134

Yale, Harry, 10
Yamagiwa, K., 107
Yellow fever, 66
Young Man Luther (Erikson), 245
Yukin, Sergei Sergeivitch, 68
Yurok Indians, 244

Zinsser, Hans, 37
Zoecon Corporation, 272
Zoll, Paul M., 175
Zondek, Bernhard, 13
Zubrod, C. Gordon, 106